REFRAMING
WOMEN'S
HEALTH

Acknowledgments

We want to thank the John D. and Catherine T. MacArthur Foundation for the generous support in making this project possible.

We would also like to thank Marilyn Fox and Jessica A. Jonikas for their invaluable editorial assistance and Zylphia L. Ford for her organizational efforts in assembling this compilation.

We would particularly like to thank the participants of the 1992 Reframing Women's Health Conference, whose energy and commitment inspired this text.

REFRAMING WOMEN'S HEALTH

MULTIDISCIPLINARY RESEARCH AND PRACTICE

EDITED BY

ALICE J. DAN

SAGE Publications
International Educational and Professional Publisher
Thousand Oaks   London   New Delhi

For information address:

 SAGE Publications, Inc.
2455 Teller Road
Thousand Oaks, California 91320

SAGE Publications Ltd.
6 Bonhill Street
London EC2A 4PU
United Kingdom

SAGE Publications India Pvt. Ltd.
M-32 Market
Greater Kailash I
New Delhi 110 048 India

Printed in the United States of America

Library of Congress Cataloging-in-Publication Data

Main entry under title:

Reframing women's health: Multidisciplinary research and practice /
    edited by Alice J. Dan.
        p.   cm.
    Includes bibliographical references and index.
    ISBN 0-8039-5773-4 (cl.)   —   ISBN 0-8039-5860-9 (pb)
    1. Women—Health and hygiene—Sociological aspects.   2. Women—
Health and hygiene—Research.   3. Women's health services—
Political aspects.   I. Dan, Alice J.
RA564.85.R44   1994
362.1'98—dc20   94-7456

    95 96 97 98 10 9 8 7 6 5 4 3 2

Sage Production Editor: Astrid Virding

Contents

Introduction

Alice J. Dan

Reframing Women's Health is intended as a sourcebook of the latest thinking in women's health from across the many disciplines involved in the development of this new field. Not only are the strongest voices from nursing and medicine represented, but also those from psychology, anthropology, social work, women's studies, sociology, legal scholarship, policy analysis, and activism appear in this volume. Together, they set out the directions in which the field of women's health will be moving in the years ahead.

Women's health is a new discipline in the process of creating itself. The recent visibility for women's health issues is no accident but is based on the growing recognition that research and practice in medicine and health care generally have been based on male perspectives, which have allowed needs and concerns of women to be neglected. Women are no longer willing to look at studies of heart disease in men and wonder whether the findings will apply to them. They are no longer willing to be considered something other than "normal," as happens when a male norm is applied to them. They want their concerns to be addressed in the mainstream of health science and practice, and this book presents important background for accomplishing that aim.

Researchers, educators, clinicians, and advocates interested in developments in women's health will find that *Reframing Women's Health* offers exciting ideas and practical strategies for implementing better health care for women. Information on women in a wide variety of situations is presented, including those most stereotyped, abused, and ignored. Although many of the writers are academics, and provide full documentation for their work, the chapters were written to communicate across disciplines, so they are accessible to a nonspecialist, educated lay audience as well.

The book is organized into six parts. Most of the chapters are based on material presented at a landmark conference held in October 1992 in Chicago. Although many conferences on women's health topics had occurred previously, this was the first to focus on the issue of defining specialization in women's health, addressing recent controversies about whether "a medical specialty" or some other approach can best serve the health needs of women.

Part I, Perspectives and Models, discusses the various shapes that a new framework in women's health might take. Although the authors by no means agree on a form, what emerges in all their discussions is a common view of women's health as a discipline freed of the old reliance on the male medical model of health and disease.

In the first chapter, Angela and William McBride present an update to their now-classic paper, "Theoretical Underpinnings for Women's Health" (McBride & McBride, 1981). They briefly review the Western tradition of medicine and philosophy that placed women in a secondary position to men's, or that ignored them altogether, using the male experience as the normative basis on which to evaluate health and disease. This view has forced feminist thinkers to begin the process of reframing by first tearing down the old framework—hence the necessity for critique to precede assertion. In exposing the old shibboleths of patriarchal thought behind which the male medical model has hidden, feminists have revealed the fallacies inherent in research, for example, when women are not included in the population under study or when women's diseases are ignored by researchers even though women constitute more than half the population.

Feminists thinkers have also questioned the intellectual habits of overgeneralization (ignoring the particular for the universal and abstract) and of reductionism (e.g., viewing women as reproductive entities only). In so doing, what has emerged is a new frame through which to view women and their place in the world: a frame that stresses *ecology,* not *gyne,* that views context as vital in understanding health and disease, that stresses the differences between women and men while acknowledging their commonalities, and that urges women to constitute themselves rather than allowing men to constitute their attributes. Such an emphasis results in new views of women's beauty, sexuality, health and fitness, and responsibilities as parents.

Lila Wallis, a physician active with the Coalition for Women's Health, next presents her case for multispecialty-generated continuing education in women's health, citing six reasons for a curriculum:

1. As presently constituted, the care of women is fragmented among medical specialties.
2. Women are different than men in a variety of ways, including hormonal, cardiovascular, gastrointestinal, immune, and psychological differences.
3. Women are the primary caregivers and channelers of their children and spouses into the health care system and resent being given second-class health care themselves.

4. Female morbidity and mortality are increased because of gender bias in research.
5. The time is propitious because there are more female physicians than ever before.
6. The most basic reason of all is to undo the damage created by gender bias in medical education, research, and clinical practice.

Wallis details the various manifestations of gender bias and then goes on to describe the American Medical Women's Association women's health curriculum, which is constructed around the life phases of women, divided into five modules from birth to advanced years, with each module discussing nine content areas. Wallis calls this 6- to 8-day course the first national attempt to teach medical providers a systematic, unbiased view of women.

Karen Johnson and Eileen Hoffman are perhaps the foremost proponents of a medical specialty in women's health; they are physicians in psychiatry and internal medicine, respectively. They maintain that medicine must "reframe its understanding and practice of women's health to reduce fragmentation and increase quality of care" by creating a new specialty devoted to women's health. Insisting that obstetrics/gynecology, internal medicine, and family practice are all limited in their focus and in their knowledge of the complexity and interrelatedness of women's health care needs, the authors argue that creating a specialty devoted to women is the only way to ensure that women's health achieves parity with men's and with children's health. Johnson and Hoffman further argue that only a specialty with a women-centered paradigm that will legitimize the consideration of such problems as violence against women, or the greater sensitivity of women to some drugs, will advance the cause of women's health. Because gender bias is so endemic to medicine, piecemeal efforts at eradicating it will not work. The medical curriculum must be transformed so that it views women as more than a pair of breasts and a uterus.

Describing how women receive health care in Canada, Gail Webber argues that family physicians should be given additional training in women's health. Because family physicians are the gatekeepers to the medical system in Canada, it is crucial that they be knowledgeable in all aspects of women's health and well-being. As a family medicine resident, the author was made aware of both the inadequacies and the power of the medical establishment vis-à-vis women's health. She was asked by Queen's University to develop a program in women's health that centered on consultation with health care providers both within and without the medical establishment. Through this consultative process, Webber developed a yearlong holistic curriculum that includes learning about the historical relationship between women and medicine, current attitudes toward women, the breadth and depth of women's health issues, learning new communication and technical skills, and, finally, learning how to become activists and advocates for women. As a Canadian

physician working within a system where the family physician screens all
health care problems, Webber says a specialization in women's health in
Canada would not be adequate to change the system at its entry point.

In their discussion of new educational paradigms, as exemplified in three
graduate nurse practitioner programs in Texas, California, and Washington,
Susan Cohen and associates reinforce the point that women's health studies
and practice must move away from the male medical model. This model both
reduces women's health to essentially reproductive health and fragments
women's care into such medical specialties as obstetrics, gynecology, endocrinology, and psychiatry. Their model proposes to care for the health of
women by recognizing the individual in context and by stressing prevention.
Caring for women is more than treatment; it includes "outreach, referral,
education, advocacy, and evaluation." The authors describe their programs
as models that incorporate a holistic, biopsychosocial approach to the care
of women, whose historically disadvantaged position in society has created
a litany of problems such as spousal abuse, poverty, and homelessness.

Jean Hamilton argues that, if physicians are truly to become incorporated
into the women's health movement, they must reframe their theory and
practice of medicine, which is currently based on the notion of "biological
primacy." This unexamined belief searches only for biological causes at the
root of an illness, reducing the human being to a concatenation of atoms,
minimizing the role of context, and serving as a strong intellectual barrier to
the improvement of women's health care.

Hamilton presents critiques of biological primacy from both feminist
theory and health psychology, finding similarities in their criticisms of its
reductionistic approach, its Cartesian split of mind and body, its inattention
to the psychological aspects of healing, and its focus on disease rather than
on prevention. Hamilton offers a way to educate physicians to turn away
from this model and their belief in their own superiority and privilege, to
embrace the importance of the contextual and the egalitarian, to view women
not as cases but as individuals of equal status whose whole person must be
cared for. She suggests that an interdisciplinary fellowship be taken by
physicians between medical school and residency to help them dismantle the
pernicious barrier of biological primacy as it operates in medicine among all
physicians, men and women alike.

Drawing on the work of Jean Baker Miller and associates at Wellesley,
Lucy Candib, a physician in family practice, posits the importance of self-
in-relation theory in understanding women's health and health care. This
theory provides a new way to view the way women behave in the world. The
traditional attributes of autonomy, separateness, and independence, described
by psychologists, almost all of whom were men, cannot simply be applied

to women. Self-in-relation theory holds up complexity, connection, and mutuality as descriptors of how human beings develop and interrelate.

Candib goes on to show how these two approaches also apply to medicine and health care. The male medical model separates the person from the disease and, in fact, teaches its students that healthy development from infancy to adulthood is characterized by progressive movement toward autonomy. In contrast, self-in-relation theory views women within the network of relationships and responsibilities in women's lives. For the clinician serving the needs of women, it allows for a caregiver-patient relationship built not on the authority of the physician but on mutuality, with both clinician and patient bearing responsibility for the course of the relationship. Candib concludes with a call not for a separate specialty in women's health but for all practitioners to apply self-in-relation theory. Arguing that women are too large and diverse a group with health care needs that span a lifetime, Candib believes that no one specialist can meet these needs.

In her call for a new academic discipline in women's health, Michelle Harrison offers yet another different approach. Although she agrees that there should be a separate specialty in women's health, Harrison believes it should include allied health professionals and advanced nurse practitioners; in this sense, it is not a "medical" specialty. According to Harrison, the debate about whether or not to create a separate specialty involves two issues: providing clinical services and creating a body of knowledge. Harrison believes both can be achieved optimally by the creation of a master's-level program, an applied academic discipline founded in theory as well as in practice. She further recommends that wellness models be developed for women, that internal medicine and family practice incorporate gynecological care, that the medical liability system be reassessed to encourage more autonomy on the part of physician assistants and nurse practitioners, that computer and video technology be used to educate women. She envisions the formation of interdisciplinary partnerships among a variety of medical, nursing, psychological, and sociological professionals to improve women's health care and to reexamine the hierarchy of power to reframe the belief that medical care is health care.

There are so many models—which one is "the best"? Discussions at the "Reframing" conference recalled the early arguments in women's studies about the issues of creating separate programs versus "mainstreaming" or integrating knowledge about women and gender into existing and core programs. This was only the first of many acknowledgments that the field of women's health has much to learn from women's studies. Strategically, we need *both/and*, not *either/or*. It is important that specialty programs be developed, so that this new discipline has a supportive home, so that the "critical mass" of committed women's health theorists, practitioners, and researchers will interact and move the field forward. But equally, these developments need to take many forms, and as the new knowledge related to women's health becomes available, existing programs need to be held accountable for including this information in non-gender-biased ways. At this moment in history, many different groups are feeling inspired to work on women's health programs to better meet the needs of the women they serve. Clearly, the answer is not a single "medical specialty" but a multiplicity of approaches. What is most central to the success of these efforts is mutual support and sharing of our energies across all of our situations.

Part II, Social and Political Issues, provides a contrast to Part I, taking the reader to some of the critical thinking on women's health *outside* the health care system. It includes chapters on international dimensions (Carmen Barroso), involving community women in women's health discussions (Sara Loevy and Mary O'Brien), national health care reform (Judy Norsigian), cautions about health care policy from a Canadian perspective (Judith Wuest), and a very personal story of health care experience, showing how much a woman's health is influenced by her sense of herself and other nonmedical factors (Ruth Behar). (A "Conference Statement" from an international women's health conference held in August 1992 was unanimously endorsed by the participants in the Reframing Women's Health conference. This statement, which reflects a unity of opinion from many countries, is found at the end of this Introduction.)

From her experience in international health, Barroso emphasizes the importance of viewing women's health from the perspectives of Third World women. Such issues as AIDS, global warming, poverty, and racism are examples of phenomena that affect health profoundly yet are often considered in isolation from our thinking on health. Viewing health globally can help women in the United States to reframe research and practice in women's health. The first lesson is the importance of prevention. Ironically, because the Third World does not have the sophisticated technology to diagnose and treat illness and injury, prevention assumes a more central role.

Barroso also points to a truly multidisciplinary approach linking economics and health. Poverty among women is directly related to health problems. Recent policies in the United States and other industrialized nations have served to reinforce the cycle of poverty in Third World countries. The reduction in economic aid for services to women and children is one example of these policies. In addition, trade barriers reflecting a protectionist posture continue to prevent developing countries from climbing out of the deep well of foreign debt that contributes to the vicious cycle of poverty and lack of health care resources for women and children.

Another lesson to be learned from developing countries is the practical impact of women's lack of power on their health status. Gender theory points to the relationship between discrimination and morbidity, but there is a need for a strong mutual support system between scholars and activists to work toward understanding how to apply theory to change the system that keeps women vulnerable.

Moving from the global to the community level, Loevy and O'Brien provide a model for incorporating the views and experiences of community women into research and program development. Focus groups provide an important context for working on women's health issues; they bring the social fabric of the community into the planning process. The authors describe their research to evaluate the system of care in Chicago that provides education and screening for poor women with regard to sexually transmitted diseases. The moving examples given are an embodiment of the admonition to "think globally, act locally."

In her chapter, Norsigian, of the Boston Women's Health Book Collective, argues for incorporating what we have learned from the Women's Health Movement into the program of health care reform. The shortcomings of the present system include overtreatment of women with medical insurance as well as lack of care for women without insurance. Long-term care coverage is neglected in favor of acute care. Perhaps most compelling is the relationship between the social structure and women's health as well as the discussion of how decisions are made and who will make them. While a single-payer system carries many advantages, the question of accountability is troublesome. When consumers do not pay directly for care, they are in a less powerful position with regard to the health care they receive.

Caregiving in families is also an aspect of women's health. Wuest presents a provocative critique of the potential risks of community influence on research. The problems of attempting to empower women within an oppressive context are discussed with insight, particulary relevant to health care reform.

Coming down again to the local level, anthropologist Behar presents the experience of one woman with the health care system. This personal and poignant story of how and why Marta has a hysterectomy brings out many aspects of health care for women and immigrants. In this example, the self-in-relation character of women's lives is illustrated in a meaningful framework.

The interplay of levels in this section, from international to community, national to individual, demonstrates the need for multiple viewpoints to fully understand the issues of the social, political, and economic context for women's health. Why should context be any more significant for women than for men? Men's lives are also lived within a context, after all. But given that the current system of health care is based on a medical model devised primarily by men, the *assumed* context is more likely to fit men than women. For this reason, special attention is needed to counter these assumptions, which may often be inaccurate for women (or for men of color).

Part III presents four significant issues in women's reproductive health and sexuality. Each of the chapters in this section makes connections between issues of reproduction, sexuality, and the social forces affecting women's lives. Nada Stotland, a psychiatrist, is concerned about the meaning of the choices available to women. Leonore Tiefer is a psychologist who challenges the medical models of sexuality, showing how far short biological theories of sexuality fall. Tiefer's more complex theoretical proposals provide important insights on sex questions. Jean Hunt and Carole Joffe consider issues in the provision of reproductive health care, specifically abortion. Whatever shape women's health care takes in the future, this review of historical background and analysis of alternate providers will be useful. And, finally, a group from the Cook County Hospital Women and Children's HIV Program (Mary Driscoll and associates) writes about women and AIDS. They view HIV as a multidimensional problem, not just as a sexually transmitted disease. As we are learning daily, HIV involves issues of poverty, race, family relationships, and female roles. Women's lack of power is a critical factor in their experience with HIV.

Part IV focuses on the impact of violence and abuse on women's health; it presents a comprehensive overview ranging from the individual level of clinician-patient interaction to the international issues of gender-based abuse. Mary Koss's chapter gives a carefully reasoned analysis of available data on use of medical services to provide a rationale to those in power for changes to the health care system. She argues convincingly that, in the current system, women who have suffered victimization lack appropriate interventions. The medical interventions they currently experience are iatrogenic, causing more problems for women following their interaction with the health care system.

Carole Warshaw's chapter helps us to understand *how* practitioners are influenced by their experiences and training to misunderstand the significance of violence in the lives of women they encounter in medical settings. Using concepts of individual pathology to explain life problems is a disempowering way to interact with victims of abuse. Warshaw's analysis leads to practical recommendations for improving clinical practice. Going even further into the experience of victimized women, Beth Richie reports on her work with African American women in prison. Her in-depth exploration with this specific group leads to understanding of more general mechanisms of power in women's lives, such as how culture affects identity and how personal, cultural, and political power are all connected.

The global context for violence against women is presented by Lori Heise, who works with the Center for Global Leadership at Rutgers University. She reports on international efforts to recognize abuse as a violation of human rights. Her overview illustrates how more specific situations are connected and how priorities for action can be set. Her description of low-violence cultures helps to clarify goals for social reform efforts for primary prevention of gender-based abuse.

Part V covers research issues, including both clinical and behavioral research as well as feminist and legal perspectives. As Sue Rosser explains, it is not only that women have been neglected as subjects of research, but the very paradigms for research have been developed from male perspectives. Available research on men cannot be simply generalized to apply to women, in part because women's experiences are not yet adequately represented in the research paradigms. Using specific examples like reproductive technology research, Rosser discusses how female perspectives might result in different paradigms. The relationship between the researcher and the researched, for example, could be different. The analysis of gender bias can be extended to understanding the significance of race and class bias in research as well.

Complicating these issues of gender bias in research are the legal implications of exposing women, particularly of childbearing age, to experimental drugs or procedures. Michelle Oberman is a lawyer with expertise in health law and ethics. Her chapter clarifies the consequences for women of their inclusion or noninclusion in drug research. Like the complex issues involved in protective labor laws, there are no simple answers to questions about the protective approach for drug research.

Moving away from traditional biomedical research, Renee Royak-Schaler reviews psychosocial health research relevant to women's health. Starting with the history of tension between policy and research, she critiques the focus of behavioral research on such concepts as "compliance," which represent a limited view of the context in which health behavior occurs. On the positive side, she identifies important advances in psychosocial research, including the use of complementary modalities and the significance of perceived control in health behavior.

The last chapter in Part V concerns guidelines for research in the area of violence against women. Nanette Silva draws from her experience to discuss the issues involved in this kind of research, which confronts the power structure supporting male violence. This research has as its goal social change, so as to lessen the risks to women's health. The long-term struggle for institutional change is necessary to a feminist methodology in research on battered women.

Part VI considers specific practice situations from a women's health standpoint. These include the provider-patient relationship, weight control, lesbian health, women with disabilities, breast cancer, and interstitial cystitis. In each chapter, insights are gained from the specific topic to contribute to the general knowledge of women's health issues.

Sue Fisher is a medical sociologist concerned with how women fare as patients with different health care providers. In this chapter, she considers the concept of "caring," as used in the nursing literature to describe differences between medical and nursing practice. She provides detailed examples of patient interactions with physician and nurse practitioner. In her analysis of these interactions, she examines the consequences for the female patients of the differences, and how the concept of caring comes into play. The complex interactions of gender, class, and professional training are explored in their historical context, going beyond the simple notion that female providers are more caring or more empowering to their female patients.

These same issues arise in many different ways throughout these chapters. Joan Chrisler, for example, points out the misogynist impact of mixed messages to young women about their bodies. What is the meaning of fat? What is its relation to health? These questions are difficult to answer in the current contradictory social context. For lesbians, as Anne Haas describes, the social context is one of invisibility and stereotyping. Women in nonreproductive roles have been ignored in the health care system. Now that there is some recognition of lesbian needs for access to health care, our awareness must go further to understand that lesbians are not a homogeneous group. Because health risks depend on individual circumstances, the practical recommendations propose a model of attention to individual experience. Women with disabilities present many similar issues, according to Carol Gill and her associates. Again, we are directed to examine the quality of the patient-provider interaction and the quality of attention granted to the female patient. Women with disabilities challenge our notions of female and feminine, of humanity and imperfection. This is also true for women with breast cancer. Using a health-belief model, Diane Lauver examines barriers to the use of preventive strategies for women with breast cancer. The final chapter in Part VI, by Denise Webster, uses the example of interstitial cystitis to return to the questions of reframing women's health. Interstitial cystitis is a painful condition experienced primarily by women, whose etiology is not well understood; nor are effective treatments readily available. Historically, treatment for this condition has reflected social ideology about women: that their complaints are psychosomatic, that somehow they are to blame for their illness, that they reject their female sexuality. Like many other conditions, no cure will soon be found for interstitial cystitis, so our focus needs to be on practice, research, and education to promote respect and compassion for women patients.

The book concludes with an epilogue chapter, which lays out the critical decisions needed to further develop the field of women's health. The groundwork is provided for building an institutional structure to support a discipline of women's health that will truly address the health needs and concerns of women. Of course such a discipline will contribute significantly to better health for *all* by incorporating women's voices into the health care system, health research, and health education.

On Saturday, October 17, 1993, a resolution was adopted unanimously by participants to affirm the statement of the "Fifth International Conference on Women's Health Issues: Environment, Daily Life, and Health." This statement holds that health is determined by economic, social, and political forces and that health is best promoted by meeting basic human needs for nutrition, rest, exercise, self-esteem, and safety. Women's roles as caregivers are recognized.

Resolution: As conference participants concerned with "reframing" women's health, we hereby recognize and support the expression of unity found in the conference statement from the 5th International Conference on Women's Health Issues, held in Copenhagen, Denmark, in August of 1992, which was attended by representatives from 31 countries. We encourage the use of this document on a continued basis for discussion in our communities. We emphasize, in particular, the responsibility of the U.S. health system, which fails U.S. women and oppresses women worldwide.

Copenhagen Conference Statement

Fifth International Conference on Women's Health Issues: Environment, Daily Life and Health—Women's Strategies for Our Common Future: Copenhagen, Denmark, August 28, 1992[1]

This Fifth International Congress on Women's Health Issues recognizes the interactive relationship between health and the environment. Participants from thirty-one countries agreed that health is first and foremost determined by adequate economic and social conditions, which assure sufficient food, water, shelter and other necessary resources for sustaining life and promoting health. Millions of persons are denied these basic life sustaining resources. It is predominantly women who are victims of health-destroying cycles of devaluation, deprivation and poor health. Poor women compose the majority of all women globally. Within all societies, the majority of poor people are women.

Health is determined by the interaction of economic, political and social forces. Understanding the significance of this interaction means an appreciation of the interconnectedness between models of development being pursued in the world and systems of domination which reduce the capacities of people, especially poor people, to sustainably lead their lives. International policies predicated on unjust economic relations and unfair trade practices have reduced the countries of the Third World to abject poverty. Policies such as Structural Adjustment, which entails among other things removing food subsidies in poor countries, now operative in about 80 countries of the world, mean that poor women, men and children bear the main burden of debt. The world debt interferes with sustainable environments protective of health. The structuring of economic systems dependent on military and technical industries reinforces violent approaches to problems, diverts resources from health enhancing development, and devalues the caring work of society on which healthy and environmentally sustainable economies should be built.

Poor people, especially women, are denied the education needed to attain control over their lives and expand the democratic structures of society. Sociocultural violence and abuse is an aspect of control over women and children, which both physically and psychologically damages their health.

All over the world women are given excessive burdens of the caring work of society. The withdrawal of the state from service provision has resulted in increasing the vulnerability of women who are the main carers for their families. Consequently, there is an erosion of women's access to food, shelter, occupation, and education resulting in deterioration of women's health. Particularly in Eastern Europe the problems of women losing long established rights has serious implications for health.

The escalation of medical treatment and technological approaches to health are not what is needed to promote the health of women, actually having become directly or indirectly damaging for the health of women in many instances. In a world of limited resources, the emphasis should not be on developing expensive technological and pharmaceutical approaches to disease, many of which have damaging effects once longterm consequences become known. Instead, the emphasis should be on promoting health by meeting basic human needs for nutrition, rest, exercise, self-esteem, and safety. For women, the central need is control over their bodies, which includes being empowered to take care of themselves and participate in the creation of more caring societies.

The following recommendations follow from these facts:

Women's health work should be based on the recognition that human health cannot be protected and improved without protecting the eco-systems that sustain all life.

Social, political and economic justice at global and national levels needs to be fundamental health policy.

Democratization and decentralization of knowledge, resources, and decision making are essential for attaining health for all.

Education for empowerment and occupational opportunity are fundamental for improving the health of women.

Health research and practice need to shift from reductionistic work to understanding the interrelationships among influences shaping health.

Practitioners and providers of health care need to pay attention to the impact of social and economic conditions on the health and safety of the women they serve, and act to increase the self determination of those women.

The fundamental health enhancing nature of care, including the unpaid health care which women provide, must be recognized in health policy and services.

Paid and unpaid work must be evenly distributed, and equitably compensated, between men and women. This would also entail putting in place mechanisms that improve women's access to and control over resources.

Women's rights must include control over their own bodies, which must be recognized at all levels of policy and practice.

All forms of coercion and violence against women must be stopped.

Women's health researchers have an important role in promoting understanding of different groups of women, recognizing that women are not a monolithic group but have diverse needs and perspectives.

Knowledge, skills, and practices of women and local communities must be revalidated and made the basis of further research in the generation of health knowledge.

Unnecessary and harmful medicalization and chemicalization of health practices need to be opposed and stopped.

Women all over the world should work against dumping of harmful and useless drugs, tobacco products, reproductive technologies and industrial and toxic waste by the industrialized countries, in less technologically developed countries.

In the present, increasingly unipolar world, UN organizations like UNEP, WHO Unicef, FAO, Unifem, and the Commission for Refugees need to be strengthened, reformed and sensitized to women's health issues worldwide. This includes greater representation of women at all organizational levels, including top leadership positions.

None of these goals can be achieved without fundamentally changing the structure of health and research systems. Therefore, women around the world need to support each other in developing alternative institutions to nurture themselves, their families, and the natural environment.

Note

1. For more information on this international congress, sponsored by the International Congress on Women's Health Issues, contact Dr. Phyllis Noerager Stern, Editor, *Health Care for Women International*, Indiana University School of Nursing, 1111 Middle Drive, NU 451, Indianapolis, IN 46202-5107.

Reference

McBride, A. B., & McBride, W. L. (1981). Theoretical underpinnings for women's health. *Women & Health, 6*(1-2), 37-55.

PART I

Perspectives and Models

Women's Health Scholarship: From Critique to Assertion

Angela Barron McBride
William Leon McBride

Women's health scholarship, as a distinct subset of women's studies, is in the process of undergoing a shift of emphasis. What began as a critique of patriarchal practices and their effects on women's well-being is evolving into a positive statement of values. Just as philosophers concerned with the concepts of freedom or power have considered both the negative and the positive meanings of these terms—*freedom from* versus *freedom for* or *power over* versus *power to*—women's health scholarship is moving from critique to assertion. This chapter provides an overview of some of the chief practices that have been called into question, touches on some current philosophical trends that may abet the shift of emphasis to which we are calling attention, and then offers examples of the new scholarship emerging in this area.

Past Practices

Although women have no doubt occupied roles of special honor as healers and been accorded adequate treatment relative to existing technology at certain times and places in past history, the same can certainly not be asserted as a generalization about the more recent past. On the contrary, women's experiences of health care have all too often been affected by a climate of practice in which male physiology and behavior have been taken as normative. Among the further effects of this stance have been a failure to include

SOURCE: This chapter originally appeared in modified form in *Journal of Women's Health,* Vol. 2, No. 1, 1993, pp. 43-47; used by permission of Mary Ann Liebert, Inc., 1651 Third Ave., New York, NY 10128.

women in much major health research, a noticeable sex bias in some treatment choices, a refusal to take seriously certain problems of special concern peculiar to women, a concomitant ignoring of those health considerations of men that are most obviously complementary to women's concerns, and a disregard for the special environmental and sociocultural factors that affect women as a group. A final effect has been the highly problematic character, in this regard as in so many others, of the health care delivery system itself.

The assumption that maleness should be regarded as the norm, from which female characteristics constitute deviations, has received sophisticated justifications from Western thinkers such as Aristotle and from much of the long, broad tradition of natural law. The lived experience of women throughout most of Western history has been one of socialization to a cultural environment in which vivacious sperm are seen as energizing the passive, virtually (or, for Aristotle and his followers, completely) inert matter that is the female egg, and women even at their wisest and saintliest have been typically expected, from the ancient Greeks through Freud to Kohlberg, to be relatively less well developed mentally and morally than their male counterparts.

The exclusion of women from many areas of research has not itself been exactly an aspect of women's lived experience—most people usually are not aware of a dearth of studies on themselves or on those significantly like them—but it has had serious, often dire consequences in millions of women's lives. For example, many of the most important alcohol and drug studies have omitted women in part or altogether (Moore, 1980); yet increased alcohol consumption is now known to be, relatively speaking, directly linked to episodes of depression and to life crises, and to occur concurrently with the use of antidepressants, more frequently in women than in men (Lex, 1991). Three of seven major studies that are the basis of standard hypertension treatment (now thought by some to be actually harmful to some women) included no women subjects (Anastos et al., 1991), and animal-model research uses females relatively rarely because of concern about the possibility of "odd" findings resulting from hormonal fluctuations.

These systematically reinforced sex biases in research, which are now finally coming under considerable public scrutiny in this country, have played themselves out in the lived experiences of most women in terms both of skewed treatment for illnesses and problems and of nontreatment of certain concerns peculiar to women that have not been taken seriously by the health care establishment. Women with breast cancer, for instance, were historically prevented or at least strongly discouraged from considering a range of treatment options (Kushner, 1975), often by means of running together the biopsy with an irreversible treatment, such as radical mastectomy, after they had been persuaded to sign a blanket release. Disproportionately little attention has been paid to certain conditions that affect women in relatively larger numbers, such as agoraphobia, urinary incontinence, osteoporosis, lupus, and autoimmune diseases in general. (It is noteworthy that approximately half of all new cases of AIDS, which only a few years ago was associated primarily with male homosexuals in the popular mind, are now women; Shayne & Kaplan, 1991.) Until recently, violence against women (rape, battering, and so on) and its concomitant physical and psychological health effects have been largely ignored (Sampselle, 1992).

Paradoxically, this kind of bias has even had adverse effects on men. For example, relatively little attention has been paid to the technical possibilities of contraception in men, because contraception has been regarded as primarily in the domain of women. Similarly, because the requirement of fulfilling multiple roles in the complex contemporary world was first seen to arise as a problem in the context of women's lives, it is only very recently that the contribution of the same requirement to serious stress in men has begun to be studied (Barnett, Marshall, & Pleck, 1992).

Mention of this last deficiency in past health care practice leads to a more general reflection on the traditional inattention, still characteristic of too much health care even today, to environmental and sociocultural factors in dealing with women's health problems. In fact, much research suggests that the fulfilling of multiple roles per se, both inside and outside the home, may be more of a solution than a problem for many women, as for many men (Baruch, Biener, & Barnett, 1987; Kritz-Silverstein, Wingard, & Barrett-Connor, 1992; McBride, 1990; Verbrugge & Madans, 1985); it all depends on the specific way in which this expectation is lived and experienced. In short, it is virtually impossible to overestimate the importance of the values of the sociocultural environment in accounting both for women's well-being and for women's illnesses and diseases major and minor, such as Third World undernourishment resulting from the vicious cycle of poverty, high infant mortality, frequent pregnancy, and exclusion of women from any but the lowest paid jobs (Nussbaum, 1992).

Theoretical Developments

These observations concerning health care treatment and research exemplify the raw material that exists to permit us to generate new theoretical frameworks for the field of women's health. A strong, though not exclusive, emphasis of theoretical efforts in this area up to now has been on *critique*: critique of health care and research practices such as those just described, complemented by the critique of a certain abstract universalism in traditional mainstream Western thought that often serves to undergird such practices. As we expressed it in our earlier contribution to this topic:

The quest for abstract universal laws remained so all-powerful a driving force
that neither Kant nor most of the other leading historical figures of Western
thought, at least until the Nineteenth Century, considered it at all important to
concern themselves with the actual condition of distinct groups, in particular those,
such as women, commonly regarded as inferior, in developing their theoretical
frameworks. They did not confront the possibility that engaging in such concrete analysis might necessitate fundamental modifications of the abstract universal laws themselves. (McBride & McBride, 1981, p. 43)

To facilitate the critique of misogynous practices, then, a theoretical refocusing away from these abstract universals and toward the notion of *lived
experience* was required; the latter implies sympathetic regard for women's
so-called subjective concerns and the sociocultural factors that we have just
discussed.

It is now both possible and desirable to place increased stress, in the
domain of theory as well as in the domains of practice and research, on developing positive, future-oriented agendas built on successful critiques of
the past. The following are a few brief suggestions about these incipient new
theoretical frameworks. One useful way of expressing the move from critique to assertion is to identify it as a shift from *gynecology* to *GYN-ecology*
(Daly, 1978), with the latter term evoking the movement known as eco-
feminism (Diamond & Orenstein, 1990; Rosser, 1991). While some of the
ecofeminists' central concerns have to do with applying feminist insights
directly to the protection of our physical environment, which is under such
intense siege from industrial interests, this movement is obviously motivated
by a recognition of the very close interconnection between hopes for a
possibly more positive, constructive approach to women's health and well-
being and fears that environmental degradation will, if unchecked, obviate
such a possibility. Ecofeminists relate the now-commonplace ethical identification of women with attitudes and practices of *caring* for other individuals
(Noddings, 1984) to the extensive scientific evidence supporting the greater-
than-ever need for global caring, that is, caring for the globe itself.

Of particular importance among other recent theoretical trends is an
enhanced emphasis on the notion of *difference* (Young, 1990). Inspired in
part by a postmodern reaction to the very idea of a systematic, "totalistic,"
or even "totalitarian" theory of society and in part by a feminist recognition
of the adverse consequences, of the sort that we have enumerated here, of
overlooking gender differences, this trend lays the theoretical groundwork
for the women's health ("GYN-ecological") practice of the future. It implies
both being sensitive to actual male-female differences while recognizing the
extent to which they are socially constructed (Jacklin & McBride-Chang,
1991) and also acknowledging differences *among* women that are attribut-

able to such factors as age, cultural background, education, sexual preference, and work experience.

One danger entailed by the welcome emphasis on *difference* in contemporary theory is that it can be used as an excuse for refraining from generalities altogether, and in practical terms for eschewing all common (sociopolitical) action in favor of strictly particular, private responses to women's health and other social needs. However, as long as we recognize that each human being, though singular, also has a universal dimension (Sartre, 1972) and that the delicate, intricate, highly interconnected ecosystem in which we all live is a reality and no mere abstraction, then it will be possible to stave off arguments for the total individualization and privatization of health care on the ground that we are all different, anyway.

A final tendency having similar positive potential among recent theoretical trends is the renewed discussion of the idea of *community*. While "communitarianism" as a set of ideas means something at least slightly different to each of its major proponents (Elshtain, 1982; Mac Intyre, 1988; Sandel, 1982) and while certain interpretations of it could actually lead to a harmful suppression of individual differences in favor of enforcing traditionalism and homogeneity, the principal motivation of this renewed discussion seems to us to be in keeping with the emphasis on environment ("GYN-ecology") and on individuals' embeddedness in their world that we see as undergirding better women's health practice in the future. There are different levels of community, from local to global; a fully adequate theory, applicable to women's health concerns, will neglect none of these.

Beyond Critique to Assertion

The theoretical frameworks touched on point the way to some of the constructions taking shape as the field of women's health moves away from critique to assertion. Ecofeminism reminds us that GYN-ecology can signify more than critique, for it represents a paradigm shift away from focusing largely on the dispositional attributes of the individual (e.g., woman as hysterical, masochistic, neurotic, orally fixated) to highlighting the extent to which the person-environment fit is important to any understandings of health. The emphasis on difference urges us to stop thinking of women as a monolithic group, while communitarianism is another reminder that one cannot understand the individual in isolation from her world.

The critique of women's health experience reflects the negative consequences of their being defined only in relation to and by men. It is a critique that builds on Beauvoir's (1949/1974) insights about women: "She is defined and differentiated with reference to man and not he with reference to her"

(p. xix). It is a critique leading to a radical thesis—"that our notions of the female body, femininity, women's nature, and the conditions that underwrite these identities are entirely masculinist social constructions" (Dietz, 1992, p. 82). The move to assertion, by contrast, takes the stance that criticizing the extent to which women have been "constituted" selves must now give way to their becoming "constituting" selves, persons who define their own experience. Women's construction of themselves vis-à-vis individual experience will necessarily recognize "the ways in which subjectivity is discursively and socially constructed" (Kruks, 1992, p. 91). Thus it will recognize both the extent to which not all women are alike and the reciprocal nature of the tensions between the person and the communities in which she is embedded (family, work, ethnic, religious, and so on).

As women constitute themselves, meanings can change profoundly. When women are asked to describe a sexually attractive woman, their answers reflect experiential descriptions—"self-confident," "having presence," "vitality"—and not just stereotypes about being "built like Marilyn Monroe with a face like Bo Derek" (Bernhard & Dan, 1986). New concepts have been formulated, such as sexual harassment and date rape (Lewin & Wild, 1991); new distinctions have been made, such as that between caring as identity and activity (Graham, 1983), with an acknowledgment that coerced caring exists (Abel, 1991; Nelson, 1990). The notion of the constituting self has led to feminist innovations in therapy—consciousness-raising, sex role resocialization, feminist psychoanalysis—that have challenged traditional categories of meaning and have encouraged "change" rather than mere "adaptation" as the therapeutic goal (Marecek & Hare-Mustin, 1991).

Awareness of health as a social construction has dramatically influenced perceptions of body image and the so-called eating disorders. Women are rejecting impossible-to-achieve standards of beauty and advocating self-love and size acceptance (Iazzetto, 1990; Wolf, 1991). Obesity has been discussed as one consequence of encouraging women to compete in the kitchen while being denied access to the athletic arena (McBride, 1988). Many everyday assumptions have been unmasked as myths—such as that the overweight overeat; that diets are the means to lose weight; that being fat is necessarily unhealthy (Rothblum, 1990). Chronic dieting is now regarded as an independent risk factor for cardiovascular disease (Bouchard, 1991) and is implicated in causing binge eating and related disorders such as bulimia (Ruderman, 1986). The more positive meanings of fat as a metaphor for women's experience are being reclaimed—fat is warm, generous, nurturing, substantive (McBride, 1989a). The notion of being fat and fit is emerging as a new view of women's possibilities that recognizes that women come in all shapes but still can be in "great shape" if fitness programs are designed for their needs (Lyons & Burgard, 1990).

Feminist critique has led to a profound rethinking of parenthood that has advocated the growth and development of mothers along with their children (McBride, 1973) and demonstrated the importance of fathers to child development (Lamb, 1981). The critical reconstitution of the meaning of women's experience as mother has resulted in renewed appreciation for the importance of commonplace thoughts and feelings, including the notion that being a parent changes one: "Becoming a parent often produces a fairly sudden enlargement of one's cognitive map" (White, 1975, p. 361). This massive rethinking of what it means to be a mother or father, in turn, has led to additional insights about parenting at various stages of the child's life (Galinsky, 1981; McBride, 1989b) and a fresh perspective on relationships between the generations as they become more reciprocal (Lenz, 1981).

As women constitute themselves, they are discovering that the distinctions Bernard once made between "his" and "her" marriage, in acknowledging that men and women may experience the world differently (Bernard, 1972), also hold for "his" and "her" health because women and men experience substantially different health trajectories over a lifetime. Women report more illness and health care use than men, but they consistently live longer too: "The data show that women have higher rates of acute illnesses and most nonfatal chronic conditions; but men have higher prevalence rates of the leading fatal conditions, which parallels their higher mortality" (Verbrugge, 1990, p. 159). This gender paradox is more than a puzzle, it underscores the extent to which *morbidity* is a key feminist issue and points the way to what should be the central focus of the next round of the women's health movement. (A further reason for focusing on morbidity as a feminist issue is that most caregivers, both formal and informal ones, are female, thus they are the ones who bear the burden of dealing with chronic conditions.)

In a society that provides better coverage generally for the acute services used more by men than for the long-term and outpatient services used more by women (Sofaer & Abel, 1990), assertion requires us to revalue morbidity and to recognize its profound importance as an area for scholarship. Women's morbidity in contemporary life is driven by social factors—"lesser employment, higher felt stress and unhappiness, stronger feelings of illness vulnerability, fewer formal time constraints (related to fewer job hours), and less physically strenuous leisure activities" (Verbrugge, 1990, pp. 183-184). The tendency has been to regard such a constellation of factors as evidence of a woman's being hypochondriacal and characterologically flawed. But men feel more mastery in their lives and have higher self-esteem; they also have less trouble taking time for care and more insurance resources to do so (Verbrugge, 1990). It is now time to excise any remaining tendencies to blame the person and instead to articulate fully the extent to which women's overall health has been constrained by the possibilities afforded them and the seemingly uncontrollable nature of the pressures on them. We must stop treating morbidity as a morbidly dull topic and use a reconfigured concept of morbidity as a springboard for actively discussing health-enhancing lifestyle possibilities where healthy choices can be the easy choices. The projection of such lifestyle possibilities, with its constructively utopian implications, should become central to the GYN-ecology of the next decade, which will also be the next millennium.

It may seem somewhat at variance with the topic to end a chapter purportedly discussing health and assertion with a plea for an innovative look at morbidity, but such a consideration will force us to confront many themes of the women's health movement in a fresh way. To begin with, it will mean reclaiming an area so often discussed pejoratively as unworthy of our most creative or intense efforts. The lifestyle issues undergirding the expression of symptoms will force us to consider the extent to which our social policies and practices encourage health. Managing chronic health problems will force us to think about health care reform—the need to demedicalize our notions of who should be included as possible health care providers; the adequacy of insurance coverage; the importance of self-help through education and support groups; and the burden of caregiving shouldered by daughters, wives, and mothers without respite care and without their work's being recognized as part of our gross national product. Morbidity is also an area where we can be exquisitely creative—in making clear the extent to which a disease label need not be a predictor of functioning or quality of life; in designing new devices that ease restrictions brought on by limitations; in studying so-called old wives' tales for suggestions about possible noninvasive treatments; in demonstrating the extent to which morbidity can be compressed until the end of life; in articulating the relationship between life span development and health as physique-based values give way over a lifetime to wisdom-based values. Though we must continue to be mindful of the range of topics that can be considered under the umbrella term *women's health*, it is in asserting the importance of understanding and limiting morbidity that we will be most likely to transform the health of real flesh-and-blood women.

References

Abel, E. K. (1991). *Who cares for the elderly?* Philadelphia: Temple University Press.
Anastos, K., Charney, P., Charon, R., Cohen, E., Jones, C., Marte, C., Swiderski, D., Wheat, M. E., & Williams, S. (1991). Hypertension in women: What is really known? *Annals of Internal Medicine, 115*, 287-293.

Barnett, R. C., Marshall, N. L., & Pleck, J. H. (1992). Men's multiple roles and their relationship to men's psychological distress. *Journal of Marriage and the Family, 54,* 358-367.

Baruch, G. K., Biener, L., & Barnett, R. C. (1987). Women and gender in research on work and family stress. *American Psychologist, 42,* 130-136.

Beauvoir, S. de. (1974). *The second sex* (Ed. and Trans., H. M. Parshley). New York: Vintage. (Original work published 1949)

Bernard, J. (1972). *The future of marriage.* New York: World.

Bernhard, L. A., & Dan, A. J. (1986). Redefining sexuality from women's own experiences. *Nursing Clinics of North America, 21*(1), 125-136.

Bouchard, C. (1991). Is weight fluctuation a risk factor? *New England Journal of Medicine, 324,* 1887-1889.

Daly, M. (1978). *Gyn/ecology: The metaethics of radical feminism.* Boston: Beacon.

Diamond, I., & Orenstein, G. F. (Eds.). (1990). *Reweaving the world: The emergence of ecofeminism.* San Francisco: Sierra Club Books.

Dietz, M. G. (1992). Introduction: Debating Simone de Beauvoir. *Signs: Journal of Women in Culture and Society, 18,* 74-88.

Elshtain, J. B. (1982, Fall). Feminism, family, and community. *Dissent,* pp. 442-449.

Galinsky, E. (1981). *Between generations: The six stages of parenthood.* New York: Times Books.

Graham, H. (1983). Caring: A labour of love. In J. Finch & D. Groves (Eds.), *A labour of love: Women, work and caring* (pp. 13-30). London: Routledge.

Iazzetto, D. (1990). Women and body image. In C. Leppa (Ed.), *Women's health perspectives: An annual review* (Vol. 3, pp. 61-76). Phoenix: Oryx.

Jacklin, C. N., & McBride-Chang, C. (1991). The effects of feminist scholarship on developmental psychology. *Psychology of Women Quarterly, 15,* 549-556.

Kritz-Silverstein, D., Wingard, D. L., & Barrett-Connor, E. (1992). Employment status and heart disease risk factors in middle-aged women: The Rancho Bernardo study. *American Journal of Public Health, 82,* 215-219.

Kruks, S. (1992). Gender and subjectivity: Simone de Beauvoir and contemporary feminism. *Signs: Journal of Women in Culture and Society, 18,* 89-110.

Kushner, R. (1975). *Breast cancer: A personal and investigative report.* New York: Harcourt Brace Jovanovich.

Lamb, M. E. (Ed.). (1981). *The role of the father in child development* (2nd ed.). New York: John Wiley.

Lenz, E. (1981). *Once my child . . . Now my friend.* New York: Warner.

Lewin, M., & Wild, C. L. (1991). The impact of the feminist critique on tests, assessment, and methodology. *Psychology of Women Quarterly, 15,* 581-596.

Lex, B. W. (1991). Some gender differences in alcohol and polysubstance users. *Health Psychology, 10,* 121-132.

Lyons, P., & Burgard, D. (1990). *Great shape: The first fitness guide for large women.* Palo Alto, CA: Bull.

Mac Intyre, A. (1988). *Whose justice? Which rationality?* South Bend: University of Notre Dame Press.

Marecek, J., & Hare-Mustin, R. T. (1991). A short history of the future: Feminism and clinical psychology. *Psychology of Women Quarterly, 15,* 521-536.

McBride, A. B. (1973). *The growth and development of mothers.* New York: Harper & Row.

McBride, A. B. (1988). Fat: A women's issue in search of a holistic approach to treatment. *Holistic Nursing Practice, 3*(1), 9-15.

McBride, A. B. (1989a). Fat is generous, nurturing, warm . . . *Women and Therapy, 8*(3), 93-103.

McBride, A. B. (1989b). *How to enjoy a good life with your teenager.* Tucson, AZ: Fisher.

McBride, A. B. (1990). Mental health effects of women's multiple roles. *American Psychologist,* *45,* 381-384.

McBride, A. B., & McBride, W. L. (1981). Theoretical underpinnings for women's health. *Women & Health, 6*(1-2), 37-55.

Moore, E. C. (Ed.). (1980). Woman and health. In *Public health reports* (September-October Suppl., pp. 1-84). Washington, DC: Government Printing Office.

Nelson, M. K. (1990). *Negotiated care: The experience of family day care providers.* Philadelphia: Temple University Press.

Noddings, N. (1984). *Caring: A feminine approach to ethics and moral education.* Berkeley: University of California Press.

Nussbaum, M. (1992). Justice for women. *New York Review of Books, 39*(16), 43-48.

Rosser, S. V. (1991). Eco-feminism: Lessons for feminism from ecology. *Women's Studies International Forum, 14,* 143-151.

Rothblum, E. (1990). Women and weight: Fad and fiction. *Journal of Psychology, 124,* 5-24.

Ruderman, A. J. (1986). Dietary restraint: A theoretical and empirical review. *Psychological Bulletin, 99,* 247-262.

Sampselle, C. M. (Ed.). (1992). *Violence against women: Nursing research, education, and practice issues.* New York: Hemisphere.

Sandel, M. (1982). *Liberalism and the limits of justice.* Cambridge, MA: Harvard University Press.

Sartre, J. P. (1972). L'universel singulier. In *Situations, IX* (pp. 152-190). Paris: Gallimard.

Shayne, V. T., & Kaplan, B. J. (1991). Double victims: Poor women and AIDS. *Women & Health, 17*(1), 21-37.

Sofaer, S., & Abel, E. (1990). Older women's health and financial vulnerability: Implications of the Medicare benefit structure. *Women Health, 16*(3-4), 47-67.

Verbrugge, L. M. (1990). The twain meet: Empirical explanations of sex differences in health and mortality. In M. G. Ory & H. R. Warner (Eds.), *Gender, health and longevity* (pp. 159-199). New York: Springer.

Verbrugge, L. M., & Madans, J. H. (1985). Social roles and health trends of American women. *Milbank Memorial Fund Quarterly, 63,* 691-735.

White, R. W. (1975). *Lives in progress* (3rd ed.). New York: Holt, Rinehart & Winston.

Wolf, N. (1991). *The beauty myth: How images of beauty are used against women.* New York: William Morrow.

Young, I. (1990). *Justice and the politics of difference.* Princeton, NJ: Princeton University Press.

2

Why a Curriculum on Women's Health?

Lila A. Wallis

Over the last several decades, the women's movement in this country led a number of women physicians to examine critically the health needs of their patients and observe the glaring disparities and gaps in research, in education/ training of physicians, as well as in clinical practice of women's health (Symonds, 1980; Wallis, 1982a, 1982b). These were voices crying in the wilderness.

The public became better acquainted with gender bias in medicine follow-ing the congressional investigation, in June 1990, of the National Institutes of Health (NIH) policies and lack of compliance with its own policies (Nadel, 1990). Public attention was further focused on the problem when an office was created within the NIH for research in women's health (ORWH) and when a woman, Dr. Bernadine Healy, was appointed as director of the NIH (Healy, 1991a). It became clear to many that the various processes of research, and of physician training and clinical practice, ignore women as patients, women as research subjects, women as doctors, and women as medical inves-tigators (Healy, 1991b).

Many papers were published proposing remedies (Harrison, 1990, 1992; Healy, 1991a, 1991b; Johnson, 1992; Johnson & Dawson, 1990; Wallis, 1992; Wallis & Klass, 1990). Women's health centers proliferated both within and outside the traditional teaching medical centers in this country.

Nevertheless, despite, or perhaps because of, the publicity, the backlash has never been more powerful (Faludi, 1992). For example, as I can attest, when-ever in the Doctors' Dining Room the conversation turns to women's health or a women's health curriculum, a few moments of strained silence are followed

SOURCE: This chapter originally appeared in modified form in *Journal of Women's Health,* Vol. 2, No. 1, 1993, pp. 55-60; used by permission of Mary Ann Liebert, Inc., 1651 Third Ave., New York, NY 10128.

by a wave of disbelief, suspicion, and ridicule: Why a women's health curriculum? What can you teach us, they say, that we don't already know? And what about men? Why not men's health? Why must you separate women from the mainstream of consumers who need and want appropriate health care?

I hope in this discussion to answer these questions of protest. First, I will present some of the reasons for a women's health curriculum. Second, I'll describe the need for a consensual multispecialty-generated curriculum, which has been launched by the American Medical Women's Association as the Advanced Curriculum in Women's Health.

Reasons for a Women's Health Curriculum

There are six basic reasons for the development of a women's health curriculum:

1. Fragmentation. Too often women's health needs get lost in the gaps between different medical specialties. Women are referred back and forth between gynecologists, internists, family practitioners, and various other specialists. A woman seldom receives thorough, comprehensive care as an individual, with attention to all her organ systems.

Fragmentation is expensive, wasteful, and generates resentment in a woman whose brother is not being referred by an internist to a urologist for male genitorectal exam. Why must women go to another specialist for a routine pelvic examination and Pap smear?

2. Differences between men and women. The second reason is that women are different than men. It is not true that "apart from reproductive function— women's health is like that of men's health" (Harrison, 1992). Differences in women's health supersede the boundaries of the reproductive tract and affect every system: cardiovascular (Becker & Corrao, 1990; Bush, Fried, & Barrett-Connor, 1988; Castelli, 1988; Corrao, Becker, Ockene, & Hamilton, 1990; Eaker, Packard, & Thom, 1989; Eaker et al., 1987; Faludi, 1992; Wallis, 1992; Wenger, 1991; Wingard, 1990), gastrointestinal (Frezza et al., 1990), immune (Grossman, 1985), resistance to infection (HIV) (Agosti, 1991; Chu, Buehler, & Berkelman, 1990; Imam et al., 1990; Maiman et al., 1990; Spence & Reboli, 1991; Stein et al., 1991), and musculoskeletal, urologic, and psychological health (Women and Health Roundtable, 1985). The physiological hormonal milieu and environmental, societal, and economic circumstances shape the course of illness and therapeutic outcome differently in women than in men. Gender differences in the metabolism of pharmaceutical agents are also well documented (Hamilton & Parry, 1983).

3. Women's dual role. The third reason is the dual role women play as receivers of health care. Women act as a distribution channel of health care to spouses, children, and parents. At the same time, women are the major source of criticism and resentment directed at the medical profession; women increasingly resent receiving second-class care (Corea, 1977/1978).

4. Morbidity/mortality. The fourth compelling reason to develop a women's health curriculum is that women suffer and die as a result of the gender bias in research and medical education. Inadequate research translates into inadequate education and training of physicians and into inappropriate clinical care.

While women succumb to arteriosclerotic heart disease later in life than men, female *mortality* after a myocardial infarction is higher than for males (Corea, 1977/1978; Dittrich et al., 1988; Fiebach, Viscoli, & Horwitz, 1990; Greenland, Reicher-Reiss, Godbourt, & Behar, 1991; Kannel & Abbott, 1987; Lerner & Kannel, 1986).

Thrombolysis therapy is associated with more side effects, including hemorrhage, in women (Becker, 1990). After an angioplasty, female blood vessels close off more readily than those of men (Cowley et al., 1985). The female mortality after bypass surgery exceeds that of men (Douglas et al., 1981; Khan et al., 1990; Lopp et al., 1983).

There have been many explanations of those gender differences. And controversies exist over whether the differences are biological or result from bias (Bickell et al., 1992; Krumholz et al., 1992; Laskey, 1992; Steingart et al., 1991; Wenger, 1990). The problem remains, however, that little or no research has been directed at the resolution of the question and no research at all directed at possible remedies.

5. Role of women physicians. Why now? The reason for developing a women's health curriculum now is the increase in the numbers of female medical students and female doctors. Women physicians have always felt responsible for the health of women and children. This advocacy is apparent in several women's professional health associations. The mission of the American Medical Women's Association (1984) also spells out, in addition to the advocacy of women in the profession, the concern about women's health care. Another organization, the National Council on Women's Health (1985), which is primarily composed of women in various health professions, has as its mission the education of the public on women's health and communication between the provider and the consumer. Increasing numbers of women physicians take on as their personal goal filling the gaps left by medical school education, which is defective in women's health issues, and the gaps left by the various specialty training programs. While there is well-documented need for further research into women's health (Healy, 1991a; Nadel, 1990; U.S. Public Health Service, 1987), there is a feeling that much that is known about women does not get communicated to practitioners and does not get incorporated into the health care of women.

6. *Gender bias.* The basic reason for the development of a women's health curriculum is to undo the damage brought on by *gender bias* in medical education, research, and clinical practice. Gender bias is inherent in a male-dominated, male-taught discipline.

There are few female role models in medical academia. Few women physicians and medical students are so fortunate as to have a female professor as their role model. An informal poll taken at a recent American Medical Women's Association meeting disclosed that the most frequently identified female role model by the gathering of women doctors was Madame Curie—a lonely, introspective scientist, not an outgoing practitioner of medicine. How odd! The dearth of female models has resulted in women turning to male role models.

We have been taught medicine by men. We have modeled ourselves after men in the field. We have learned to think like men, as if this were the greatest compliment they could bestow on us. Hence gender bias, which manifests itself in medical thinking, research, education, and care, is even perpetuated by women who have been trained to think like men.

In constructing the classification of gender bias in medicine, I have used the schema first proposed by Drs. Eichler, Reisman, and Borins (1988; Eichler, 1988) for assessing medical research for gender bias, and I have expanded it to cover all activities in medicine (education, research, training, and practice) as well as adding another manifestation, that of failure of identification.

The five main manifestations of gender bias are as follows:

1. *Androcentricity*—a view of the world from a man's perspective: In medical education it can take various forms, including female invisibility or use of a male frame of reference. For instance (Table 2.1), first-year medical students are taught that women are different than men. In physiology classes, they are told that the average weight of a human being is 70 kg and, parenthetically, that of an aberrant species (women) is 50 kg. Similarly, the blood values for women indicate, by male standards, a mild anemia.

Now, contrasting this presentation with the next one (Table 2.2), one finds that the difference between the sexes indicates relative mild polycythemia in

TABLE 2.1   Physiology Data

Weight	average 70 kg
	(women average 50 kg)
Hematocrit	range 44%-52%
	(women range 40-45%)
Hemoglobin	range 14-18 gm%
	(women range 12-16 gm%)

TABLE 2.2.   Physiology Data, Alternative Presentation

Weight	average 50 kg
	(men average 70 kg)
Hematocrit	range 40-45%
	(men range 44%-52%)
Hemoglobin	range 12-16 gm%
	(men range 14-18 gm%)

men. But by constantly using the male frame of reference, the professor teaches the student that women are a minor aberration of the species *Homo sapiens.* This engenders an attitude toward women patients that is both alienating and patronizing.

2. *Overgeneralization* occurs when a study includes only one sex but presents itself as if it were applicable to both sexes. For example, in the February 15, 1992, issue of a respected medical journal, a paper appeared titled "Chronic Chlamydia Pneumoniae Infection as a Risk Factor for Coronary Heart Disease in the Helsinki Heart Study" (Saikku et al., 1992). The gist of the study was that chronic Chlamydia infection may be a significant risk factor for developing coronary heart disease.

The gender of the patients was not mentioned in the title or in the structured abstract. It was not until well into the discussion that the reader discovers that only men were tested. Women were not tested even though chronic infection with a related species Chlamydia trachomatis is prevalent in women. More important, not including the gender of subjects in the title or abstract was another example of assuming that the male is the generic human.

Perhaps the editors did not wish to irritate the authors of the paper with a reminder that gender of subjects should be mentioned. After all, "everybody should know that only men were part of the Helsinki study." Or perhaps the editors, themselves, forgot. That is not unusual. Female patients are frequently not included in observational studies or in interventional trials—the cause: androcentricity and overgeneralization.

3. *Gender insensitivity* consists of ignoring sex as a socially or medically important variable. Lack of knowledge of sex differences and similarities impedes appropriate progress in subsequent research, making it impossible to devise gender-sensitive treatments for women and men. Many psychotropic medications were tested on the males of the species even though these medications are clinically used mostly in women (Hamilton & Parry, 1983).

Of course, studies done on men do not necessarily apply to women at all. Women are different biological entities, with different hormones, different patterns of health and disease, and different responses to stress. No one does a study on a group of women and then assumes the results apply to men, but the reverse happens again and again.

The famous concept of the type A personality, the ambitious aggressive workaholic, was developed from a study of 4,000 California businessmen (Rosenman et al., 1976). "Type A behaviors" were associated with an increased incidence of coronary heart disease in men. Promptly, pundits began to warn that women, as they penetrated into the higher echelons of the working world, would sacrifice serenity, develop the type A personalities that their new jobs demanded, and pay the price in heart attacks. The male investigators assumed that women would follow the male pattern. This attitude reflects both overgeneralization and gender insensitivity.

Women patients were not studied until recently. Actually, when focusing on women in the Framingham Heart Study, Susanne Haynes (Haynes & Feinleib, 1980) found that, overall, working women as a group did not have significantly higher rates of coronary heart disease than housewives. Specific stresses found to be associated with heart disease in women were feelings of suppressed hostility, having a nonsupportive boss, decreased job mobility, and being married to a blue-collar worker.

Women clerical workers had twice as much coronary disease as women who stayed home. They experienced a lack of autonomy and control over the work environment, underutilization of skills, and lack of recognition of accomplishments.

Working married women were at even greater risk if they had three or more children, imputing role multiplicity as a risk factor. Single working women had the lowest incidence of coronary heart disease. So the stress of holding down a job per se is not solely responsible for higher rates of heart disease. Married men tend to live longer than single men. Marriage is protective of men's health. Does employment protect coronary arteries of single women?

How would the risk factors operate, for women and for men, when one holds a powerful, decision-wielding position. Will it turn out that, instead of paying the type A personality price, women would thrive on a balanced mixture of high-powered work and family? Would they be even healthier than if they married and stayed home? These studies are lacking. Gender insensitivity in research impairs our ability as clinicians to care for and advise our women patients.

4. *Double standards* involve evaluation, treatment, or measurement of identical behaviors, traits, and situations by different means. Women have repeatedly complained that doctors do not take them seriously, that their symptoms are waved aside as imaginary. In San Diego, a research team investigated the way that physicians responded to five medical complaints common in both men and women: chest pain, back pain, headache, dizziness, and fatigue (Armitage, Schneiderman, & Bass, 1979). They examined the extent of the workup ordered on patients with these complaints and found that, across the board, men received a more extensive workup than women for all complaints studied. The difference could not be explained in terms of medical facts alone and suggested that (perhaps), in fact, physicians did not take complaints as seriously when they came from women.

This double standards attitude may also explain the results of the classical Tobin et al. (1987) study of sex bias in considering coronary bypass surgery. The investigators looked at patients with abnormal cardiovascular radionuclide exercise scans: 40% of the men but only 4% of women with abnormal test results were referred by their physicians for cardiac catheterization. This 10:1 ratio was independent of age. Once again, for the same symptoms, and even for the same abnormal test results, women got less medical attention. The authors raised the question of whether coronary artery bypass surgery is underused in women. A similar study at another institution confirmed the findings (Ayanian & Epstein, 1991) and provoked further soul searching (Council on Ethical and Judicial Affairs, 1991).

Recent studies and an editorial acknowledge the discrepancy but attribute it to the overuse of procedures in men (Bickell et al., 1992; Krumholz et al., 1992; Laskey, 1992). Whichever it is, women get less attention, and less treatment.

5. *Failure of identification* leads to *failure of interest.* Medicine has been a male preserve for centuries and still is, despite the increasing numbers of female medical students and residents. Perhaps male doctors have tended to be more interested in those with bodies like their own, in how their own habits and preferences might affect their health and longevity. Medical research depends on grant money, which also depends on the prejudices of those in power, on what they think is interesting, important, mainstream. In addition, men have traditionally been the wage earners. The society is hypnotized by the image of the "hot-shot" businessman, struck down in his vigorous prime by a sudden heart attack. Health risks to those at the top of the social heap, those who are visible and important, successful and respected, have been a powerful impetus to research, and those who fund the studies, and those who carry them out, are looking for information about the

dangers that threaten close to home. The health risks of the housewife just have not seemed as pressing.

A failure of identification says that, *if we don't feel it, it doesn't exist.* Failure of identification leads to that pervasive stereotype of the woman as complainer, as someone who manifests her mental woes in physical symptoms, such as the hysteric, the neurasthenic, about whom the physician does not have to be too concerned; her headaches or her chest pains are imaginary. Dysmenorrhea and PMS are written off as psychosomatic.

But even when faced with scientific evidence that physical disease exists, physicians react differently to that evidence in men, taking it more seriously. Heart disease became a male disease; in the eyes of those physicians: "The 70-kg man needs bypass surgery."

Nevertheless, cardiovascular disease is still the foremost killer of American women, responsible for about 500,000 female deaths in the United States (Healy, 1991a). The same reluctance to identify with the female patient has led to rough, painful, inconsiderate, uncommunicative, hurried, incompetent pelvic exams and superficial and incompetent breast exams. It wasn't until 1979 when we started the Teaching Associates Program at Cornell, followed by many other medical schools, that we determined that pelvic exams need not be painful, insensitive, and embarrassing (Guenther, 1984; Wallis, 1984; Wallis & Jacobson, 1984; Wallis, Tardiff, & Deane, 1984).

Why are mammograms so painful to many women? If it were a routine procedure for male patients, somebody would have long ago modified the equipment to prevent the pain.

A paradigm based on male needs does not serve women patients well; women have different patterns of health and disease. Complications of hypertension, for example, appear an average of 10 to 15 years later in women than in men. Diseases such as rheumatoid arthritis and lupus erythematosus are much more common in women. Anxiety disorders and depression are much more common in women, while men have at least twice the rates of antisocial personality and alcohol abuse/dependency. Alcohol abuse in men leads most commonly to violence; in women, to depression.

Urologists, who are almost exclusively men, have spent much of their time dealing with prostate problems. Women have urologic problems too, such as cystitis, urethritis, the "honeymoon pyelitis," the poorly understood "interstitial cystitis," and the various forms of urinary incontinence, problems that have received less medical attention and less interest in research. One reason is that there are few female urologists to identify with the female patient.

Or consider feet. Women have always had foot problems, stemming from foot-binding to spike heels, often engendered by male-directed notions of female beauty and attractiveness. Orthopedics, a surgical specialty that has historically been almost entirely male, has not accorded a great deal of prestige to the study of foot problems. The emphasis has been on heroic surgical procedures such as total hip and knee replacements.

Medical school education and physician training programs have over the centuries reflected male attitudes and interests and many of women's health needs are left unattended or fragmented. Hundreds of individual women physicians, having confronted the unmet needs of their patients, went on to take additional courses and informal preceptorships to fill the gaps in their training. This process has been largely haphazard, intuitive, and unorganized and guided by the individual physician's perception of the needs.

AMWA's Project on a Women's Health Curriculum

Over the last 4 years, AMWA leaders, along with various multidisciplinary and multispecialty groups, have been compiling lists of the health needs of women. In November 1990, a group of women, representing a number of medical societies and women's health consumer organizations, drafted the First Core Curriculum on Women's Health, a 20-page list of skills and knowledge that primary physicians should possess to meet health needs of women.

In November 1991, an ad hoc committee was formed on a women's health curriculum. In 1992 we formulated our vision of designing and offering physicians an Advanced Curriculum in Women's Health to improve and integrate the care of women patients, heighten physicians' awareness of the psychosocial aspects of women's treatment, improve the physician-patient partnership, and increase the physicians' understanding of the differences and unique qualities of women's health.

It was believed that the participation of various specialties was necessary for outlining a comprehensive curriculum. With the help of an educational grant, AMWA arranged for a 3-day retreat in August with official representatives of 17 medical specialty societies to brainstorm the content and structure of the course.

It was the consensus of physicians attending the retreat to structure the curriculum around the life phases of the woman. We felt that the life-phase structure was more organic and unique to women than a division by specialties, diseases, or organ systems. The curriculum is divided into five modules:

Early years (birth to 18)
Young adult (19-39)
Midlife (40-64)

Mature years (65-79)
Advanced years (80 and beyond)

Nine content areas are addressed to varying degrees in each module:

Sexuality and reproduction
Women and society
Health maintenance and wellness
Violence and abuse
Mental health and substance abuse
Transition and changes
Patient-physician partnership
Normal female physiology
Abnormal female physiology, including diagnosis and management of conditions
    common to the age groups

The course incorporates lectures along with interactive and hands-on workshops and problem-solving learning techniques. A curriculum specialist and a meeting planner have been hired. The Task Force on Women's Health Curriculum is an AMWA group that provides assistance to the three-person executive team: Course Director, Lila A. Wallis (M.D., F.A.C.P.); Curriculum Consultant, Nancy Wolf-Gillespie (Ph.D., D.); and Meeting Planner, Marge Adey.

The course consists of two parts, 3-4 days each. Part I, which addressed the Midlife and Mature Years, took place October 29 to November 1, 1993, at the Marriott-Marquis Hotel in New York City to a record audience, which included physicians representing 37 states and 23 specialties; internal medicine, gynecology, and family medicine vied for the most represented specialty. The feedback from the registrants was overwhelmingly enthusiastic. A comprehensive handbook added permanence to the learning experience. Part II will address Early Years, Young Adult, and Advanced Years and is being planned for fall 1994.

Plans are being discussed to incorporate the Advanced Curriculum in Women's Health into the curricula of medical schools and training programs.

Discussion

The Advanced Curriculum in Women's Health (ACWH) has been long in coming. It is the fruit of the cooperation of various disciplines and various specialties including the insights of organizations representing the woman patient. It is the first national attempt to teach medical providers a systematized, unbiased view of the woman, the female patient, within a structure that is specific to women's health, namely, the life-phase related issues.

It is difficult to predict the future course of the developing discipline. Despite the official moratorium on creation of new specialty boards, despite the open and covert backlash, it is possible that public opinion will exert enough pressure to ratify the effort as leading to a new multidisciplinary specialty of women's health. But this is not the present goal of the American Medical Women's Association. Its leaders will be satisfied if the ACWH leads to better care of women patients.

Should medical schools and training programs adopt the ACWH into their own curricula, the pressure to create a new specialty in women's health may abate. In the meantime, two groups continue to clamor for a separate specialty: women patients and women medical students who are eager to learn about, train in, and practice women's health.

References

Agosti, J. M. (1991). HIV infection in women: Diverse approaches to a growing problem. *Journal of General Internal Medicine, 6,* 380-381.

American Medical Women's Association. (1984). *Mission statement.* Alexandria, VA: Author.

Armitage, K. J., Schneiderman, L. J., & Bass, R. A. (1979). Response of physicians to medical complaints in men and women. *Journal of the American Medical Association, 241,* 2186-2187.

Ayanian, J. Z., & Epstein, A. M. (1991). Differences in the use of procedures between women and men hospitalized for coronary heart disease. *New England Journal of Medicine, 325,* 221-225.

Becker, R. C. (1990). Coronary thrombolysis in women. *Cardiology, 77*(Suppl. 2), 110-123.

Becker, R. C., & Corrao, J. M. (1990). Cardiovascular disease in women: Scope of the problem. *Cardiology, 77*(Suppl. 2), 6-7.

Bickell, N. A., Pieper, K. S., Lee, K. L., et al. (1992). Referral patterns for coronary artery disease treatment: Gender bias or good clinical judgement? *Annals of Internal Medicine, 116,* 791-797.

Bush, T., Fried, L., & Barrett-Connor, E. (1988). Cholesterol, lipoproteins and coronary heart disease in women. *Clinical Chemistry, 34*(8B), B60-B70.

Castelli, W. P. (1988). Cardiovascular disease in women. *American Journal of Obstetrics and Gynecology, 158,* 1553-1560.

Chu, S. Y., Buehler, J. W., & Berkelman, P. T. (1990). Impact of the human immunodeficiency virus epidemic on mortality in women of reproductive age, United States. *Journal of the American Medical Association, 264,* 225-229.

Corea, G. (1977). *The hidden malpractice: How American medicine treats women as patients and professionals.* New York: William Morrow. (1978, New York: Jove [Harcourt Brace Jovanovich])

Corrao, J. M., Becker, R. C., Ockene, I. S., & Hamilton, G. A. (1990). Coronary heart disease risk factors in women. *Cardiology, 77*(Suppl. 2), 8-24.

Council on Ethical and Judicial Affairs. (1991). Gender disparities in clinical decision making. *Journal of the American Medical Association, 266,* 559-562.

Cowley, M. J., Mullin, S. M., Kelsey, S. F., et al. (1985). Sex differences in early and long-term results of coronary angioplasty in the NHLBI PTCA Registry. *Circulation, 71,* 90.

Dittrich, H., Gilpin, E., Nicod, P., Cali, G., Henning, H., & Ross, J., Jr. (1988). Acute myocardial infarction on women: Influence of gender on mortality and prognostic variables. *American Journal of Cardiology, 62,* 1-7.

Douglas, J. S., Jr., King, S. B., III, Jones, E. L., Carver, J. M., Bradford, J. M., & Hatcher, C. R., Jr. (1981). Reduced efficacy of coronary bypass surgery in women. *Circulation, 64*(Suppl. 2), II-11, II-16.

Eaker, E. D., Packard, B., & Thom, T. J. (1989). Epidemiology and risk factors for coronary heart disease in women. *Cardiovascular Clinics, 19,* 129-145.

Eaker, E. D., Packard, B., Wenger, N. K., et al. (Eds.). (1987). *Coronary heart disease in women.* New York: Haymarket-Doyma.

Eichler, M. (1988). *Nonsexist research methods: A practical guide.* Boston: Allen & Unwin.

Eichler, M., Reisman, A., & Borins, E. (1988, November 5). *Gender bias in medical research.* Paper presented at the Conference on Gender, Science and Medicine, Toronto, Ontario, Canada.

Faludi, S. (1992). *Backlash: The undeclared war against American women.* New York: Anchor.

Fiebach, N. H., Viscoli, C. M., & Horwitz, R. I. (1990). Differences between women and men in survival after myocardial infarction: Biology or methodology? *Journal of the American Medical Association, 263,* 1092-1096.

Frezza, M., Padova, C., Pozzeto, G., Terpin, M., Barano, E., & Lieber, C. S. (1990). High blood alcohol levels in women: The role of decreased gastric alcohol dehydrogenase activity and first-pass metabolism. *New England Journal of Medicine, 322,* 95.

Greenland, P., Reicher-Reiss, H., Godbourt, U., & Behar, S. (1991). In-hospital and 1-year mortality in 1,524 women after myocardial infarction; comparison with 4,315 men. *Circulation, 83,* 484-491.

Grossman, C. J. (1985). Interactions between the gonadal steroids and the immune system. *Science, 227,* 257-261.

Guenther, S. M. (1984). There is no excuse . . . *Journal of the American Medical Women's Association, 39,* 40-42.

Hamilton, J., & Parry, B. (1983). Sex-related differences in clinical drug response: Implications for women's health. *Journal of the American Medical Women's Association, 38,* 126-132.

Harrison, M. (1990). Woman as other: The premise of medicine. *Journal of the American Medical Women's Association, 45,* 225-226.

Harrison, M. (1992). Women's health as a specialty: A deceptive solution. *Journal of Women's Health, 1,* 101-106.

Haynes, S. G., & Feinleib, M. (1980). Women, work and coronary heart disease: Prospective findings from the Framingham Heart Study. *American Journal of Public Health, 700,* 133-141.

Healy, B. (1991a). Women's health, public welfare. *Journal of the American Medical Association, 26,* 566-568.

Healy, B. (1991b). The Yentl syndrome. *New England Journal of Medicine, 325,* 274-276.

Imam, N., Carpenter, C. C., Mayer, K. H., Fisher, A. S., Stein, M., & Danforth, S. B. (1990). Hierarchical pattern of mucosal candida infections in HIV-seropositive women. *American Journal of Medicine, 89,* 142-146.

Johnson, K. (1992). Women's health: Developing a new interdisciplinary specialty. *Journal of Women's Health, 1,* 95-99.

Johnson, K., & Dawson, L. (1990). Women's health as a multidisciplinary specialty: An exploratory proposal. *Journal of the American Medical Women's Association, 45,* 225-226.

Kannel, W. B., & Abbott, R. D. (1987). Incidence and prognosis of myocardial infarction on women: The Framingham study. In E. D. Eaker, B. Packer, N. K. Wenger, T. Clarkson, & H. A. Tyroler (Eds.), *Coronary artery disease in women* (pp. 208-214). New York: Haymarket-Doyma.

Khan, S. S., Nessim, S., Gray, R., Czer, L. S., Chaux, A., & Matloff, J. (1990). Increased mortality of women in coronary artery bypass surgery; evidence for referral bias. *Annals of Internal Medicine, 112,* 561-567.

Krumholz, H. M., Douglas, P. S., Lauer, M. S., et al. (1992). Selections of patients for coronary angiography and coronary revascularization early after myocardial infarction: Is there evidence for a gender bias? *Annals of Internal Medicine, 116,* 785-790.

Laskey, W. K. (1992). Gender differences in the management of coronary artery disease: Bias or good clinical judgement? *Annals of Internal Medicine, 116,* 869-871.

Lerner, D. J., & Kannel, W. B. (1986). Patterns of coronary heart disease morbidity and mortality in the sexes: A 26-year follow-up of the Framingham population. *American Heart Journal, 111,* 383-390.

Lopp, F. D., Golding, L. R., Maximillian, J. P., Cosgrove, D. M., Lytle, B. W., & Sheldon, W. C. (1983). Coronary artery surgery in women compared with men: Analysis of risks and long-tern results. *Journal of American College of Cardiology, 1,* 383-390.

Maiman, M., Fruchter, R. G., Serur, E., Remy, J. C., Feuer, G., & Boyce, J. (1990). Human immunodeficiency virus infection and cervical neoplasia. *Gynecological Oncology, 38,* 377-382.

Nadel, M. V. (1990, June). *National Institutes of Health: Problems in implementing policy on women in study populations.* Washington, DC: Government Accounting Office, National and Public Health Issues Human Resources Division.

National Council on Women's Health (Formerly National Council on Women in Medicine). (1985). *Mission statement.* New York: Author.

Rosenman, R. H., Brand, R. J., Jenkins, C. D., et al. (1976). Coronary heart disease in the Western Collaborative Group Study: Final follow-up experience of 8½ years. *Journal of the American Medical Association, 233,* 872-877.

Saikku, P., Leinonen, M., Tenkanen, L., et al. (1992). Chronic chlamydia pneumoniae infection as a risk factor for coronary heart disease in the Helsinki Heart Study. *Annals of Internal Medicine, 116,* 273-278.

Spence, M. R., & Reboli, A. C. (1991). Human immunodeficiency virus infection in women. *Annals of Internal Medicine, 115,* 827-829.

Stein, M. D., Leibman, B., et al. (1991). HIV-positive women: Reasons they are tested for HIV and their clinical characteristics on entry into the health care system. *Journal of General Internal Medicine, 6,* 286-289.

Steingart, R. M., Packer, M., Hamm, P., et al. (1991). Sex differences in the management of coronary artery disease. *New England Journal of Medicine, 325,* 226-230.

Symonds, A. (1980). Women's liberation: Effects on physician-patient relationship. *New York State Journal of Medicine, 80,* 211-214.

Tobin, J. N., Wassertheil-Smoller, S., Wexler, J. P., et al. (1987). Sex bias in considering coronary bypass surgery. *Annals of Internal Medicine, 107,* 19-25.

U.S. Public Health Service. (1987, October). *Women's health: Report of the Public Health Task Force on Women's Health Issues* (Vols. 1, 2; DHHS Publication 88-50206). Washington, DC: Department of Health and Human Services. (Also in Women's Health; Report of the Public Health Services Task Force on Women's Health Issues, *Public Health Reports, 100,* 85, January-February 1985)

Wallis, L. A. (1982a). Medical education and women's health. In J. I. Boufford & L. A. Wallis (Eds.), *Spotlight on women in medicine: Vol. 2. Selected papers from the 2nd Regional Conference on Women in Medicine, 1981* (pp. 71-75). New York: Regional Council for Women in Medicine.

Wallis, L. A. (1982b). The patient as a partner in the pelvic exam. *The Female Patient, 7* (February—OBGYN), 3662-3667 (March—Primary care), 2804-2807.

Wallis, L. A. (1984). A quiet revolution [Guest editor's page]. *Journal of the American Medical Women's Association, 39,* 46-48.

Wallis, L. A. (1992). Women's health: A specialty? Pros and cons. *Journal of Women's Health, 1,* 107-108.

Wallis, L. A., & Jacobson, J. S. (1984). The hundred years are up. *Journal of the American Medical Women's Association, 39,* 59-62.

Wallis, L. A., & Klass, P. (1990). Toward improving women's health care. *Journal of the American Medical Women's Association, 45,* 219-221.

Wallis, L. A., Tardiff, K., & Deane, K. (1984). Changes in students' attitudes following a pelvic Teaching Associate program. *Journal of the American Medical Women's Association, 39,* 46-48.

Wenger, N. K. (1990). Gender, coronary artery disease, and coronary bypass surgery. *Annals of Internal Medicine, 112,* 557-558.

Wenger, N. K. (1991). Cardiovascular drugs: The urgent need for studies in women. *Journal of the American Medical Women's Association, 46,* 117-120.

Wingard, D. L. (1990). Sex differences and coronary heart disease: A case of comparing apples and pears? *Circulation, 81,* 1710-1712.

Women and Health Roundtable. (1985). Women and health roundtable. In N. F. Russo (Ed.), *The status of women's mental health needs.* Washington, DC: American Psychological Association.

3

Women's Health and Curriculum Transformation: The Role of Medical Specialization

Karen Johnson
Eileen Hoffman

Present-day medical specialization reflects an outdated understanding of women's health. Physicians wishing to specialize in the care of women have inherited a surgical specialty with a narrow focus on reproduction that is inconsistent with a contemporary understanding. Our worldview of women's health has changed and medicine must change to reflect it.

Background

Medicine was unsophisticated when it created the specialty of obstetrics and gynecology almost a century ago (Eiler & Pasko, 1988). In the context of the social and scientific beliefs of the day, physicians considered women and men biologically identical except for reproduction. A specialty in women's reproductive health was seen as a sufficient complement to general training in adult medicine.

Times have changed. Although the precise definition of women's health is still in debate (Dan, 1993), there is little doubt that women's health no longer translates to reproductive health. Yet, *no medical specialty provides exclusive and comprehensive training in the care of women* (Johnson, 1992). Instead, components of women's medical care are widely distributed among existing specialties. This might merely be an expensive inconvenience if such fragmentation did not contribute to inadequate care for women (Lurie et al., 1993).

No existing primary care medical specialty assumes responsibility for all the basic preventive, diagnostic, and treatment procedures that are required to provide comprehensive care for women (Rosenthal, 1993). This flaw in the structure of medical specialties may cause unnecessary morbidity and mortality among female patients (Anastos et al., 1991). Medicine must reframe its understanding and practice of women's health to reduce fragmentation and increase quality of care.

Gaps and Fragmentation

Multidisciplinary women's health centers are a step in the right direction (Johnson, 1987; Looker, 1993). However, women's health means more than simply offering a variety of services at one location. Clinical medicine is the application of science to the care of patients. To provide the best care for women, medicine must change the lens through which scientific information about women is learned and applied. Although internal medicine, obstetrics-gynecology, and family practice provide the majority of primary medical care to women, none meets the broad health concerns of women (Henrich, n.d.).

Internal Medicine

The female reproductive tract is the only organ system deleted from the repertoire of competency among internists. Yet, we are increasingly aware that ovarian hormones interact and overlap with all other organ systems. Insulin has gonadotropic functions (Barbieri, Smith, & Ryan, 1988; Poretsky & Kalin, 1987). Polycystic ovarian syndrome is a risk factor for coronary artery disease. Endothelin levels vary with sex steroid exposure. This may be significant in the pathogenesis of hypertension and atherosclerosis (Polderman et al., 1993). If estrogen enters the internists' pharmacopoeia of cardioactive drugs, they need to know how to prescribe it, to whom, and by which protocol.

Obstetrics-Gynecology

The one specialty that is devoted exclusively to women is obstetrics-gynecology, but its scope is narrow because of its surgical orientation. Unless the specialty is willing to radically transform its mission and training to qualify as a true primary care specialty in women's health (Johnson & Hoffman, 1993), obstetrics-gynecology should become a consultative specialty. Primary care physicians can refer patients to obstetrician-gynecologists in much the same way they refer them to urologists, ophthalmologists, and other surgical specialists.

Family Practice

The exclusion of women from clinical trials makes family physicians as handicapped as all other physicians in acquiring sufficient information to make informed and wise recommendations to female patients. The biopsychosocial approach of family practice is an improvement over the biomedical model more characteristic of internal medicine and obstetrics-gynecology, but it does not help if the psychosocial data are inadequate or unreliable—or if the psychological or behavioral interventions are inappropriate for women (Johnson, 1991).

Medicine as a Male Paradigm

No physician can ethically assume that clinical research or drug trials with men yield results that safely and accurately apply to women. At best, women's health is a "patchwork quilt with gaps" (Clancy & Massion, 1992) and, at worst, redundant and inadequate. Reliance on multiple physicians is expensive and antithetical to the principles of primary care. Women must coordinate their own care among physicians, if they can afford it at all. Some receive duplication of services while few receive attention to major psychological issues that reside outside the conventional framework of medicine.

Fragmentation of services within the traditional biomedical model makes it impossible to adequately treat complex medical problems such as domestic violence. In the current system, each caregiver attends to a piece of the problem: the blackened eye, the broken bone, the social work referral, the police complaint, the court system. Domestic violence is decontextualized in a male paradigm. Our diagnostic acumen, differential diagnosis, evaluative process, and management plan are off the mark.

If medicine had evolved with women rather than men as the standard, violence would have long ago been identified as a problem of epidemic proportion and the science of ovarian function would always have been an integral component of every physician's training. Instead, medical problems that present differently (e.g., AIDS), exclusively (e.g., fibroids), or with greater frequency (e.g., migraine headaches) in women are often misdiagnosed, inadequately researched, or inappropriately treated. An androgynous view of the nonreproductive aspects of medicine has kept women invisible (Healy, 1991).

Small Changes

If medicine's response to the deficiencies in women's health is a partial accommodation, it will create the illusion that women are being fully served. Internal medicine fellowships, family practice subspecialties, and primary care tracks in obstetrics-gynecology are modest improvements. Furthermore, they are congruent with the belief that few meaningful differences exist between women and men (Harrison, 1992). More important, they are consistent with the cultural expectation that women are not supposed to demand anything explicitly for themselves. They are to accept limited changes in the male paradigm—and be satisfied.

Toward a Woman-Centered Paradigm

Women's medical problems are described and understood as deviations from the norm. When there is no male paradigm from which to deviate, the system simply does not respond effectively. Like blind men examining individual parts of an elephant, each relies on his own limited experience without grasping the whole.

Perhaps medicine has been better able to deal with child abuse than violence against women because children have a medical specialty. Pediatricians study and treat children in the context of their whole lives. To address women's health in an equally responsible and comprehensive way, we must reframe our approach. The woman and all her medical concerns must become the focus.

Just imagine how the problem of violence against women will be handled in a woman-centered paradigm. It will be seen as the primary etiology of disturbances we now categorize as dissociation, borderline personality, eating disorders, substance abuse, somatization, chronic pelvic pain, and frequent use of health services. Male aggression will become a leading *DSM* diagnosis and million of dollars will be spent researching the causes and treatments of this life-threatening disorder.

Taking a Stand

Medicine was in error when it made men the standard. A specialty in women's health—in contrast to the current structure or partial accommodations—is the first demand women have made of a health care system that has been unrepresentative of and unresponsive to their needs (Johnson & Massion, 1991). In contrast to the women's health movement of the 1970s, this demand reflects a new political conviction among women that social institutions should take them into account. They do not expect to resort to lay-controlled clinics outside mainstream medicine as they did a generation ago (Ruzek, 1979).

Medicine must correct its earlier mistake and bring the power of science to the medical care of women. This requires an integrated database that suspends the arbitrary boundaries between existing specialties. The separation of the abdomen from the pelvis is a professional, not an anatomic, boundary; both are influenced by the brain. The bowel can reach down into the pelvis and form fistula in the vagina. Endometriosis can extend up to the diaphragm and cause pleuritic pain. Neurotransmitters have been implicated in menstrually linked affective disturbances (Hamilton & Jensvold, 1992). For many of the standard medical therapies, there are simply no definitive data on women (Montgomery & Moulton, 1992a). This is inexcusable when women are the majority of medical patients.

Resistance

Opposition to a specialty in women's health takes many forms. Change provokes anxiety; anxiety stimulates resistance. In this case, the anxiety is fueled by forces as divergent as economics, fear of devaluation, disinformation, mistrust of physicians, and alliances with existing specialties.

Cost

Economic challenges to a new specialty are voiced as concerns that such efforts will be too costly. The argument is that medicine cannot afford new training programs. One humorous counter is this: "Men have come first for 500 years. We can direct all our resources to women, if there is not enough for both sexes" (S. V. Rosser, personal communication, October 1992). Of course, it is as ludicrous to focus primarily on women as it has been to do the opposite, but it makes a point. If physicians are to provide the appropriate health care to women, they must have an opportunity to do so based upon explicit training in women's health.

Marginalization

Worries that a specialty in women's health will cause marginalization are ill-founded. It is the current arrangement that marginalizes women's health. The lesson of "separate versus integrated" has already been taught by women's studies scholars (Rosser, 1993). Those colleges and universities that have most successfully integrated scholarship about women into the broader curriculum have separate departments of women's studies. Here new knowledge about women is generated and then distributed to other departments. Institutions without women's studies programs have been far less successful in these endeavors.

No Differences

It is worrisome that even some feminists believe that there are no substantial differences between women and men (Harrison, 1993a). Except for organs associated with reproduction and breast-feeding, women and men do appear to be anatomically similar. This may explain some physicians' beliefs that women and men are physiologically similar. However, for medical scientists, this is a peculiar assumption given that the same one is not made about animals.

Scientists working with animals carefully differentiate between the male and female of any species because differences are meaningful. For example, it has long been recognized that the duration of action of many drugs is dependent on the sex of the animal under study (Skett, 1988). Yet, until the federal government mandated that women be included in drug trials, most drugs were never studied in women. In 1990 the General Accounting Office reported that, even under this mandate, most drug manufacturers were still not including women in Phase III clinical trials. These drugs were, however, prescribed to women.

It is disturbing that medicine has been less rigorous in the study of humans than other scholars have been in the study of animals. Researchers and clinicians studying women's health report many areas of medicine in which women and men are not the same. Whether it is the hepatic, cardiovascular, gastrointestinal, connective tissue, or immune systems, they find differences. Furthermore, these differences are often interrelated.

A Medical Specialty Is Antifeminist

Some argue that women's health care should be excluded from the hierarchical system of medicine and instead be delivered by nurse practitioners or physician assistants. Training nonphysician clinicians in women's health, without also training physicians, limits the ability of the health care delivery system to provide comprehensive care to women.

Physicians assess and treat pathology. It will not do women a great service if women's health focuses only on prevention or leaves out physicians. Unless physicians have medical training in women's health, women with illnesses will have no one to evaluate and treat their problems from a pro-woman perspective. Women will continue to have undiagnosed or misdiagnosed abdominal pain because their symptoms do not match the physician's specialty bias; doctors will continue to miss the etiology of gastrointestinal bleeding that is secondary to purging; chest pain will escape investigation or be inappropriately managed if physicians only know how to evaluate and treat coronary artery disease in men.

A feminist approach requires that clinicians from all areas of health care work to flatten the system's hierarchy. Each member of the women's health team brings unique training, experience, and talent to the care of women.

Too Many Specialties

Debating the future of medical specialties in general is beyond the scope of this chapter. It is enough to point out that the divisions among medical specialties have always been arbitrary. The recent decision to close the profession to new specialties is recognition of a process gone awry.

Perhaps there are too many specialties. However, this should not interfere with the development of a needed one. Reevaluating the structure of medical specialties makes more sense. Medicine could discontinue specialties no longer needed or reduce the number of residency positions in overdoctored specialties. "Too many specialties" is no reason to thwart the development of one for patients currently underserved.

Women's Health and Health Reform

This call to restructure medical specialties is occurring in the context of other pressures for health care reform. The cost-effective delivery of medical services is addressed by a women's health specialty. One physician who can care for all of a woman's needs is a sensible response, but there is a more important reason for streamlining women's health care. The health status of women is intimately connected to their political and economic subordination. "Because they are more likely than men to be poor and working part-time or not at all, women are . . . less likely to have access to needed medical care than men" (News release from the Commonwealth Fund's Commission on Women's Health, July 14, 1993).

Inadequate or incomplete care is also more common among women who are disabled, elderly, lesbian, or non-Caucasian as well as uninsured. According to the Commonwealth Fund's Commission on Women's Health (News release, July 14, 1993), 36% of uninsured and 13% of insured women do not receive needed care. More than one third of women do not seek or receive Pap smears, mammograms, pelvic exams, breast exams, or complete physical examinations. The rate is even higher for elderly women.

Many women have significant risk factors for heart disease, lung cancer, and osteoporosis, but no knowledge about risk reduction. These failures in preventive health occur in a setting of reported dissatisfaction with physicians: 41% of women report changing physicians within a year, and the leading reason is poor communication; 25% report "being talked down to" or being treated like a child.

It is "all in their head" is the explanation 17% of women hear when they describe symptoms they think are due to medical conditions. Although 40% of women report depression, physicians often neglect the relationship between physical and psychological health. Depression is twice as common in women as men. Yet, it is underdiagnosed and undertreated. Of the women in this study, 30% report childhood physical or sexual abuse. Due to discomfort with this topic, 90% did not discuss this with their physician. This is particularly unfortunate given the strong correlation between a history of childhood abuse and medical complaints (Bolen, 1993). The system as it currently exists will fail women no matter how women's health is structured if access remains hampered, mental health is dismissed, or sexism colors doctors' professional behaviors.

Reframing Women's Health

No one medical specialty is accountable for assuring women comprehensive care (Lurie et al., 1993). The consequences of inadequate knowledge and fragmented care are serious. Imagine a physician trained to offer women— and only women—comprehensive care. It is a difficult notion to grasp because we often focus on the programs already in existence rather than considering new possibilities.

Gender bias is embedded in medicine. Correcting this bias will not be simple. Incomplete solutions have already been put forward: nursing programs in women's health; the Office of Research on Women's Health at the NIH; the Women's Health Initiative, which will conduct large clinical trials in women; a remedial curriculum for physicians with insufficient training in women's health (Wallis, 1992); and lay groups and professional lobbyists for individual issues such as breast cancer, interstitial cystitis, osteoporosis, and menopause. Nevertheless, even those already working in women's health must realize that piecemeal efforts will not transform medicine in a way that includes women fully.

The focus must shift from individual organ systems to the whole woman. A woman-centered medical paradigm is the only way to ensure that physicians learn to care for women within the context of their lives. The failure to develop medical specialties in such a way that women obtain appropriate care was not intentional, but it happened. Correcting this error is imperative. *The most powerful and effective political strategy to (a) bring women's medical care to parity with men's and (b) guarantee that students and residents receive the pertinent training is to create a medical specialty in women's health.*

There are already self-designated specialists in women's health, but they have had to customize their training. These physicians have a deep commitment to women and a passionate interest in improving their medical care. As physicians with less altruistic motives enter the field, calling oneself a specialist in women's health will carry less meaning unless a formal specialty ensures standardized and supervised training. Beyond this, a specialty will be an explicit acknowledgment from the medical profession to women that it will no longer use men as the standard. This is an excellent way for medicine to regain the trust it has lost among women. Women are clear about their preference. They would like one physician to provide all their primary medical needs (Atkinson, 1993).

Transforming the Medical Curriculum

A specialty in women's health will legitimize the field. Without it, physicians interested in women's health must pursue it as a sideline. Their first obligation is to an existing specialty or department.

Moreover, physicians do not take a field seriously or even learn much about it unless it is an integral part of their training. Consider nutrition. No physician questions the value of good nutrition in maintaining maximum health and speeding recovery from medical and surgical problems. However, physicians cannot specialize in nutrition and most medical students have little or no nutritional training. The same fate awaits women's health unless it becomes a medical specialty.

Currently, students and physicians interested in women's health must make a personal effort to learn about the field—sometimes at considerable cost to their reputations and career advancement—because it is not in the standard curriculum. Indeed, women's health is inadequately represented within undergraduate and residency curricula (Montgomery & Moulton, 1992b). Less than 25% of medical schools teach women's health and much of what they do offer is elective and nonstandardized. Medical students must have education and training in all aspects of women's health. Graduates deserve residencies in women's health without having to invent their own, become double-boarded, or compromise by entering the specialty with the closest approximation.

Departments of women's health within medical schools will provide a setting in which medical educators, clinicians, and researchers can accelerate the task of filling the gaps in our clinical knowledge about women and distributing this information to students and physicians. They will foster the development of faculty committed to advancing a women's health agenda at all levels of medical education (Henrich, n.d.). Physicians will be able to apply for grants, seek tenure, and receive promotions—all in women's health. Without departments, alternative strategies are less likely to become permanent or to ensure that all physicians learn women's health.

A specialty in women's health means that medicine will have a group of physicians continually adding to the field and in turn receiving intellectual and emotional sustenance from like-minded colleagues. Both are critical to the full and permanent integration of women's health in the medical curriculum. Until women reach parity with men in all areas of life, discrimination against medical specialists in women's health remains a risk—even with a specialty. However, much as women's studies has acquired increasing respectability and prestige over the 20 or so years of its existence, a formal specialty in women's health will eventually reduce the devaluation of the field.

The Relationship Between Women's Health Specialists and Others

The presence of specialists in women's health will not eliminate the need for other primary care providers. Family physicians can continue their role as providers to the family. For women, family physicians will rely on the knowledge and expertise of specialists in women's health in much the same way they rely on pediatricians for expertise in children's health. General internists can continue to provide health care for adults of both sexes. However, in consultation with specialists in women's health, internists will finally acquire reliable information upon which to base their clinical evaluation of women. Innovative programs in women's health outside the standard medical curriculum, such as an interdisciplinary master's degree (Harrison, 1993b) and an interdisciplinary fellowship (Hamilton, 1993), will provide opportunities for physicians who do not specialize in women's health to gain exposure to the field.

Conclusion

Women suffer needlessly because medicine has consigned their health care to a reproductive surgical specialty. Let's stop quarreling over issues of territory, accept our mistake, and correct it. All primary care physicians must deliver sex- and gender-aware medicine to female patients. However, it is insufficient to train internists to perform pelvic exams and Pap smears or to instruct obstetrician-gynecologists in interpreting EKGs or thyroid function tests.

Women's health is much more than blending internal medicine with office gynecology. Neither is it simply approaching women from a biopsychosocial perspective based on research and clinical experience drawn from existing specialties. Although family practice currently comes closest to encompassing the requisite skills necessary for the comprehensive care of women, we should not be satisfied by family physicians' insistence that they already provide comprehensive women's health care (Tobin, 1992). Family physicians cannot provide adequate care for women because they have no source of specialized knowledge on which to base this care. Furthermore, because of their broad mandate, family physicians are unlikely to fully advance a research and educational agenda in women's health (Henrich, n.d.).

It is time to discontinue the genitalized focus of women's health and reeducate both physicians and patients. Women's health is not limited to breasts and uteri. Lung cancer is the most frequent cancer in women; colon cancer kills more women than any gynecological malignancy; domestic violence is the etiology of most women's injuries; abuse and poverty are the two main contributors to depression in women (McGrath, Keita, Stickland, & Russo, 1990).

We must transform medicine and the medical curriculum to reflect women as whole human beings with minds, bodies, and spirits—separate and distinct from men's—and worthy of an equal investment in scientific study, clinical education, and medical services. Departments of women's health will provide environments in which medical students and physicians can focus on the female organism instead of female organs.

Nineteenth-century American physicians

> saw woman as the product and prisoner of her reproductive system. It was the ineluctable basis of her social role and behavioral characteristics, the cause of her most common ailments; women's uterus and ovaries controlled her body and behavior from puberty through menopause. The male reproductive system, male physicians assumed, exerted no parallel degree of control over man's body. (Smith-Rosenberg, 1984, p. 13)

Medicine stands on this sexist foundation. With such a flawed beginning, remodeling is inadequate. The building needs to be torn down and rebuilt. An interdisciplinary medical specialty in women's health is the best strategy for reframing women's health to reflect our new worldview.

References

Anastos, K., et al. (1991). Hypertension in women: What is really known? *Annals of Internal Medicine, 115,* 287-293.

Atkinson, H. (1993, August 12). [Television presentation on women's health]. *Today.*

Barbieri, R. L., Smith, S., & Ryan, K. J. (1988). The role of hyperinsulinemia in the pathogenesis of ovarian-hyperandrogenism. *Fertility and Sterility, 50,* 197-212.

Bolen, J. (1993). The impact of sexual abuse on women's health. *Psychiatric Annals, 23,* 446-453.

Clancy, C. M., & Massion, C. T. (1992). American women's health care: A patchwork quilt with gaps. *Journal of the American Medical Association, 268,* 1918-1920.

Dan, A. J. (1993). Integrating biomedical and feminist perspective on women's health. *Women's Health Issues, 3,* 101-103.

Eiler, M. A., & Pasko, T. J. (1988). Obstetrics and gynecology. In *Specialty profiles* (pp. 297-298). Chicago: American Medical Association.

Hamilton, J., & Jensvold, M. (1992). Personality, psychopathology and depression in women. In L. S. Brown & M. Ballou (Eds.), *Personality and psychopathology: Feminist reappraisals* (pp. 116-143). New York: Guilford.

Hamilton, J. A. (1993). Feminist theory and health psychology: Tools for an egalitarian, women-centered approach to women's health. *Journal of Women's Health, 2,* 49-54.

Harrison, M. (1992). Con: Women's health as a specialty. *Journal of Women's Health, 1,* 101-106.

Harrison, M. (1993a, June 3). *Con: Women's health: A medical specialty?* Presentation at the First Annual Conference on Women's Health, Washington, DC.

Harrison, M. (1993b). Women's health: New models of care and a new academic discipline. *Journal of Women's Health, 2,* 61-66.

Healy, B. (1991). The Yentl syndrome. *New England Journal of Medicine, 325,* 274-276.

Henrich, J. B. (n.d.). *The status and future of academic medical programs in women's health.* Unpublished manuscript.

Johnson, K. (1987). Women's health care: An innovative model. *Women and Therapy, 6,* 305-311.

Johnson, K. (1991). *Trusting ourselves: The complete guide to psychological well-being for women.* New York: Atlantic Monthly Press.

Johnson, K. (1992). Women's health: Developing a new interdisciplinary specialty. *Journal of Women's Health, 1,* 95-99.

Johnson, K., & Hoffman, E. (1993). Women's health: Designing and implementing an interdisciplinary specialty. *Women's Health Issues, 3,* 115-120.

Johnson, K., & Massion, C. T. (1991, November/December). Why a women's medical specialty. *Ms.*, pp. 68-69.

Looker, P. (1993). Women's health centers: History and evolution. *Women's Health Issues, 3,* 95-100.

Lurie, N., Slater, J., McGovern, P., Ekstrum, J., Quam, L., & Margolis, K. (1993). Preventive care for women: Does the sex of the physician matter? *New England Journal of Medicine, 329,* 478-482.

McGrath, E., Keita, G. P., Stickland, B. R., & Russo, N. F. (Eds.). (1990). *Women and depression: Risk factors and treatment issues.* Washington, DC: American Psychological Association.

Montgomery, K., & Moulton, A. W. (1992a). Medical education in women's health. *Journal of Women's Health, 1,* 253-254.

Montgomery, K., & Moulton, A. W. (1992b, May). Undergraduate medical education in women's health. *Women's Health Forum,* pp. 1-2.

Polderman, K. H., Stehouwer, C. D., van Kamp, G. J., Dekker, G. A., Verheugt, F. W., & Gooren, L. J. (1993). Influence of sex hormones on plasma endothelin level. *Annals of Internal Medicine, 118,* 429-432.

Poretsky, L., & Kalin, M. F. (1987). The gonadotropic function in insulin. *Endocrine Reviews, 8,* 132-141.

Rosenthal, E. (1993, October 13). Does fragmented medicine harm the health of women? *The New York Times,* pp. A1, B7.

Rosser, S. V. (1993). A model for a specialty in women's health. *Journal of Women's Health, 2,* 99-104.

Ruzek, S. B. (1979). *The women's health movement: Feminist alternative to medical control.* New York: Praeger.

Skett P. (1988). Biochemical basis of sex differences in drug metabolism. *Pharmacotherapy, 38,* 269-304.

Smith-Rosenberg, C. (1984). The female animal: Medical and biological views of woman and her role in 19th century America. In J. Leavitt (Ed.), *Women and health in America.* Madison: University of Wisconsin Press.

Tobin, M. (1992, December 28). Point/counterpoint: Should women's health be a new specialty? *Physician's Weekly,* p. 1.

Wallis, L. (1992). Women's health: A specialty? Pros and cons. *Journal of Women's Health, 1,* 107-108.

4

Women's Health and Family Medicine: A Canadian Perspective

Gail Webber

> Currently, when a woman seeks medical care her body is arbitrarily divided among specialists. (Johnson & Massion, 1991, p. 68)

The image of a severed woman with body and mind strewn among different members of the medical establishment is a familiar one to advocates of women's health. It is also the real experience of many women in countries known to be the healthiest in the world and is the basis of the argument for a new multidisciplinary specialty in women's health (Johnson, 1992). While not disputing that a women's health specialist would be an invaluable addition to our current health care system, Canadians need and deserve a change at the primary care level. In Canada, family physicians have initial and ongoing contact with the general population; specialists are usually reserved for consultation only. More than 50% of visits to family physicians are by women. Postgraduate education in family medicine therefore cannot be considered complete without a good understanding of women's health issues.

This chapter will address the philosophy of Family Medicine in Canada as well as the role for training in women's health within this discipline. In particular, the creation of an optional third-year program dedicated to training in Women's Health at Queen's University in Kingston, Ontario, will be discussed. Emphasis is placed on the consultative process in the development of the curriculum. Program objectives and course content will also be

AUTHOR'S NOTE: I would like to recognize the significant contributions of others to the development of the Queen's University curriculum. Specifically, I would like to thank Drs. Brian Kain, Ruth Wilson, and Susan Phillips, as well as the members of WHISCC (Women's Health Inter-School Curriculum Committee) and all those who offered ideas and resources to the program.

discussed. Finally, ongoing initiatives in women's health medicine will be presented.

Family Medicine in Canada

To understand the impact that education in women's health care within family medicine residencies would have upon women in general, American readers need to understand the health care system of their northerly neighbors. Whitcomb and Desgroseilliers (1992) have summarized the differences in primary care in Canada and the United States. In Canada, unlike the United States, primary health care is almost solely provided by family physicians or general practitioners (GPs), who constitute about 50% of the physician population of the country. The Royal College of Physicians and Surgeons of Canada has defined criteria and educational objectives for specialist training, and as a political body they have been influential in informing government policy such that specialists are financially rewarded for acting in a consultant role. That is, to be referred to any specialist, a patient generally first must be attached to a family physician or GP. It is these physicians who both provide and coordinate the health care for Canadians.

Postgraduate clinical education for Canadian physicians is funded by provincial governments. Thus these governments can and do control the number and types of residency programs available across the country. They exercise this control to meet the perceived needs of the population. Regardless of the controls, family medicine residency programs are among the most popular and competitive in the country. This trend will only increase as the new 2-year licensure requirement took effect in July 1993. (To practice anywhere in the country, physicians are required to have a minimum of 2 years of acceptable training; many will wish to ensure they have a license to practice by completing a residency in family medicine.)

The College of Family Physicians of Canada regulates the training programs across the country. According to their guidelines, family medicine residencies must consist of 2 years of training in which at least 8 months is to be spent in a family practice setting. The college also requires a minimum of 1 year of in-hospital experience in medicine, surgery, obstetrics, emergency medicine, and pediatrics.

Women's Health Within Family Medicine

The College of Family Physicians of Canada (1985) has defined the "four pillars of family medicine"; it is to these that all residents should aspire:

1. First and foremost, family physicians should be good clinicians.
2. Family medicine is a community-based discipline.
3. The family physician is a resource to a defined practice population.
4. The responsibilities and tasks of the family physician arise out of the physician's personal relationship with the patients who choose him or her as their physician.

Of interest, when women's groups were asked what they expected of physicians, they identified four roles that correlate with the pillars described above. The women felt physicians had the following roles in the community: medical expert, gatekeeper (entry point to the health care system and access to other services), partner in health care (both physician-patient and physician-community partnership), and advocate for women's health care needs ("Some Views on Women's Expectations of Physicians," 1992). Thus the philosophy of women's health care as defined by women is compatible with how family physicians define themselves. What remains is a greater realization of these goals.

The Canadian College of Family Physicians has recently recognized the need for improved training of family medicine residents in both reproductive health and illness, and "other health issues" for women (under which they include mental health, impact on health of roles and relationships, health care concerns of special groups, violence against women, occupational health, and conditions more common in or specific to women) (Report of the Joint Working Group, 1990). The residency programs have followed these guidelines to varying degrees (McCall & Sorbie, in press), and some are actively trying to improve their curricula in these areas. The Department of Family Medicine at Queen's University in Kingston, Ontario, hired the author to develop an optional third-year specialization in women's health for their residency program. It is this program that will be the focus of the discussion to follow.

Queen's University Women's Health Program: Development

In January 1991, the director of the Family Medicine Residency Program chaired a meeting of women interested in women's health issues about the need for specialized training in women's health for family medicine residents. This initial meeting was the impetus for the department to hire me to develop this program in fall 1991. As a feminist and family medicine resident, I was acutely aware of both the inadequacies of the medical model in the treatment of women and the power the medical establishment possessed. I used this opportunity of program development to consult those involved in women's health care delivery (defined in the broadest sense) both inside and outside the medical profession. They were asked what they felt family doctors should know about women's health and how they could act as resources in the education process. Thus, in addition to discussing these needs with interested family physicians and members of the Department of Obstetrics and Gynecology, I also sought out advice from feminist academics, social workers who worked closely with women, and other service providers such as those working in shelters and crisis centers, in alcohol and drug education and referral centers, and with women in conflict with the law.

The concept of community consultation in curriculum development within medical education is a radical one. In the past, the medical establishment has generally determined what its members should be taught. Changes in this patriarchal process are being made, however; those involved in creating women's health curricula need to develop strategies for effective community consultation. In developing the Queen's program, "key providers" (i.e., caregivers) were consulted; time constraints required this. Ideally, diverse groups of women who will ultimately be served by the caregivers should be involved in the consultation process. Only in this way will family physicians be adequately trained to meet the health care needs of all women, including lesbians, women of color, poor women, differently abled women, immigrant women, Native women, older and younger women.

Some may question such an emphasis on consultation, maintaining that experienced clinicians are well aware of the health care issues facing women. However, this consultative process of curriculum development is crucial for several reasons. First, it demonstrates a commitment to sharing power, moving away from the elitist model of "doctor knows best." Indeed, often an important step to regaining health is control. Women are empowered by having input into what their doctors learn.

Second, community consultation provides opportunities for others to take an active role in physician education. This is desirable in a women's health curriculum for there are many "experts" who are not physicians. Thus social workers and staff from shelters and sexual assault crisis centers, among others, have valuable contributions to make to the education of physicians, contributions that were often missed in traditional curriculum designs. Individual women can also be identified as resources when given the opportunity to take part in the process; their stories may prove to be useful instruction to medical students and residents. Thus community consultation proves not only to share power but also to reveal resources for education.

A third benefit of consulting the community about women's health care issues is the opportunity to model feminist principles for the residents. A

significant objective in women's health care education is understanding the
power imbalance in society that women experience, and how this relates to
the physician-patient relationship. By recognizing the value of patient input
in curriculum development, residents may learn to give more consideration
to patients' wishes and concerns in their everyday interaction. I hope that this
will contribute to a more equalitarian partnership between doctor and patient.
In addition, the use of a multidisciplinary team in resident education demonstrates to the residents the contribution other health care providers make to
women's overall health. This further encourages sharing of physician power
(i.e., control over patients) with others by referral to appropriate resources
in the community.

Program Objectives and Content

Health for women is much more than absence of disease. In the development of the Queen's program, the following definition of women's health,
created by the Women's Health Office at McMaster University, Hamilton,
Ontario, was a guide:

> Women's health involves women's emotional, social, cultural, spiritual and physi-
> cal well-being, and is determined by the social, political, cultural and economic
> context of women's lives, as well as by biology. In defining women's health,
> we recognize the validity of women's life experiences, and women's own beliefs
> about, and experiences of, health. We believe that a woman should be provided
> with the opportunity to achieve, sustain and maintain health, as defined by
> the woman herself, to her full potential. (*Women's Health Office Newsletter,*
> 1991, p. 1)

The objectives of the Queen's program were written to reflect this all-
encompassing and true-to-life-experience view of women's health, both in
general and in specific terms. The general objectives describe desired
changes in knowledge, skills, and attitudes in the residents to benefit their
women patients. They include an understanding of both the historical relationship of medicine and women as well as reflection on the current attitudes
held by the medical establishment and themselves toward women, including
women of differing race, class, sexual orientation, age, and abilities. The
program aims to raise residents' consciousness to how broad women's health
is and to improve their knowledge base and skills in women's health care
from communication skills to technical procedures. Another key objective is
for the residents to have a greater appreciation for the skills and expertise of
other health care personnel and community workers such that they will be
better able to access these resources and work as team members.

The final two general objectives of the Queen's program concern the wider impact we hope the program will have. The program is intended to create a group of physicians who will both work as activists and serve as resources in women's health issues, for the health care system, medical education, and the community. Finally, it is a primary goal of the program to encourage incorporation of women's health issues into the core family medicine residency and undergraduate medical education. It is expected that, during the initial years, the women's health program would have few members, thus its impact on the core residency program is particularly important to broaden its effect.

The specific objectives of the program are grouped into eight headings (though these are far from all-inclusive). These objectives would be met in teaching rounds, clinical interactions, and informal discussions as well as through elective time and readings. In brief, the specific objectives of the program concern reproductive health (normal processes, common problems), mental health (factors that contribute to "mental illness" in women, recognizing presentation, counseling skills), violence against women (prevalence, spectrum, presentation, skills in dealing with survivors, community resources), and health promotion (how to counsel about healthy behaviors, screening procedures, encouraging patient responsibility for health). Residents are also expected to develop their critical appraisal skills, applying principles of feminist research (e.g., Are gender, class, and race differences recognized to limit generalizability? Does it focus on women's experience, and is empowerment one of its goals?) (Clarke, 1992). Reflection on their role as physicians is also anticipated (e.g., power issues with patient and other providers). The residents are expected to think about the stress in their own lives and ways of taking care of themselves and their colleagues. Finally, opportunities will be made for the residents to participate in medical education through organizing rounds and conferences about women's health issues.

The content of the women's health program is organized to meet these objectives, providing the maximum amount of flexibility such that residents can pursue particular areas of interest or educational need. An outline of the curriculum appears in Table 4.1. Essentially, the first and last 10-week blocks of the 1-year program are elective time. Suggested elective experiences include family practice-based obstetrics (low intervention, high contact), a research project, geriatrics, and various out-of-town rotations. During the first elective block, residents also can begin to develop a relationship with their mentor/program director and do directed readings.

The remaining 10 months of the program form the core component, consisting of a variety of "horizontal" or simultaneous learning opportunities. These experiences are both "medical" and "nonmedical." Not unlike traditional residency training programs, the women's health residents will

TABLE 4.1. Curriculum Outline

First 10 weeks	—July 1 to mid-September: ELECTIVE
	—Required reading
	—Establishment of relationship with mentor

Seven months   —mid-September to mid-April: CORE ROTATION
                   "Horizontal learning"
  Continuing care family medicine 1-2 days/week
  Gynecology clinics (reproductive technology, PMS, endocrinology, sexual medicine,
    gynecological cancers, incontinence)
  Eating disorders clinic
  Counseling with supervision (adult survivors of child sexual abuse, women experiencing
    domestic violence, and so on)
  Women's clinic at Kingston General Hospital (assisting with TA counseling and procedure)
  Sexual assault call
  Prison for women clinics
  Community placements (see Table 4.2)
  Women's studies courses
  Teaching rounds
  Feminist critical appraisal
  Support group

Last 10 weeks   —mid-April to end of June: ELECTIVE
                   Extension of core, research, other
                   Evaluation of program by resident

spend part of their week in a family practice setting and attending clinics to gain specialized medical knowledge of women's health (included here would be reproductive technology, PMS, endocrinology, sexual medicine, gynecological cancers, and incontinence). Other potential clinics that residents may wish to participate in are the eating disorder clinic, women's clinic (TAs), and Prison for Women clinic.

Residents will also take part in teaching rounds; the topics that could be covered are, of course, endless. Suggestions for topics are grouped under transitions through childhood and adolescence, transitions through adulthood, common problems for women, and the physician role. Transitions through childhood and adolescence include normal physical and emotional development, sex role socialization, implications of puberty and menarche, sex education and contraception, sexuality and sexual identity, teenage pregnancy, and childhood sexual, physical, and emotional abuse. Adult transitions that may be useful topics for rounds are relationships/marriage, choice of remaining single or having lesbian relationships, pregnancy and childbirth, parenting, work, and aging. Common problems that could be discussed are premenstrual syndrome, sexually transmitted diseases and AIDS, therapeutic abortions, sexual assault and other violent acts toward women, addictive behaviors,

TABLE 4.2. Community Placements

Sexual Assault Crisis Centre
Interval House and Dawn House (Women's shelters)
Community Support Program (helping women who have left the shelter)
A.W.A.R.E. (Action on Women's Addictions—Research and Education)
Alcohol and Drug Referral Centre
Independent Living Centre (for disabled adults)
C.A.S.C.A. (Citizens Against Sexual Child Abuse provides housing for abused adolescents)
Elizabeth Fry Society (works with women in conflict with the law)

---

financial stresses, depression, eating disorders, sexual dysfunction, infertility, breast cancer, and osteoporosis. Finally, a discussion of physician role could include reflection on the history of the medical profession's treatment of women, the power of the physician role, physicians as healers, prescription drugs, sexual abuse of patients by physicians, the stresses of being a physician, and continuing education responsibilities.

Other components of the Queen's Women's Health Program include community placements, women's studies course work, supervised counseling, feminist critical appraisal, and a support group. Potential community placements are listed in Table 4.2. The residents are given the opportunity to work as volunteers in an organization of their choice, thus learning more about specific community resources. For the residents to grasp the fundamentals of feminist theory, it is expected that they will enroll in at least one women's studies course. The "Women's Health Issues" course offered jointly through nursing and women's studies is recommended, as it addresses women's experiences within the Canadian health care system from a social, economic, and cultural perspective. Counseling supervision is provided by therapists who have experience working with women. The amount of supervision is dependent both on resident interest and on availability of financial resources to reimburse the therapist.

The residents in the program will also meet regularly with their mentors/ supervisors for "feminist critical appraisal" and mutual support. Feminist critical appraisal, like "journal club" in traditional postgraduate programs, provides the residents with the opportunity to examine and critique medical research articles. Women's health residents should use the principles of feminist research in their critique, as discussed earlier. The support element of the program is very important, for, to adequately care for others, one must also take care of oneself. As feminists are acutely aware, working within a system that does not support one's value system can be exceedingly stressful; residents will no doubt wish to meet regularly to share concerns and ideas and, in the process, develop coping strategies for the future.

Conclusion

The Queen's University Women's Health Program is just one initiative among many in Canada. Family medicine residencies across Canada are taking serious looks at their curriculum content for women's health issues. The University of Toronto has developed a 1-year fellowship in Women's Health for family physicians, and others are attempting to incorporate women's health issues into their core curriculum. In Ontario, a group of physicians have been meeting to discuss objectives for women's health in medical education. This Women's Health Inter-School Curriculum Committee (WHISCC) has members from the five medical schools in the province and aims to develop useful material for undergraduate medical education.

Women's health issues must no longer be dismissed or overlooked because of lack of interest or ignorance on the part of physicians. All physicians have a responsibility to their female patients to learn more about their health care needs. As Monique Begin (1991), former Canadian federal minister of health and a well-known feminist, has said: "The time has come for a new medical 'specialization': women's health" (p. B3). However, we need more than a few women's health specialists to make a significant difference. Those of us committed to the health of women must use this opportunity of increased interest to ensure that women's health is high on the agenda of all medical curriculum planners. Women deserve to have complete primary health care by practitioners who are familiar with the social, political, and economic forces influencing their health as well as the physical (Lempert, 1986). The time has indeed come for women's health in medical education: Let us listen to what women want from their health care providers and then work with dedication to meet these needs.

References

Begin, M. (1991, November 25). Women in medicine: Males, practising a male-created science unilaterally impose their views on female patients. *Montreal Gazette*, p. B3.

Clarke, J. (1992). Feminist methods in health promotion research. *Canadian Journal of Public Health, 83*(1), S54-S57.

College of Family Physicians of Canada. (1985, April). *Report of the Task Force on Curriculum Section of Teachers of Family Medicine*. Mississauga, Ontario, Canada: Author.

Johnson, K. (1992). Women's health: Developing a new interdisciplinary specialty. *Journal of Women's Health, 1*(2), 95-99.

Johnson, K., & Massion, C. (1991, November/December). Why a woman's medical specialty? *Ms.*, pp. 68-69.

Lempert, L. B. (1986). Women's health from a woman's point of view: A review of the literature. *Health Care for Women International, 7*, 255-275.

McCall, M., & Sorbie, J. (in press). Educating physicians about women's health: Survey of Canadian family residency physicians. *Canadian Family Physicians.*

Report of the Joint Working Group on Family Medicine in Obstetrics, Gynecology, and Women's Health. (1990). In *The Report of the Postgraduate Family Medicine Joint Committee on Residency Training in Family Medicine.* Mississauga, Ontario, Canada: College of Family Physicians of Canada.

Some views on women's expectations of physicians. (1992, April). *Educating Future Physicians for Ontario Working Paper, 9,* p. i.

Whitcomb, M. E., & Desgroseilliers, J. P. (1992). Primary care medicine in Canada. *New England Journal of Medicine, 326,* 1469-1472.

Women's Health Office Newsletter. (1991, October). Hamilton, Ontario, Canada: McMaster University, Faculty of Health Sciences.

5

From Female Disease to Women's Health: New Educational Paradigms

Susan M. Cohen
Ellen O. Mitchell
Virginia Olesen
Ellen Olshansky
Diana L. Taylor

The changes that are evolving in women's primary health care within nursing have broad impact for its future directions. The evolution/revolution is occurring due to forces of academic, clinical, and consumer views. At the master's level, advanced practice means holistic care. Therefore a number of faculty involved with women's health care nurse practitioner programs have worked separately and collectively to broaden the educational process beyond reproductive health care.

While medical practice has arbitrarily divided a woman's body among medical specialties, so too has nursing practice in women's health followed a biomedical model. However, over the past 20 years, graduate nursing education has moved beyond the medical model to develop curricula that provide a biopsychosocial approach to women's health and illness. In particular, graduate nursing programs preparing nurse practitioners have developed curricula that create links between medical specialties that fragment the individual woman (e.g., obstetrics, gynecology, endocrinology, and psychiatry) as well as add the perspectives of health and wellness across the life span.

This chapter addresses the current state of curricular development at the University of Washington, the University of California, San Francisco, and the University of Texas—Houston. We have been developing nurse practitioner program revisions that combine a biopsychosocial, multicultural, life span, political, and gendercentric framework. The foundation for this new paradigm is characterized by a feminist style incorporating the values of humanism, sensitivity to diverse views, personal concern, and collaboration. Critical to this foundation is the meaning of women's experiences as women live through them presuming the integrity of the woman/client as a complex, perceptive, and healthy individual. A curriculum for clinical practice must incorporate disease management specific to women but must expand far beyond the biomedical framework to include primary prevention, health promotion, healing, caring, and facilitating health across the life span to diverse populations of women. Health policy and its impact on access to and quality of care are integral to the graduate program.

Historically, nurses have recognized the need for management of client health services (care management), and the underlying principles are incorporated into community health nursing practice, advanced practice specialties, primary care practice, school nursing, as well as acute care nursing practice. The goals of care management are an integral part of nursing practice and nursing education: to reduce the incidence of disease, premature death, discomfort, and disability and to increase or maintain health and the quality of life. Nurses' leadership in care management reflects nursing's tradition of coordinating resources to meet clients' multiple health service needs.

University of California, San Francisco

The curriculum at the University of California, San Francisco, is designed to increase knowledge and skills for advanced practice in the provision of primary health care to women. The graduates are prepared to:

a. determine the primary health care needs of the individual woman within the context of her family and community,

b. apply the relevant knowledge base in providing women's health care needs,

c. intervene by assisting the woman to meet her primary health care needs,

d. evaluate primary health care outcomes related to the individual woman's health and illness status,

e. demonstrate a sensitivity to the effect of culture and ethnic background as they relate to women's health care,

f. collaborate with multiple disciplines and the woman's family in determining and managing primary health care needs, and

g. facilitate necessary change in the delivery of women's health care.

The program balances the generalist focus of primary health care with the needs particular to women and their health. The curriculum is centered in a conceptual framework of women's adaptation to health and illness with the core model of health protection and health promotion.

Primary health care provides direct care services, personal health services, and illness/disease management. Further, the student is taught prevention including primary, secondary, and tertiary prevention, risk screening, and disease prevention. Health promotion includes increasing health status and increasing the level of wellness. Inherent in the program are case coordination and managed care. Case coordination content includes outreach, referral, education, advocacy, and evaluation. Managed care, a major component of health care reform, encompasses cost containment and outcome evaluation.

Content specific to the needs of women is taught within a series of specialty seminars. The specialty begins with a critique of women's health research to prepare the students for a clearer understanding of the relationship between practice and research. The students explore the physiology of women and the enormous changes that occur during pregnancy. Nutrition, health, and healing courses add to the specialty content. There are four seminar courses that examine health promotion and maintenance as well as the management of diseases common in women.

Also available to students in the UCSF advanced practice program are a wide range of classes taught in the Women, Health and Healing Program in the Department of Social and Behavioral Sciences. These classes include women and work, the sociology of women's reproductive health, sociohistorical issues, and the sociology of health of women of color.

University of Washington School of Nursing

In 1991 we implemented the Women's Health Care Nurse Practitioner (WHCNP) program at the University of Washington School of Nursing. This program is part of a larger Primary Health Care (PHC) program in nursing. Before 1991 the Family Nurse Practitioner (FNP) program and Pediatric Nurse Practitioner (PNP) program existed as two distinct programs. Now our nurse practitioner programs are organized within a "core" primary health care program that encompasses the specialty pathways of FNP, PNP, WHCNP, and Adult/Geriatric Nurse Practitioner (A/GNP).

The strong PHC core has allowed us to develop the WHCNP program so that it focuses on women as adults rather than only in terms of their reproductive organs. Our students learn reproductive health care, but they also learn primary care of women (from adolescence through post menopause). While this comprehensive view of women's health care is exciting, a challenge exists to promote and maintain a strong identity as women's health care providers because much of the "core" program is historically rooted in the FNP program. We have therefore developed two specialty women's health care courses to ensure that our students are learning content and concepts that are "core" to women's health. We are fortunate to have the strong influence of the Center for Women's Health Research directed by Nancy Fugate Woods (Ph.D,. R.N., F.A.A.N.).

In developing these curricular changes, we have had to clearly explicate our philosophical basis for the program. This philosophical basis includes the following:

1. Women's health is more than reproductive health.
2. Women's health is more than a focus on women as organisms but also emphasizes women as persons who experience their lives in varied ways and create their own meanings of their experiences.
3. Women's health exists within a socio/cultural/political context that includes racism, sexism, classism, and homophobia.

At this stage in the development of our program, we are working on developing this philosophical basis and on meeting the challenge to do so on several levels.

1. Within nursing. We need to clearly delineate the uniqueness of women's health care within a core primary health care curriculum.

2. Within health sciences and beyond. We need to work collaboratively across disciplines (including, but not limited to, biomedical sciences, social sciences, environmental sciences, psychological sciences). While the biomedical context is a critical component of women's health, we need to increase the visibility of other components, such as the social sciences.

3. Within the larger social context. We need to identify our voices as women (as health care providers and as recipients of health care). In so doing, we need to recognize and celebrate diversity among women, while continuing to search for commonalities within our diversity. This means creating a safe environment for diversity and learning from our diversity.

The University of Texas—Houston

The Women's Health Care graduate track is based in a feminist framework centered in women's life experience and health and illness care needs. The faculty believe that human beings, health, and nursing are interrelated and exist in a dynamic environment. Humans are viewed as holistic beings. The inherent dignity and worth of humans gives them the right and responsibility to participate as actively as they are able in decisions that affect their state of health. These decisions are influenced by individual values, beliefs, and perceptions.

The Women's Health Care track prepares graduates to be specialists in the multidimensional care of women. Health promotion, health maintenance, and health restoration are studied across the life span within a holistic developmental focus. Emphasis is placed on the effects of gender on women's lives, health, health care access, and health policy.

Courses concentrate on the application of physiological, developmental, psychosocial, and cultural theories to advanced clinical decision making. Women are studied within the context of the female life cycle, adolescence through late maturity. Content centers on the primary health care of women with gender providing the lens to focus on the individual. The flow of classes begins with the women in healthy states and defines health promotion and disease detection throughout life. Subsequent courses provide the basis for health maintenance and illness management in both physical and psychological arenas. Special emphasis is placed on the incorporation of health care policy information and activism. Graduate students carry out group policy projects across the year. Recently, students completed projects focused on access to care for women who use hospital emergency care departments to meet primary health care needs, improving chances for adolescent parents by working with a school system to establish school-based clinics, and decreasing violence toward women by instituting a violence-prevention curriculum in a large urban school. The students identify public policy, develop the projects, and then evaluate the impact of the policy projects on the community.

The graduates are educated to provide a wide range of services to women. The feminist framework of the program provides a constant mechanism to evaluate the impact of the graduates on women, their lives, and health as well as the influence of nursing on public policy.

The importance of moving from a fragmented view of women to a holistic vista is based in a belief system that involves the importance of gender and its influence in our society. All of this requires a reframing of our approach to women's health, incorporating feminist principles. Physical/health assessment and disease management are certainly important components of women's health, but understanding women's subjective experiences within their social contexts is also important. We must emphasize more clearly the social issues and conditions that are critical to the health of women. Examples of such issues include violence against women, homelessness, women and the criminal justice system, substance abuse, and poverty. We must include socio/political activism as part of this vision of reframing women's health by recognizing that we cannot prepare our students to intervene with women on a one-to-one basis only but instead must seriously consider the context under which women experience their lives and their health.

6

Feminist Theory and Health Psychology: Tools for an Egalitarian, Woman-Centered Approach to Women's Health

Jean A. Hamilton

There is increasing interest in creating a new medical specialty focused on women's health (Harrison, 1992; Johnson, 1987, 1992; Johnson & Dawson, 1990; Lewin, 1992). Medicine came to the modern U.S. women's health movement relatively late and it is important for it to catch up with other fields. Early leadership in the women's health movement had come from the lay women's community in the late 1960s and the 1970s (Zimmerman, 1987). When professional groups got involved, leadership first came from the nonmedical health professions, most notably including nursing, psychology, and other social sciences and public health.[1]

This is not to say that women in medicine are unimportant to the advancement of women's health. There were early pioneers in the late 1800s and early 1900s, including Dr. Mary Putnam Jacobi, who demonstrated that women were not generally fatigued by menstruation and Dr. Elizabeth Blackwell who spoke out against the surgical mutilation of women (Roy, 1992). Recently, several women in medicine have worked over the past decade to advance the field of women's health (Hamilton & Parry, 1983; Johnson, 1987). An especially powerful advocate emerging in the past few years has been Dr. Florence

SOURCE: This chapter originally appeared in modified form in *Journal of Women's Health,* Vol. 2, No. 1, 1993, pp. 49-54; used by permission of Mary Ann Liebert, Inc., 1651 Third Ave., New York, NY 10128.

AUTHOR'S NOTE: I am grateful to the faculty and administration of Duke University and its medical center for providing a supportive and intellectually nourishing environment for this type of inquiry. I am also grateful to Karen Johnson for her thoughtful comments on an earlier draft of this chapter, for her colleagueship as a feminist physician, and for her leadership on this important issue.

Haseltine, the driving force behind the Society for the Advancement of Women's Health; Dr. Bernadine Healy (1991) has also played an important role at the National Institutes of Health (NIH), along with Vivian Pinn.

It is critical that women in medicine join in the women's health movement to an even greater extent. Medicine has long been considered the premier health-related field and physicians continue to dominate the hierarchy at health-related institutions, such as the NIH. The high status of medicine is one reason that it has taken women in medicine so long to gain power in the profession. Yet the power and privilege associated with having a medical degree is one reason that it may be difficult for women in medicine to join in egalitarian efforts to advance women's health. Particularly if one is interested in a feminist—in the sense of woman-centered—approach to women's health, an egalitarian relationship between disciplines is crucial. Even though women physicians may add a more humane dimension to medical care (e.g., tending to listen more to their patients; Roter, Lipkin, & Korsgaard, 1991), they also practice in a historically patriarchal field. The high-status degree and powerful social role is a mixed blessing, coming at the price of considerable "extra baggage."

In this chapter, I explore two negative aspects of that baggage: (a) An implicit theory, central to most of our training that is antithetical to feminism; and (b) the ways we learn to cope with trauma, our privileged social role, and structural aspects of many of the institutions in which we train and practice interfere with humane, compassionate care and impede forming egalitarian relationships with other health care professionals. Little progress will be made by physicians seeking to join in the women's health movement unless cognitive, emotional, and structural barriers to our fuller participation are better understood and addressed.

In the long run, what is needed is not just mild reform but a direct challenge to the current model for health care research and practice. In the meantime, a women's health specialty is one way for medicine to begin catching up with other fields. It now appears that health care reform will occur in the United States in the near future. If so, then it is critical that women's health issues be addressed, but even more important that they be addressed in appropriate ways. One of women's "chief complaints" about health care has been that we are too often not listened to and that we are misunderstood and treated callously—without regard for the social context of our actual lives. Just as health care financing tends to give mental health issues short shrift, it is likely that emotional aspects of health care will be neglected. In raising issues such as these, it is important to clarify that I am not criticizing earlier proposals. Instead, I am attempting to broaden the debate by raising new issues for discussion.[2] Feminist scholarship and the *social* "health sciences" provide critically needed tools for conceptualizing and implementing more fundamental, humanistic change in health care research and practice. As in reform movements in the past, women leaders—coming from diverse health-related fields—will improve health care for all, male as well as female.

Cognitive Extra Baggage:
The Implicit Theory

Most physicians would deny that medicine is "theoretical." Instead, medicine might be described as "scientific," pragmatic, and eclectic. Despite these claims, I argue that modern medicine embodies an implicit theory: "biological primacy" (Fausto-Sterling, 1985). That is, even when psychosocial or situational factors are known to play a role in a phenomenon, if a biological factor can be identified, then it will be assumed to be causal. Biological primacy inevitably fosters "reductionism" and the mind-body dichotomy. For example, adherents of biomedical primacy tend to explain illness by reduction of complex issues in the lives of human beings to much simpler explanations grounded in biochemistry or molecular genetics (Friedman & DiMatteo, 1989; Taylor, 1991)—hence their support for projects like mapping the human genome (Fausto-Sterling, 1992). Psychologists studying social cognition have studied the error in thinking committed by adherents of biological primacy: the "fundamental attribution error" (Jones & Harris, 1967; Ross, 1977). It consists of the tendency to underestimate the role of situations (context) as determinants of a person's behavior and to overestimate the importance of internal (or, in this version, biological) factors. The error functions as an invisible cognitive barrier to changing the health care system. By better understanding its roots, however, we may learn to overcome it.

One problem with failing to recognize theory is that you use it without reflecting upon it. The theory of biological primacy tends to become part of the invisible background of our everyday thinking and functioning. In major medical research centers, so-called basic science research (typically using nonhuman animals) is generally more highly valued than clinical research (using humans); and basic science is narrowly construed, referring to the physical or biological sciences, but not, for example, to psychology. Thus the biomedical model narrowly defines and constricts the range of inquiry as well as the range of acceptable explanations. It is problematic not because it simplifies but because it is overly simplistic, dampening true interdisciplinary scholarship. It functions as a zero-sum game: When the biological sciences are overvalued, the psychosocial sciences are devalued.

Of course, not all physicians subscribe to the biomedical model. Those trained in psychiatry, family practice, community medicine, and public health are probably the most likely to escape its grip. It is interesting that many of the physicians most involved in the women's health movement trained in psychiatry. But it is also, perhaps, no accident that psychiatry, the only medical specialty with an explicit claim to social science expertise, rests at the bottom of the hierarchy of medical specialties when it comes to pay and status.[3]

Feminist scholarship (Fausto-Sterling, 1985, 1992) and health psychology research (Friedman & DiMatteo, 1989; Taylor, 1991) nonetheless describe the biomedical model and document its pervasive and insidious effects (Mizrahi, 1988).[4] That a gulf generally exists between scientific and other intellectual (e.g., humanistic) traditions has been even more widely recognized, however, dating back to Snow's (1964) classic discussion of "two cultures." The theory of biological primacy ultimately discourages appreciation of unique aspects of using humans, much less gendered persons, as research subjects (Hamilton, 1992).[5] It operates, cognitively, as extra baggage, creating barriers to offering "humane" health care, in general, and even more so when it comes to understanding and addressing women's health needs in particular.

Critiques of Medicine and Biological Primacy: Feminism, Health Psychology, and Barriers to Change

Mary Zimmerman (1987) has observed that "the Women's Health Movement is not the only current challenge to modern medicine, but it is the most *deeply rooted historically* as well as the most *analytically sophisticated*" (p. 442, italics added). Yet an empirically based critique of the biomedical model has come from the relatively new discipline of "health psychology."

There is a great deal of overlap between the feminist and health psychology critiques. Both recognize, for example, that gender is socially constructed. The social construction of gender implies that women's health can only be understood by a better appreciation of psychosocial aspects of women's lives, along with more integrative biological research. Indeed, every health discipline—with the notable *exception* of medicine—recognizes that psychology and the social sciences must be *central to* and at the very *core of* a woman-centered women's health movement. A related critique has come from health care consumers more generally, that is, the need to humanize medical care.

A Feminist Critique

A feminist critique of medicine is concerned with issues of power, both as it shapes health, illness, and recovery and as it determines forms of and access to health care and research. A feminist approach will address how organized medicine relates to patients, to its own practitioners, and to other health care professionals. And, finally, a feminist approach will address how to change health care to better meet the needs of women, both as patients and as caregivers.

The feminist critique of medicine begins with recognition of dominant and subordinate social roles in society: Male and female social roles are unequal, and men's gender role is more highly valued than women's. Gender roles inevitably influence health and health care, though not necessarily in ways that the biomedical model would recognize. As examples, the victimization of women, as women, is rooted in unequal gender roles and has had profound and enduring effects on women's physical and mental health. The hierarchy present in the rest of society is mirrored in medicine, where physicians, who have been mostly male, have enjoyed the highest status educational degree and greatest income of all health professionals; whereas nurses, who have been mostly female, have enjoyed much less status and income. At home, at work, and in the doctor's office or hospital, women have too often felt devalued and disbelieved, with our concerns either trivialized or overly pathologized. As lay caregivers, women's health-related work for family and friends has remained unpaid (Boston Women's Health Collective, 1992; Zimmerman, 1987).

The feminist critique embodies a substantial challenge to traditional power relationships in the medical profession. But perhaps more important, it challenges the "biomedical model." The flip side of overvaluing biology is devaluing emotional aspects of healing. For example, the biomedical model generally neglects the role of communication and empathic relationships, including the physician-patient relationship, in healing; it does so in favor of an apparent ethic of (short-term) "efficiency," leading to lessened time spent with patients and a controlling and, too often, a dismissive and demeaning interview style. The biomedical model also trivializes the effects of social roles and social context on health and illness.

The Health Psychology and
Related Humanistic Critiques

The health psychology critique centers on the biomedical model's reductionism and the mind-body split, such as its viewing the body as a machine, its inattention to psychological and emotional aspects of healing, its devaluation of psychosocial contributors to health and illness, as well as its predominant focus on disease as opposed to health and primary prevention (Friedman & DiMatteo, 1989; Taylor, 1991).

The health psychology critique is echoed by consumers and others seeking to more generally humanize the practice of medicine ("Dartmouth Redesigns," 1992; Hendrie & Lloyd, 1990; Mizrahi, 1988). When patients are objectified and the body is seen as a machine, then there is little reason to be humane ("Dartmouth Redesigns," 1992; Mizrahi, 1988): Why be humane to a machine?[6]

Because of its focus on psychosocial factors, health psychology has recently come to specifically address effects of gender on health. Important reviews by psychologists have included the following: Bonnie Strickland's (1988) article in the *Psychology of Women Quarterly* and Judith Rodin and Jeannette Ickovics's (1990) article in the *American Psychologist*. Sheryle Gallant and a colleague have prepared an article highlighting the contribution of health psychology to the women's health movement, which will appear shortly (S. Gallant, Medical Psychology, Uniformed Services University of Health Sciences, Bethesda, MD 20814, personal communication, November 5, 1992).

On the Overlap Between These Critiques:
Why Psychosocial Perspectives Are Critical
to Advancing Women's Health

In the face of differences by sex in rates of illness and recovery, adherents of biological primacy will tend to assume that the effect is due to biological factors such as genes or hormones. In contrast, feminists or health psychologists—and some of us who are both—will tend to assume that psychosocial factors, including poverty and victimization, may play an important role in determining the apparent effects of sex on health. These assumptions lead to differing research, clinical training and practice, and public policy priorities. These differences are illustrated using the example of depression.

Research. Mary Koss and colleagues (1991) have demonstrated that victimization has substantial and often chronic effects on physical and mental health. Among the serious mental health effects is depression (Council on Scientific Affairs, 1992; Hamilton & Jensvold, 1992). According to a recent study, childhood sexual abuse history may account for as much as a third of the excess of depression occurring in women compared with men (Cutler & Nolen-Hoeksema, 1991). Moreover, the latter finding suggests that *gender roles*, not biological sex per se, may be a critical determinant of depression.

Clinical training and practice: Emotional and structural barriers. The Council on Scientific Affairs of the American Medical Association recently recognized the need for medical practitioners to attend to domestic violence

(Council on Scientific Affairs, 1992). Carole Warshaw (1992) has recognized that there are emotional and structural barriers to asking the right clinical questions, and thereby to providing appropriate care. For example, emergency room physicians feel more comfortable fixing a woman's broken arm than in learning about the domestic abuse leading to the injury. The former leads to a sense of efficacy in the physician, whereas exploring the latter can lead to a sense of helplessness and despair. As long as cognitive, emotional, and structural factors are ignored in physician training, many, if not most, physicians will be emotionally unable to tolerate doing what feminists, health psychologists, and others would like them to do.

As physicians, emotional and structural aspects of our training encourage us to use denial and avoidance as methods for coping with the extreme traumas we are exposed to. Yet these ways of coping can interfere with appropriate empathy for our patients (Murphy, 1992; Weiner, 1990). That is, if we can't recognize and express our own feelings, we won't be able to recognize or tolerate hearing what our patients are feeling. Time pressures also inhibit opening up emotional and contextual aspects of injury. It is seemingly more "efficient" to quickly record: "Patient hit in face by fist" than to spend 20 minutes taking an abuse history (Warshaw, 1992). For reasons such as these, it can't be enough to merely instruct medical students and trainees to ask about victimization. Such instructions are contradicted by *structural* aspects of training that have led some interns to cynically brag about their efficiency in doing "two-minute" intake histories ("Dartmouth Redesigns," 1992; Dickstein, 1990). Ignoring emotional and structural factors such as these may lead to physicians sending an abused woman home, rather than referring her to a battered woman's shelter, and may lead to ignoring depression, which can, among other things, result from head injury (Brown, 1989; McGrath, Keita, Strickland, & Russo, 1990) suffered during domestic violence.

Only recently have physicians begun to acknowledge that structural aspects of training and conditions of clinical practice have impeded our efforts to be compassionate and caring physicians.[7] Issues such as these will be critical to consider as health care delivery and payment are subject to reform. Moreover, outright "abuses" in medical training have recently been documented (Mizrahi, 1988; Richman, Flaherty, Rospenda, & Christiansen, 1992). These abuses are expected to have direct consequences for patient care, leading to less humane treatment (Hendrie & Lloyd, 1990).[8]

Public policy. Many social and economic factors affect health, yet public policy tends to recognize only certain interventions as health related and essential. There is typically less reimbursement for "talking" specialties and primary prevention than for technical interventions, even when the latter are of questionable merit. This bias in policy continues even though psychosocial factors, such as depression and social support, appear to affect prognosis for illnesses such as heart disease (Friedman & DiMatteo, 1989) and breast cancer (Spiegel, Bloom, Kraemer, & Gottheil, 1989). The economics of health care financing may appear to be "cost efficient" in the short run but may do so at the price of shortchanging women and men in the long run when it comes to receiving appropriate, effective, and humane care.

Shedding Extra Baggage: Using the Tools of Feminist Scholarship and Health Psychology for a More Egalitarian Model

Medical training can be so all-consuming that it becomes isolating, so steeped in biological primacy that it becomes parochial and anti-intellectual, and so "practical" and seemingly efficient that it becomes, ultimately, inefficient. For reasons such as these, it will take a determined effort for many of us trained in medicine to shed unwanted, extra baggage. An additional problem is the privilege that physicians generally enjoy in our society. To put it succinctly, many of us are, as *physicians* (whether we are male or female), situated like *men* with respect to the women's movement: No one finds it easy to give up power.

We can look to women's studies programs for help with this dilemma. Women's studies offers a proven model for interdisciplinary study and collaboration; such programs are strong in many university settings, though not at traditional medical centers. By seeking new tools for dealing with entrenched barriers to change, we will be better able to *join with*, rather than "lead," other health professionals in a more explicitly feminist, egalitarian, and collaborative effort to advance women's health.

Women's health, at its best, will be based in the recognition of gender, not just sex, effects on health. As such, it will inherently challenge biological primacy. The practice of women's health must involve the *education* of health care providers, including physicians. Education in women's health must be strongly rooted in the social, as well as biological, health sciences.[9]

Notes

1. To the extent that physicians were involved, they most often worked as part-time paid employees for community-based gynecology clinics. Some gynecologists also did volunteer work, such as for Planned Parenthood.

2. In particular, I am not suggesting that Karen Johnson or her proposals for a woman's health specialty would in any way adhere to or support the extra baggage. I am generally seeking to

elucidate; neither am I suggesting her support for any of the barriers to change. In fact, I know full well that she is both an advocate and a practitioner of woman-centered, egalitarian, contextualized, and humane health care. Rather, I am throwing *additional* considerations into the pot, so to speak. In a sense, her original proposals are now taking on a life of their own. While she, of course, remains a leading spokesperson on the issue, it may be useful to flesh out practical considerations that have previously not been made explicit.

3. Similarly, pediatrics and family practice, both of which acknowledge family context, are also low in pay and status.

4. By way of illustration, a university professor I know was recently visiting her sister, who is studying for an advanced degree in biochemistry at Johns Hopkins University, a renowned bastion of the biomedical model. At the lab, she was introduced to her sister's boss, a male physician-scientist, as an anthropologist. He asked, "What's your organism?" She answered "humans." He responded with a look of dismay, saying, "But they're so *complicated*, I didn't know anyone *did them* anymore; you'll never get anywhere that way" (italics added). This attitude is, unfortunately, not idiosyncratic; instead, it is indicative of a broader problem: Within medicine—at least at elite academic research-oriented institutions—higher status is associated with less direct patient contact, such as by "getting rid of patients" (Mizrahi, 1988).

Also by way of illustration, in the mid-1980s I was speaking with a respected male colleague at the NIMH, also a physician-scientist, about the link I hypothesized between depression and rape (Hamilton & Jensvold, 1992; McGrath et al., 1990). It must be understood that this man is generally quite sensitive to women's issues and also highly supportive of women in science. He responded that rape was "a terrible social problem, but [that] it couldn't cause depression." "Why not," I asked? He answered: "Depression is a medical illness." Thus rape could lead women to be "demoralized," but because biology lies at the root of biomedical illness, depression couldn't be caused by a social problem. I believe that this type of misunderstanding of our lives as women has led some physicians, not all certainly but too many and too often, (a) to discount women's actual experiences of abuse, along with the associated pain and distress (e.g., "It's all in your head") and (b) to overlook important psychosocial research questions (e.g., the link between abuse and depression) in favor of biologically based questions (e.g., the effect of hormone changes on depression in women, though not in men).

5. While there are clearly some physicians who actively resist it, myself included, I for one can testify to the smothering effects of the model on trying to do woman-centered research. The struggle became so draining (Hamilton, 1992) that I eventually chose to leave a career in academic medicine, per se (happily, I was able to find a nourishing intellectual environment elsewhere). I realize that for other physicians the indoctrination may not have been so great or the struggle to resist it so oppressive.

6. The humanistic critique, often coming now from physicians themselves, clearly does *not* suggest that physicians are somehow innately callous people who are generally uncaring. However, leaders in medicine, including former U.S. Surgeon General Everett Koop, have identified the need to inspire future physicians to pay more attention to the human side of the doctor-patient relationship. According to Dr. Koop ("Dartmouth Redesigns," 1992), there is widespread agreement that the health care system isn't working and needs change; not only patients but also medical faculties are dissatisfied with the status quo. While Koop does not speak to effects on women per se, Mizrahi (1988) observes that the dehumanization that many patients experience is "exacerbated for the poor, the elderly, the working class, minority groups, and *women*" (p. 13, italics added).

7. I personally know of several caring physicians who have felt compelled to leave certain health organizations because the quality of care they chose to deliver was not consistent with management quotas dictating 15 minutes per patient.

8. An additional consideration is this: It may also be true that, developmentally, physicians may reach their prime relatively later in life—like social scientists. Perhaps a certain amount of lived experience, if not personal tragedy, and professional security are needed to heighten the capacity for complexity, ambiguity, and relatedness that humane care requires.

9. An idea that would complement Johnson's suggestion for a women's health specialty and address some of Harrison's concerns, as well, is this: an interdisciplinary women's health "fellowship [*sic*]," to occur between medical school and the internship and residency, or as a postdegree fellowship (e.g., after an M.P.H. or Ph.D.). That is, the fellowship would include fellows (*sic*) having different educational backgrounds and degrees, a method used previously in human development and aging programs (e.g., the clinical postdoctoral fellowship in adolescence at the University of Chicago and Michael Reese Medical Center). Education in women's health might occur as a sort of "fifth year" at the medical school, except that it would be cosponsored by and housed elsewhere at the university, and it might eventually culminate in a women's studies "certificate" or a terminal master's-level degree. Alternatively, the combined M.D.-Ph.D. might be sought in the usual 6 years but with a primary emphasis on the Ph.D. in a social, rather than a biological, health science, along with a graduate women's studies certificate.

References

Boston Women's Health Collective. (1992). *The new our bodies, ourselves*. New York: Simon & Schuster.

Brown, L. (1989, August). *The contribution of victimization as a risk factor for the development of depressive symptomatology in women*. Paper presented at the annual convention of the American Psychological Association, New Orleans.

Council on Scientific Affairs, American Medical Association. (1992). Violence against women: Relevance for medical practitioners. *Journal of the American Medical Association, 267*, 3184-3189.

Cutler, S. E., & Nolen-Hoeksema, S. (1991). Accounting for sex differences in depression through female victimization: Childhood sexual abuse. *Sex Roles, 24*, 425-438.

Dartmouth redesigns medical training to give future doctors a human touch. (1992, September 22). *The New York Times*, Education sec., p. 7.

Dickstein, L. (1990). Communication. In H. Hendrie & C. Lloyd (Eds.), *Educating competent and humane physicians* (pp. 54-71). Bloomington: Indiana University Press.

Fausto-Sterling, A. (1985). *Myths of gender*. New York: Basic Books.

Fausto-Sterling, A. (1992). Building two-way streets: The case of feminism in science. *NWSA Journal, 4*(3), 336-349.

Friedman, H. S., & DiMatteo, M. R. (1989). *Health psychology*. Englewood Cliffs, NJ: Prentice Hall.

Hamilton, J., & Jensvold, M. (1992). Personality, psychopathology and depressions in women. In L. S. Brown & M. Ballou (Eds.), *Personality and psychopathology*. New York: Guilford.

Hamilton, J. A. (1985). Avoiding methodological and policymaking biases in gender-related research. In *Report of the Public Health Service Task Force on Women's Health* (Vol. 2, pp. 54-64). Washington, DC: Government Printing Office.

Hamilton, J. A. (1992). Biases in women's health research. *Women & Therapy, 12*, 91-101.

Hamilton, J. A., & Parry, B. (1983). Sex-related differences in clinical drug response: Implications for women's health. *Journal of the American Medical Women's Association, 38*(5), 126-132.

Harrison, M. (1992). Women's health as a specialty: A deceptive solution. *Journal of Women's Health, 1,* 101-106.

Healy, B. (1991). Women's health, public welfare. *Journal of the American Medical Association, 266,* 566-568.

Hendrie, H., & Lloyd, C. (Eds.). (1990). *Educating competent and humane physicians.* Bloomington: Indiana University Press.

Johnson, K. (1987). Women's health care: An innovative model. *Women & Therapy, 6,* 305-311.

Johnson, K. (1992). Women's health: Developing a new interdisciplinary specialty. *Journal of Women's Health, 1,* 95-99.

Johnson, K., & Dawson, L. (1990). Women's health as a multidisciplinary specialty: An exploratory proposal. *Journal of the American Medical Women's Association, 45,* 222-224.

Jones, E. E., & Harris, V. A. (1967). The attribution of attitudes. *Journal of Experimental Social Psychology, 3,* 1-24.

Koss, M. P., Koss, P. G., & Woodruff, W. J. (1991). Deleterious effects of criminal victimization on women's health and medical utilization. *Archives of Internal Medicine, 151,* 342-347.

Lewin, T. (1992, November 7). Doctors consider a specialty focusing on women's health. *The New York Times,* pp. 1, 9.

McGrath, E., Keita, G. P., Strickland, B. R., & Russo, N. F. (1990). *Women and depression.* Washington, DC: American Psychological Association.

Mizrahi, T. (1988). *Getting rid of patients.* Rutgers, NJ: Rutgers University Press.

Murphy, L. B. (1992, November 7). *The education of physicians: Impact on humanity and patient care.* Paper presented at the Women's Studies Graduate Seminar, Duke University, Durham, NC.

Richman, J., Flaherty, J., Rospenda, K., & Christiansen, M. (1992). Mental health consequences and correlates of reported medical student abuse. *Journal of the American Medical Association, 267,* 692-694.

Rodin, J., & Ickovics, J. (1990). Women's health: Review and research agenda as we approach the 21st century. *American Psychologist, 45,* 1018-1034.

Ross, L. (1977). The intuitive psychologist and his shortcomings: Distortions in the attribution process. In L. Berkowitz (Ed.), *Advances in experimental social psychology* (Vol. 10). New York: Academic Press.

Roter, D., Lipkin, M., & Korsgaard, A. (1991). Sex differences in patients' and physicians' communications during primary care medical visits. *Medical Care, 29,* 1083-1093.

Roy, J. M. (1992). Gynecological surgery. In R. D. Apple (Ed.), *Women, health, and medicine in America* (pp. 173-196). New Brunswick, NJ: Rutgers University Press.

Snow, C. P. (1964). *The two cultures: and a second look.* Cambridge: Cambridge University Press.

Spiegel, D., Bloom, J. R., Kraemer, H. C., & Gottheil, E. (1989). Effects of psychosocial treatment of patients with metastatic breast cancer. *Lancet, 2,* 888-891.

Strickland, B. R. (1988). Sex-related differences in health and illness. *Psychology of Women Quarterly, 12,* 381-399.

Taylor, S. E. (1991). *Health psychology.* New York: McGraw-Hill.

Warshaw, C. (1992, October 16). *Multidisciplinary approaches to violence against women.* Presentation at the conference "Reframing Women's Health," Chicago.

Weiner, H. (1990). Facts and values in medical education. In H. Hendrie & C. Lloyd (Eds.), *Educating competent and humane physicians* (pp. 3-23). Bloomington: Indiana University Press.

Zimmerman, M. K. (1987). The women's health movement: A critique of medical enterprise and the position of women. In B. B. Hess & M. M. Ferree (Eds.), *Analyzing gender: A handbook of social science research* (pp. 442-472). Newbury Park, CA: Sage.

7

Self-in-Relation Theory:
Implications for Women's Health

Lucy M. Candib

In this chapter, I will briefly review self-in-relation theory and suggest why it is important for understanding women's health and health care.

Many readers will be familiar with self-in-relation theory through the work of Jean Baker Miller and her associates at the Stone Center at Wellesley. Baker Miller's pathbreaking book, *Toward a New Psychology of Women*, originally published in 1976, shows how women's strengths lie in our relationships with others, relationships that inevitably bear the marks of our oppression at both social and interpersonal levels. Baker Miller is clear not to see women's relational capacities as inherent or genetic, and she is explicitly clear about the power dynamics that constrict us in our relational tasks. More recently, self-in-relation theory has been made available with the publication of a new book: *Women's Growth in Connection* (Jordan et al., 1991), a collection of writings by Baker Miller as well as Judith Jordan, Irene Stiver, Jan Surrey, and Alexandra Kaplan. This group has hammered out the basis of a new way of looking at ourselves and our relationships through lenses far less distorting than those of conventional psychology.

Traditional approaches to human development and psychology have used male views and imagery about development and adulthood as the framework to understand *human* development. These models emphasize autonomy, separateness, and independence as the ideals of development. We all recognize how these themes imply that healthy childhoods and adulthoods should be characterized by degrees of separateness and autonomy that have little to do with the lived realities of our lives. Until now women could only see themselves or be seen by others as failures from the point of view of autonomy.

AUTHOR'S NOTE: This chapter draws on material from a forthcoming book on the subject to be published by Basic Books in 1994.

Our involvement with others was denigrated with the use of such terms as *immature ego development* or *inadequate boundaries* or, for lesbians, *failure to achieve adequate separation.* The converse possibilities—overdeveloped ego, failure to allow penetration of others into one's boundaries, or inability to tolerate intimacy—never achieved the status of psychological jargon, perhaps because these terms would apply largely to the men who generated and perpetuated that jargon.

In contrast to traditional psychological theory, self-in-relation theory considers children, adolescents, and adults from the perspective of relationships, using an understanding that development means increasing complexity, connection, and mutuality in those relationships. This relational approach allows clinicians to focus on the importance of relationships to women rather than to dismiss their involvement as pathological. Being-in-relation theory has dramatically altered how feminist mental health practitioners in various fields (psychology, social work, counseling, family therapy) approach the care of women patients.

Some readers may accept that being-in-relation theory is important for our psychological health but wonder what it has to do with our health or health care. Let me reveal my bias that I do not think our mental health and our physical health are truly separable. Our illnesses are the complex result of all that we experience socially and interpersonally, interpreted by our bodies, which are affected by all the foods, substances, toxins, bacteria, viruses, and trauma that life may expose us to. Even when we are sick primarily in our bodies, that sickness is interpreted, modulated, and altered by our reality as lovers, parents, daughters, coworkers, and so on. A cold is not just a cold, it is Cindy's cold, Cindy who was supposed to drive Molly to day care, talk to her mother's lawyer about a health care proxy, respond to her partner's worries about overextension at work, and attend to her own responsibilities as an administrator. This seems like a trivial example, but if it is true of a person with a cold, how much more so of a person with rheumatoid arthritis, angina, or breast cancer!

Although we are aware that illness creates an intensely personal and unique interference in our connectedness with others, the traditional medical model is based on the opposite assumption—the need to distinguish the disease from the person. The medical model separates out each symptom and turns it into an element that, with adequate matching, lines up with abstract notions of disease. In other words, if one has a runny nose, headache, low grade fever, and muscle aches, one has a virus. It is not sinusitis, strep, pneumonia, or any other more serious condition that might warrant medical intervention. Cindy has nothing to do with it, much less her lover, her child, or her mother's lawyer.

The medical model creates several kinds of distance—between the person and her illness, between the clinician and the person, and between the clinician and the illness. If the illness is chronic or disabling, the medical model requires and maintains a distance between the ill person and those defined as healthy, including the person's family members and the health care workers involved in her care. Sickness is isolating, as any narrative from those affected will testify.

But the medical model is not the only explanation for the emphasis on human separateness and distance in medical thought. Let's turn to an area where separateness and autonomy would not be our initial assumption: infant and child development. Although the study of development does not constitute a large part of training in most health care disciplines, assumptions about infant, child, and adolescent development are central to fields that deal with children and families. Freud imagined that the infant, initially seen as fused with the mother, gradually separated from the inchoate enormity of the mother. The path of infant development moved from fusion to independence, with a negative emphasis on the pathology of fusion with the female figure. The infant gradually pulls away from this primitive union with the mother. Herein lies the notion that dependence is synonymous with what is pathological, not manly. Dependence is synonymous with closeness; independence is the goal.

The themes of separation and independence from the mother persist today as the centerpieces in the understanding of development offered to students of medicine. Medical teachings about infant and child development unabashedly describe infant and child development as a trajectory of autonomy. Let me give you some quotes:

From Gesell in 1940:

Whether boy or girl, the 2-year-old is especially prone to dramatize the mother-baby relationship through dolls and otherwise. In a dim way he is beginning to understand this relationship which means that he himself is becoming somewhat detached from his mother. Only by increasing this detachment can he achieve an adequate sense of self. (p. 40)

From Brazelton (1974):

It must be difficult for a mother to see why a child needs to be punished or rejected to establish himself as a separate person, but perhaps it is as simple as that—when he is intensely loved, it is even more difficult to separate. When his behavior creates even a temporary ambivalence in his parent, then he can more easily feel his separateness. (pp. 102-103)

From *Nelson,* a standard pediatrics textbook:

> The demands on mother and infant during the first year are for the development
> of comfortable interactions which will lead to the infant's movement from a
> position of dependency to one of independent activity. . . . Failure of achieve-
> ment of the developmental goals of the first year leads to emotional dissatis-
> faction or to chronic anxieties on the part of the infant, which may be the root
> of life-long personality disorders. (Vaughan & McKay, 1975, p. 24)

Once we recognize the underlying assumptions in these quotes—that
dependence must give way to independence and attachment to separation—
then we begin to see that this view of development itself contains an ideological
bias. Jan Surrey (1991a) identifies this bias in the underlying belief "that the
person must first disconnect from relationship in order to form a separate,
articulated firm sense of self or personhood" (p. 36). Of interest, research on
infants by Daniel Stern (1985) shows that within the first 2 months of life infants
demonstrate the ability to initiate, maintain, and break off social interactions
through the control of gaze. This ability could be construed as the preliminary
gestures of autonomy; we could also describe it as the infant setting a pace
of interaction with the parent. What is at issue here is the focus: on separateness rather than on *being in relation to.* I use this awkward-sounding term to
call attention to the fact that the emphasis on separateness ignores the infant's
growing abilities to be an active participant in creating the connection with
parents. From the very beginning, infants can actively shape their relationships through engaging or disengaging in eye contact. A change in focus allows
us to see infant development differently: Disconnection is not primary; rather,
the ability to relate is primary.

I would like to make one further point about the medical conception of infant
development: the discussion appears devoid of gender. The meaning of autonomy in the context of infancy appears gender neutral. Nevertheless, under
scrutiny, autonomy itself emerges as a highly *gendered* concept, specifically
in this instance as strongly influenced by ideas about male identity. For instance,
the idea that separateness must precede identity is not a gender-neutral idea.
Chodorow (1978) argues that identity rooted in sameness may be more typical
of girls' experience while boys may differentiate themselves through separation. Certainly, social expectations of children reinforce these gendered
constructions of what it means to be a girl or boy. Separateness, independence, and autonomy are characteristics stereotypically attributed to male
identity. Later these same attributes are linked to accepted images of mental
health (Broverman et al., 1970). Thus the bias in the portrayal of infancy
above lies in the preferential designation of these male-gender-identified quali-

ties as the goal of development. The masculine template of separation has become the standard for the medical understanding of all infant development, and stereotypical male attributes—autonomy, separateness, and independence —are translated backward onto infant development. Thus the notion of separateness as a goal of development derives from a gendered construction of what development means.

In contrast to this autonomy model, self-in-relation theory

> makes an important shift in emphasis from separation to relationship as the basis for self-experience and development. Further, relationship is seen as the basic goal of development: i.e. the deepening capacity for relationship and relational competence. The self-in-relation model assumes that other aspects of self (e.g. creativity, autonomy, assertion) develop within this primary context. . . . There is no inherent need to disconnect or to sacrifice relationship for self-development. (Surrey, 1991b, p. 53)

Let's turn for a moment to adolescence. Here, as with infancy, the language of autonomy and separation dominates descriptions of the developmental tasks of this period. Here is the section on adolescence from the 12th edition of the *Nelson Textbook of Pediatrics*:

> At adolescence the child goes through a second and more definitive emergence as a person separate from his or her parents, as he or she strives for an identity as an independent adult. The adolescent has many advantages over the 4 yr old . . . but periodic regressions again reflect the underlying tension between needs for dependence and for autonomy. (Behrman & Vaughan, 1983, p. 51)

Using autonomy as the focus of our lens on adolescence prevents us from seeing how deeply these same adolescents cherish their connections to their parents. An alternative view of individuation in adolescence sees it as a dimension of relationships. For instance, adults often consider a teenage girl's sexual activity as a symbol of rebellion or independence; it can also be seen as part of the search for relatedness and intimacy, occurring within the network of relationships important to the girl herself. The relational perspective may seem foreign to parental (and clinical) adults who have long interpreted the struggles of the teenage years in terms of Eriksonian autonomy, but attention to teenagers' accounts of their own experience supports its usefulness. Research on college women reveals the importance to them of their relationships with their mothers. While classical teachings about adolescence might regard such mother-daughter ties as pathological, in self-in-relation theory, adolescence is a time of maturation of the relational self. Kaplan and Klein (1991) describe this growth among college age women as including:

1. increased potential for entering mutually empathic relationships with sharing of one's own empathic states and responsiveness to the affect of others;
2. relational flexibility, allowing relationships to evolve and change;
3. ability and desire to work out conflicts in relationships while maintaining the emotional connection;
4. feeling empowered through relational connection with others, including mothers. (p. 131)

If clinicians were to step away from the autonomy view of infancy, childhood, and adolescence, how would our clinical approach to patients be different? Infants and small children might be examined in a parent's lap, making the child feel safe and keeping parent and practitioner comfortably seated at the same level. A mother bringing her child for a health problem can be asked what other family members think about the problem, to situate the symptom and the visit within a perspective that recognizes that the woman lives in a world composed of relationships and that the opinions of those family members may be more influential than anything a practitioner says or does to the contrary. Clinicians can begin direct conversations with children, recognizing them as persons whose viewpoints count. As they get older, portions of the visit can be conducted with them alone, demonstrating that they have their own relationship with the practitioner, that they can begin to have relational competency. (This is a different assumption from seeing them as autonomous or completely in charge of their own health care.) Teenagers can be viewed in terms of the importance to them of their relationships with their parents and their sense of themselves as young people able to participate in caring connections with parents, siblings, friends, and extended family as well as with potential romantic partners.

Let's turn now to look at how medical thought has approached women's adult development. We are all familiar with medicine's violations against women patients, the use of surgery, drugs, and shock therapy to control us, and the categorization of our ailments as the result of our poor adjustment to our feminine roles. (See, for instance, Scully & Bart, 1973, for a description of these assumptions in gynecological textbooks and Scully, 1980, for the explicit nature of these beliefs in specialty training in obstetrics and gynecology.) This approach is not merely the accidental accumulation of the acts of individual chauvinist males. That might be easier to fix! Instead, medicine has a theoretical understanding of adult development that is based solely on men's view of their own development and their view of women's development. Medicine has no other theory of women's adult development.

Contemporary medical understandings about men's development derive from three sources: Erikson (1968), who viewed women as holding their spaces open for the men they would marry; Vallaint (1977), a psychiatrist who studied several hundred male Harvard graduates; and Levinson, who studied a small number of men in his well-publicized book, *Seasons of a Man's Life* (Levinson, Darrow, Klein, Levinson, & McKee, 1978). In these sources, the commonly accepted views of adult development are based on discussions of men's developmental trajectory toward presumed autonomy. Written by men primarily about men, they define men's identity or male development in terms of separateness instead of relationships. The very limited mention of women's development is only in terms of their heterosexual and reproductive functions in relation to the men studied.

Surprisingly the story of development is almost absent from medical texts about adults. This omission is all the more striking because development is central to medical thinking about children and adolescents. When adult development is mentioned, Erikson, Vaillant, and Levinson are the sole sources named. The scant literature on women's development in medical texts draws on these authors to restrict women's growth to heterosexual and reproductive roles. Other texts consider development as a feature of the family life cycle, a framework that places two wobbly cornerstones under adult development: heterosexuality and reproduction. Even in the 1990s common expectations of women's and men's gender roles in the family life cycle remain remarkably familiar: men the achievers, women the nurturers; men accomplishing out in the world, women caring for others in the bosom of their families; men agentic, women communal; men instrumental, women relational (Candib, 1989).

Take for instance the topic of paid work, considered a central feature of men's adult development; in men's development studies, work appears primary and family life secondary. In the absence of an explicit study of women's development, medical texts have ignored the meaning of work outside the home for women and instead made the implicit assumption that the family life cycle *is* women's development. Taking the family life cycle for women's development reinforces stereotypical gender roles and creates a constricted view of women centered on their reproduction.

If men's development is adult development, what is women's development? The scant references in the medical literature leave the reader with an unstated group of pernicious false conclusions: that women's development is inconsequential; that women's development does not differ significantly from men's; that women's development is obvious, that is, it is the family life cycle; that all women's development is the same, obscuring differences of race and class; or, most insidiously, that women's development is *complementary* to men's development.

No thoughtful look at development can fail to recognize how these assumptions limit the full range of possibilities for both sexes. Racism as well constrains what people of color can accomplish, both by limiting opportunity in the world at large and by creating self-doubt and despair within individuals. A more adequate model would take into account how racism and sexual oppression produce a set of developmental problems not addressed in the standard approach to adulthood. For women, such oppressive conditions include experiences of child sexual abuse, date rape, wife battering and marital rape, chronically reduced educational and occupational opportunities, excess household and caregiving responsibilities, and limited options to determine their own health care. Given these realities, it is not surprising that adult women show well-documented excess medical and psychiatric morbidity when compared with men. A basic question we can ask of any description of adult development is this: Does it recognize how racism and gender roles circumscribe developmental options? Does it recognize, for instance, how customary expectations of gender roles play directly into cultural prescriptions of men's violence and women's acquiescence (Kaplan, 1988)? The study of human development should not be merely a study of what is but, instead, a study of what can be.

The contribution of being-in-relation theory to adult development is that healthy selves are constituted by relations and that such persons at some level recognize that they are so defined. This recognition is one of the real accomplishments of adult development. Self-definitions in terms of subservient relations or relations in which a person is not free to express herself represent an oppressed or unhealthy condition. When women define themselves entirely through taking care of others and assume that such caring constitutes a relational self, they fail to take care of themselves and thus accept a subservient definition of their adulthood. Baker Miller shows how such sacrifice makes women feel depressed and angry without a clear formulation of why they feel that way. The challenge of being-in-relation theory for women's development is to envision development in affiliations or relations that do not compromise the potential for women's autonomy *as women define it*. (See Yanay & Birns, 1990, and Griffiths, 1992, for discussions of the need for a relational understanding of autonomy.)

What are the implications of these understandings for how we conduct women's health care? Self-in-relation theory offers us the insight that women's health cannot be narrowly confined to the study of diseases unique to females or to specific time periods in women's adult lives. Women's health must be viewed within the network of relationships and responsibilities in women's lives and understood within the broader frameworks of racism and oppression that characterize the world in which women conduct those relationships and carry out those responsibilities. Our look at mother-infant relationships, mother-daughter relationships, balancing work and family responsibilities, menopause, aging, and sexuality all require revisioning from a being-in-relation perspective.

Here are a few glimpses of what such revisions might look like: A relational approach allows us to consider the strengths and needs of women in abusive relationships and the kinds of relationships with health care providers that could help them put an end to the abuse. Another example: Because women arrange and participate in most of the health care for their children, a relational understanding is helpful in approaching women's work in the care of infants and children. Women's role as caregivers extends further to caring for sick and frail adults in their families. Caring for others is part of relationships but also work; overresponsibility for the care of others forms a major element of women's oppression. How racism constricts women's abilities to care for themselves and others is another element central to considering women's health. Being-in-relation theory offers a perspective on women as caregivers that places health within the network of connections women maintain with and for others. Clinicians who work with adults of all ages in the complexity of relationships with friends and family should find the assumptions underlying a relational picture of development more compatible with clinical work.

This brief chapter is obviously too short to develop these themes in detail. Rather, I would like to make one further point: the relevance of being-in-relation theory to the conduct of clinical relationships. In *Women's Growth in Connection,* Jordan (1991) has written most explicitly about the nature of empathy in clinical relationships. Just as autonomy prescribes a clinical approach based on distance and separateness, a relational perspective advises *mutuality* in clinical work. The clinician joins with the patient in seeing the world from her viewpoint. Taking into consideration a woman's relational and social context, the clinician can join with the woman patient in trying to understand her health and her needs for health care. She makes herself open to the patient and is willing to be changed by the patient. Both parties hold some responsibility for the course of the relationship, but the clinician can use her understanding of women's disempowerment in most settings as a focus for empowerment in the clinical relationship.

Given the male-dominated models of development that pervade medical understandings of infancy, childhood, adolescence, and adulthood; given the sexism inherent in limiting a view of women to heterosexuality and reproduction; given the need for a feminist approach to clinical relationships for the empowerment of women; what then are the implications of being-in-relation theory for women's health care? Some readers might argue that my critique argues for the creation of a women's health specialty. After all, if we train highly selected clinicians in this model as well as in properly scrutinized health care practices, wouldn't the resulting women's health specialists be the ideal clinicians for women? My answer is *no*.

Here are some of my reasons. First, women perform the vast majority of caring work for the dependent and ill, young and old, in their families. In the course of this work, women obtain the bulk of medical care for children and for their families. They have innumerable encounters with health care professionals in doing this work. All of these interactions need to be informed by a feminist approach both to the identified patient and to the woman who brings that patient. If only the practitioners who do women's health care itself are trained to care for women, then all the other clinicians whom women will meet in the course of their caring work for their families will follow the traditional medical approach, which emphasizes the separateness of persons rather than their relatedness. This is inadequate. All clinicians need to change.

Second, there are too many of us. A specialty for half the people is not a specialty, which by definition is appropriate for a select group. My fear is that the select group who would benefit from a women's health specialty would be exactly that group of educated upper-middle-class white women who are already able to make critical choices about their health care. An overweight black woman on welfare from the South Side of Chicago who cares for her grandchildren because their parents are strung out on crack cocaine—who is sick with diabetes and hypertension, with no Pap smear for 5 years and no mammogram ever—this woman won't be on the top of the appointment list when a women's health specialist nails up her shingle. Yet this woman and the millions like her are precisely those who could most benefit from a relational approach to their health care.

Third, health care for women spans a lifetime. A 5-year-old girl, a 10-year-old girl, a 15-year-old young woman, a 20-year-old woman—each of them needs a women's health specialist, yet the skills involved in their care span several existing specialties—similarly for 40-, 60-, and 80-year-old women. When and if a woman chooses to get pregnant, she needs a practitioner, or several practitioners, to provide prenatal care, attend her delivery, and look after her baby. And when that baby and the ones that follow grow up, she needs a clinician who knows what it means when her daughter starts to become a sexual being, and can help that daughter enter the world of sexual activity in as safe and healthy a way as possible. The tasks involved in her health care span her lifetime and the lifetime of the clinician who chooses to provide that care. Only one medical specialty, as I see it, can offer that breadth—and that is family practice.

But a single medical specialty is not the answer either. Nurse practitioners and physicians' assistants are already providing women's health care in innumerable settings. And among women who choose to go to doctors, many will elect kinds of specialists other than family practitioners. And not all practitioners wishing to do women's health will find themselves suited by interest or temperament to the work of family practice. So women's health will need to be practiced by *all* kinds of practitioners. And *all* kinds of practitioners will need to learn about being-in-relation theory so as to provide appropriate health care to women in a variety of settings. Rather than arguing for a women's health specialty, or for all women to go to family practitioners, we need to struggle for all clinicians to gain an understanding of the needs of women at all points in the life cycle and in all the work of caring that they do for others in their families. Being-in-relation theory offers an opening to reshape our developmental understandings of infants and children, adolescents and grown-ups, to see the connectedness of persons in sickness and in health, and to enable clinicians to join patients in clinical relationships characterized by mutuality and empathy. Limiting our goals to a mere specialty falls short of the mark. We need to transform the entire clinical endeavor.

References

Baker Miller, J. (1976). *Toward a new psychology of women.* Boston: Beacon.

Behrman, R. E., & Vaughan, V. C. (Eds.). (1983). *Nelson textbook of pediatrics.* Philadelphia: W. B. Saunders.

Brazelton, T. B. (1974). *Toddlers and parents: A declaration of independence.* New York: Delta.

Broverman, I. K., Broverman, D. M., Clarkson, F. E., et al. (1970). Sex-role stereotypes and clinical judgments of mental health. *Journal of Consulting Clinical Psychology, 34,* 1-7.

Candib, L. M. (1989). Family life cycle theory: A feminist critique. *Family Systems Medicine, 7,* 473-487.

Chodorow, N. (1978). *The reproduction of mothering: Psychoanalysis and the sociology of gender.* Berkeley: University of California Press.

Erikson, E. H. (1968). *Identity: Youth and crisis.* New York: Norton.

Gesell, A. (1940). *The first five years of life: A guide to the study of the preschool child.* New York: Harper.

Griffiths, M. (1992). Autonomy and the fear of dependence. *Women's Studies International Forum, 15,* 351-362.

Jordan, J. V., et al. (Eds.). (1991). *Women's growth in connection: Writings from the Stone Center.* New York: Guilford.

Kaplan, A. G. (1988). How normal is normal development? Some connections between adult development and the roots of abuse and victimization. In M. B. Strause (Ed.), *Abuse and victimization: A life span perspective.* Baltimore: Johns Hopkins University Press.

Kaplan, A., & Klein, R. (1991). The relational self in late adolescent women. In J. V. Jordan et al. (Eds.), *Women's growth in connection: Writings from the Stone Center* (pp. 122-131). New York: Guilford.

Levinson, D. J., Darrow, C. N., Klein, E. B., Levinson, M. H., & McKee, B. (1978). *Seasons of a man's life.* New York: Knopf.

Scully, D. (1980). *Men who control women's health: The miseducation of obstetrician-gynecologists.* Boston: Houghton Mifflin.

Scully, D., & Bart, P. (1973). A funny thing happened on my way to the orifice: Woman in gynaecology textbooks. *American Journal of Sociology, 78,* 1045-1050.

Stern, D. N. (1985). *The interpersonal world of the infant: A view from psychoanalysis and developmental psychology.* New York: Basic Books.

Surrey, J. L. (1991a). The relational self in women: Clinical implications. In J. V. Jordan et al. (Eds.), *Women's growth in connection: Writings from the Stone Center* (pp. 35-44). New York: Guilford.

Surrey, J. L. (1991b). The "self-in-relation": A theory of women's development. In J. V. Jordan et al. (Eds.), *Women's growth in connection: Writings from the Stone Center* (pp. 51-66). New York: Guilford.

Vaillant, G. E. (1977). *Adaptation to life.* Boston: Little, Brown.

Vaughan, V. C., & McKay, R. J. (Eds.). (1975). *Nelson textbook of pediatrics.* Philadelphia: W. B. Saunders.

Yanay, N., & Birns, B. (1990). Autonomy as emotion: The phenomenology of independence in academic women. *Women's Studies International Forum, 13,* 249-260.

8

Women's Health: New Models of Care and a New Academic Discipline

Michelle Harrison

The debate as to whether there should be a specialty of women's health has been primarily limited to the question of whether there should be a formally structured separate specialty of women's health within medicine (Harrison, 1990, 1992; Johnson, 1992; Johnson & Dawson, 1990; Wallis, 1992; Wallis & Klass, 1990). The debate attempts to solve two separate problems: One is that of improved clinical care of women; the other is how to create and institutionalize a body of knowledge about women's health. This chapter will first address the clinical care of women and then propose a framework for interdisciplinary research and education in women's health, at the level of a master's degree.

The need for new models of clinical care evolves from a growing awareness of ways in which the current medical system has failed to meet the needs of women. Recent literature has addressed differential treatment of women with cardiac symptoms (Bickell et al., 1992; Krumholz, Douglass, Lauer, & Pasternak, 1992) and other complaints (Armitage, Schneiderman, & Bass, 1979). Women have been excluded from clinical trials (Gurwitz, Col, & Avorn, 1992) and little research has been done, for example, on the effects of the menstrual cycle on various medications—ones that are then prescribed for women. Marketing research has shown that women are concerned about issues such as nutrition and preventive care and "they just wanted a doctor who was personal with them and willing to answer their questions" (Boscarino, 1987).

SOURCE: This chapter originally appeared in modified form in *Journal of Women's Health,* Vol. 2, No. 1, 1993, pp. 61-66; used by permission of Mary Ann Liebert, Inc., 1651 Third Ave., New York, NY 10128.

The debate as to a medical specialty assumes that the solutions to women's health care needs lie within the scope of medicine and clinical practice. However, the reframing of women's health requires that the question be changed from this one: "Should some physicians specialize in women's health?" to this: "What model of women's health best meets the needs of women as patients?" Answering the latter question places the emphasis on the woman rather than the provider and requires that the health care industry overcome its traditional historic roots to adapt to contemporary social structures and values with regard to class, race, and gender.

Origins of Contemporary Medicine

The current organization of women's health care with its bifurcation of reproductive from nonreproductive women's health has its historic roots in the nineteenth century. Medicine, as a specialty, was founded on the model of a male body, with woman as "other" (Harrison, 1990). With the development of obstetrical instrumentation and gynecological surgery, female midwives were replaced by male obstetrician/gynecologists. While, in theory, these new specialists could meet the medical needs of women, they could not replace the more complex and social role of midwives in the lives of women. Midwives did not just deliver babies but attended to a vast array of "female conditions," often becoming friend and confidant to the women they served and passing on the lore of conception, contraception, childbirth, menstruation, sexuality, lactation, and mothering. Attending women at home, living within the same social class and community, they were often trusted friends, counselors, and healers, roles that were not replicated by the male obstetrician/gynecologists.

Medicine, in attempting to address women's needs, was further burdened by the legacy of nineteenth-century sexist attitudes toward women that appeared in medical textbooks into the 1970s (Walsh, 1992). Women had been defined by their reproductive organs and roles. Dr. Charles Meigs, in a series of 1859 medical lectures, wrote: "Her mere human or generic nature is modified by her sexual or female nature . . . she demands a treatment adapted to the very specialties of her own constitution, as a moral, a sexual, germinferous, gestative, or parturient creature" (p. 55). Describing differences between men and women, he wrote: "*He* enters on the path of ambition, that dark and dangerous, or broad and shining road. . . . She sits at home to adorn the tent or the cottage with wreaths of flowers. . . . All rude, boisterous, and immodest speech or action unsexes and disgraces woman" (Meigs, 1859, p. 63, italics added). Rudiments of such attitudes are found today in myths about premenstrual syndrome and hormonal explanations of women's anger (American Psychiatric Association, 1987; Harrison, 1989).

The early twentieth century saw yet another development that affected the current organization of care with respect to gender, class, and race. The "Flexner Report of 1910" (*Medical Education in the United States and Canada*) and its use by state licensing and accreditation boards catalyzed the process of eliminating the less well established and less endowed medical schools (Hudson, 1992, p. 12). However, these schools were less expensive and accepted more women and minority students. While Flexner's assessments of schools may have been valid with regard to inadequate facilities, *the decisions of the accreditation bodies to close these schools rather than improve them* led to markedly fewer schools and students, with even fewer women and minorities matriculating.

The late nineteenth century also saw the influence of German science and technology on American medicine. Hudson (1992, pp. 3-4), in *Abraham Flexner in Historical Perspective*, describes three major effects of the German influence on American medicine: The idea of research became important; medicine developed specialties, based in part upon technology and surgical procedures; and innovations in American medical education with the establishment of Johns Hopkins included many features of German medical education. The increasing cost of medical education, and the exclusivity of the education and skills, often influenced physicians to enter more lucrative surgical and technology-related specialties.

These changes, along with Flexner's strong recommendation that all faculty be full-time, hospital-based physicians (Flexner, 1910, p. 106), strengthened the medical model of health care. The changes mirror what Kiesler (1992) describes as the current medical system, in which "short-term, acute care hospitals are the cornerstone of health care . . . and . . . the hospital is regarded as the doctors' workshop—which others pay for but physicians control" (p. 1077).

The legacy of this history of changes in the past 100 years is a medical system heavily weighted toward private enterprise (Hillman et al., 1992; Mitchell & Scott, 1992) with substandard care for those who lack money or insurance (Burstin, Lipsitz, & Brennan, 1992). For the poor, the nearest hospital emergency room is often the primary care site. It is estimated that as many as 31 to 37 million Americans under 65 lack health insurance (Fuchs, 1990). These combined characteristics of medicine, the cost, the emphasis on technology and procedures, and the ingrained stereotypical views of women have created a vacuum, one being met by the development of new groups of practitioners to address unmet health care needs of women.

Allied Health Professionals
and Nursing Advanced Practice

Physicians' assistant (PA) programs grew initially out of the return from Vietnam of a sizable force of medically trained midlevel professionals with no comparable role outside the military. Their success in the military led to a movement to use them and similarly trained professionals in civilian settings. Soon after, partly emboldened by the PA success and partly as a result of the women's health movement (Mulligan, 1983) with its focus on bringing midwives back to childbirth and to women's health, nursing expanded the training and roles of nurses. Three major groups evolved: nurse practitioners, nurse clinicians, and midwives. In 1991 the American Nursing Association formed the Council of Nurses in Advanced Practice and created standards for membership (Hawkins & Rafson, 1991).

The combined groups—PAs, nursing advanced practitioners (APs), and nurse-midwives (CNMs)—have established programs and provided services in a wide variety of settings. The expanded role of nurses has been found to be acceptable to consumers (Olade, 1989) and effective in providing quality care (Spitzer et al., 1974). A 10-year review showed that "nurse practitioners and physician's assistants provide office-based care that is indistinguishable from physician care" (Cox, 1979). The acceptability and effectiveness of nurse practitioners were further documented in a 1987 comprehensive review and analysis of published studies (Feldman, Ventura, & Crosby, 1987). Care has been provided in rural settings (Reid, Eberle, Gonzales, Quenk, & Oseasohn, 1975), in urban settings in conjunction with community groups (McElmurry et al., 1990; Reeves, Dan, Keys, & Hennein, 1989), for the elderly (Lamper, Goetz, & Lake, 1983; Utley, Hawkins, Igou, & Johnson, 1988), the chronically ill (Igou, Hawkins, Johnson, & Utley, 1989), in screening for Pap smears (Clay, 1990), and in community education to reduce cardiovascular and cerebrovascular risk among women (Bjorkelund & Bengtsson, 1991).

The granting of prescriptive privileges in some states to nurse practitioners (Mahoney, 1992b) has enhanced their value in medically underserved communities (Mahoney, 1992a). In a study of prescribing patterns, nurse practitioners were more likely than physicians to ask more questions of the patient and to take a sleep history and less likely to prescribe psychoactive drugs for insomnia in the elderly (Everitt, Avorn, & Baker, 1990). Programs administered by PAs and APs tend to be based upon a "wellness" model (Utley et al., 1988), to emphasize education (Fenton, Rounds, & Anderson, 1991) and communication (Alexander, 1987), and to be sensitive to issues of access to care (Graham & Pierce, 1989). Such primary care programs have tended to recognize the woman in the context of her environment, focusing on emotional well-being and prevention (Nagel, 1988).

The current health care system operates within the premise that physicians are the best providers of medical care. However, different characteristics and motivations characterize students who enter medicine, nursing, and the allied health professions. Students applying to medical schools learn that "wanting to combine practice with research" is a more acceptable motivation than "wanting to help people" (Harrison, 1982, p. 5). Medical students must successfully master the basic sciences to enter and remain in medical school, and yet those skills are not the ones best suited to the interpersonal requirements of comprehensive care of patients. In contrast, PAs and nursing students enter their respective clinical fields with an emphasis on caretaking, education, and preventive care. They are able to give quality care that is experienced by patients as acceptable, for considerably less cost than that of a physician, often in underserved communities that are unable to attract physicians (Reid et al., 1975).

Shifting the Focus to Patient Needs

The creation of a model of care based upon patient need requires first that those needs be identified. Consider the health care needs of two women, one in her twenties, the other in her sixties, the former in her reproductive years, the latter postmenopausal. What are the *health* services needed by each? Who can best provide those services? Who can do so in the most cost-effective way?

Examination of Table 8.1 makes it clear that, for the vast majority of primary care needs, a physician is an optional choice. Although internal medicine, family medicine, and obstetrics/gynecology have fought with each other for designation of "primary care physicians" for women with regard to third party reimbursement, in fact, most primary care does not require a physician, other than for consultation and referral. Once a physician is needed, the question of women's health as a specialty diminishes. Gender differences in health care are matters of degree, not of type. In other words, cardiac illness of women is a variation of cardiac illness in men. Women's hearts may be smaller, but so are those of some men. Health care continues to function as if women were always the exception to the rule. Regular (male) hearts are the normal size; women's are smaller. However, women use proportionally more services than men in almost every area of health care (*Why Women's Health?* 1990). Therefore health care, as such, is about women's health, while it functions as if it were not. In health care, women are the invisible majority. How do we bring the majority back into the health care model?

TABLE 8.1. Representative Health Care Needs of Women: Provider Options

Type of Care	Needed Care	Physician: Needed or Optional	Advanced Practitioner
Woman in Her Twenties:			
Routine care	Yearly physical and Pap smear	Optional	Yes
	Health education on nutrition, exercise, sports injuries, smoking, alcohol	Optional	Yes
	Breast care, self-examination	Optional	Yes
	Sexuality concerns, education about contraceptive options, sexually transmitted diseases, AIDS, possible diaphragm fitting	Optional	Yes
Pregnancy	Education counseling regarding effects of working, weight gain or loss, exercise, harmful agents, fertility changes in relation to age	Optional	Yes
	Prenatal care	Optional	Yes (midwives)
Potential illnesses	Cold/flu	Optional	Yes
	Allergy	Needed for diagnoses, optional for ongoing treatment	Yes for ongoing care
	Fractured arm in accident	Needed	No
	Abdominal pain, uncertain as to gastrointestinal or gynecological etiology	Needed, internist and gynecologist for differential	No
	Depression, eating disorder	Physician, psychologist, social worker	If has psychiatric training
Woman in Her Sixties:			
Routine care	Yearly physical with Pap smear	Optional	Yes
	Breast care, self-examination, mammography	Radiologist for reading	Yes for teaching self-exam
	Health education on nutrition, exercise, information about osteoporosis, information about cardiovascular health, hormone replacement therapies, information about vitamins, smoking, alcohol, habituating medications, like sleep medications	Optional	Yes
	Sexuality information, changes with aging	Optional	Yes
Potential illnesses	Cold/flu	Optional	Yes
	Pneumonia	Needed	No
	Cardiac ischemia	Needed	No
	Depression, concerns about aging	Physician, psychologist, social worker	With psychiatric training

A Master's Degree in Women's Health

Women's health has been defined as "the field of practice, education and research that focuses on the physical, social-emotional and political-economical well-being of women, and encompasses women's internal and external worlds of reality" (Mulligan, 1983, p. 2). The creation of master's programs in women's health acknowledges and legitimizes the study of women's health; it provides a focus for research on women's health; and it produces teachers in women's health. Established as an applied discipline, it places the field in an academic context, ensuring that it is founded in theory as well as practice. Linkages between schools and departments could form the basis for master's programs that would combine disciplines of public health, nursing, allied professions, psychology, medical sociology, gender studies, management studies, health policy, and so on.

Here, the establishment of master's level programs in medical ethics may serve as a model. Ethics programs vary by institution, in that the degree may be granted by a school of public health, a department of philosophy, or a center for medical ethics. What they have in common is the knowledge base, applied to clinical situations, thus bridging the strictly philosophical with the strictly clinical. Students in medical ethics may be clinicians, sociologists, epidemiologists, lawyers, and so on, who then take back the perspective of medical ethics to their respective disciplines or specialties. The production of master's level experts in ethics does not free the rest of medicine from acting in an ethical manner. It does, however, provide a group of experts to whom one can turn in making decisions, developing programs, designing research, examining the impact of legislation on women's health, and so on. Likewise, a discipline in women's health does not exempt the rest of medicine and health care from addressing the needs of women, but it does create a body of experts who can be called upon to develop programs, design research, develop curriculum, and teach a varied student constituency.

Curriculum for a Master's Degree in Women's Health

A curriculum in women's health at a master's level could include some of the following: history of women's health; cross-cultural women's health; research in contemporary women's health; models of user-friendly women's health care; developing curriculum in women's health; theories of women's psychological development; women and health care financing; models of wellness and prevention; women's health in relation to family and to society;

feminist theory in women's health; access to care for women; societal violence in relation to women's lives; women's sexuality; history of reproductive health issues; the menstrual cycle in relation to women's health; women's health and employment; women and AIDS, STDs, and so on.

Women's health is a legitimate area for research, study, and teaching. The creation of master's level programs will help bridge the gap between clinicians and behavioral scientists by creating channels of communication between clinicians, theorists, and educators. Its placement within academic institutions and in partnership with health care institutions would facilitate cross-listing of courses in public health, medical sociology, economics, medicine, nursing, political science, women's studies, and so on. It would further facilitate communication between individuals in respective fields and create networks nationally and within universities for collegial communication and collaboration in women's health.

Directions for the Future

The creation of user-friendly models of women's health care and the development of master's level educational programs in women's health are complementary solutions to the identified problems in women's health. It is essential that work continue on both fronts, that direct impact on design and implementation be felt, and that the body of knowledge about women's health be legitimized, developed, and expanded. The following "actions list" indicates the steps necessary for achieving the outcomes of making health care adaptive to women's needs and establishing the applied discipline of women's health with training at the master's level.

Creation of models of primary care for women that are based upon wellness and preventive health, with attention to the complexity of the psychosocial roles of women. Allied health professionals and nursing advanced practitioners would provide primary care to women, with continued emphasis on wellness and prevention. Women's health is not reproductive health. It may include reproductive health, but it is not limited to it. A recent "needs analysis" showed women's health priorities to be those of breast cancer, use of tranquilizer drugs, stress, other cancers, incest, and physical violence. The same study, however, showed that the areas in which women also would have most appreciated help were weight problems, stress, money problems, smoking, caring for elderly and sick relatives, menstrual problems, and the cost of medical care (Redman, Hennrikus, Bowman, & Sanson-Fisher, 1988).

Restructuring of medical specialties so that women do not need two primary care providers. Gynecology and reproductive health belong in the body of internal medicine and is to remain in the body of family medicine. Obstetrics/gynecology is to be the consultative, referral specialty for reproductive disease and obstetrical and gynecological surgery (Harrison, 1992).

Reassessment of the issue of liability in health care, including questions of consumer responsibility and practitioner responsibility. Physicians cannot be expected to relinquish control as long as they carry full liability for the decisions of other practitioners. Nor can physicians be held responsible for patients who don't follow their advice. Increased consumer education must be matched with increased consumer responsibility.

Use of technology to expand women's access to health education and services. Women's health must reconcile itself to an increasingly technological society. The question must be asked: "How can management information systems (MIS) assist in the health care of women?" If not addressed, this will remain one more area in which women's health concerns are left out of health inventories or are only included when there is a product to sell. Home computers and interactive video programs may be an ideal source of information and consultation for women isolated at home with children. Television is an ideal means of providing women with access to and education in health care. Women ought not to be left out of the revolution in information and technology.

Creation of partnerships across disciplines. An interdisciplinary organization constituted by medicine, nursing, and allied health professions—fused with psychology, social work, sociology, public policy and health, and women's studies—is needed to address the social, psychological, economic, and specifically gender-related aspects of women's health. Currently there is little communication across health-related disciplines. For instance, a literature search for primary care of women in Medline reveals little information because the extensive literature that does exist resides in a nursing data bank and therefore is only accessible if one knows to look there. In medicine, there is a professional disincentive to look in the data banks or quote literature from other disciplines. Forging links between medicine and the other health-related disciplines involved in women's health will require new values, attitudes, and leadership.

Reexamination of the hierarchy of power within health care. Medicine has tended to see other disciplines as competitors rather than partners in providing health care. *There is an underlying assumption in the United States that medical care is health care*, that all services exist in a hierarchy in which medicine is positioned at the peak. Battles have been fought over prescribing privileges, hospital privileges, licensing laws, and reimbursement. When, in the late nineteenth century and early twentieth, the male physicians drove out midwives instead of establishing partnerships, a pattern was set that has defined medicine's current relationship to all other health-related professionals. This fundamental assumption that medicine should remain alone at the apex of the health care hierarchy must be examined and challenged.

Several forces appear to have combined to bring attention to deficits in women's health. There is growing attention on women's leadership. Increasing numbers of women are entering medicine. Women in nursing are moving away from their role as doctors' helpers and defining their own contributions and skills. The paucity of research on women's health has been acknowledged. The women's health market, from an economic perspective, has not been fully tapped.

A call for action is needed to explore, within each university setting, what interdisciplinary links may be made with an eventual goal of creating relevant master's programs. An institutionalized, interdisciplinary, applied field of study has the potential to create innovative models of care and to begin, in health care at least, to give to women the attention their numbers warrant. It is time for the invisible majority to become visible. It is time for clinicians, social scientists, and behavioral scientists to take their places, along with physicians, in the creation of wellness models of health, user-friendly services, and a strong grounding in applied theory. In an earlier time and another place, it was said that "women's health care will not improve until women reject the present system and begin instead to develop less destructive means of creating and maintaining a state of wellness" (Harrison, 1982, p. 259). The present call is not a new one. Historical movements result from hard work, dedication, and seizing the moment. This may well be the time to "seize the moment" in women's health care.

References

Alexander, L. M. (1987, July-August). Women and their health care providers: A matter of communication. In *Patient education: The role of the physician assistant and other allied health professionals* (Public Health Reports Supplement, pp. 145-146). Washington, DC: Government Printing Office.

American Psychiatric Association. (1987). Late luteal phase dysphoric disorder. In *Diagnostic and statistical manual of mental disorders* (3rd ed., rev.). Washington, DC: American Psychiatric Press.

Armitage, K. J., Schneiderman, L. J., & Bass, R. A. (1979). Response of physicians to medical complaints in men and women. *Journal of the American Medical Association, 241,* 2186-2187.

Bickell, N. A., Pieper, K. S., Lee, K. L., et al. (1992). Referral patterns for coronary artery disease treatment: Gender bias or good clinical judgement? *Annals of Internal Medicine, 116,* 791-797.

Bjorkelund, C., & Bengtsson, C. (1991). Feasibility of a primary health care programme aiming at reducing cardiovascular and cerebrovascular risk factors among women in a Swedish community, Stromstad. *Scandinavian Journal of Primary Health Care, 9,* 89-95.

Boscarino, J. A. (1987). Successfully marketing women's health care services: A realistic approach to segment marketing. *Health Care Strategic Management, 5,* 16-18.

Burstin, H. R., Lipsitz, S. R., & Brennan, T. A. (1992). Socioeconomic status and risk for substandard medical care. *Journal of the American Medical Association, 268,* 2383-2387.

Clay, L. S. (1990). Midwifery assessment of the well woman: The Pap smear. *Journal of Nurse Midwifery, 35,* 341-350.

Cox, H. C. (1979). Quality of patient care by nurse practitioners and physician's assistants: A ten-year perspective. *Annals of Internal Medicine, 91,* 459-468.

Everitt, D. E., Avorn, J., & Baker, M. W. (1990). Clinical decision-making in the evaluation and treatment of insomnia. *American Journal of Medicine, 89,* 357-362.

Feldman, M. J., Ventura, M. R., & Crosby, F. (1987). Studies of nurse-practitioner effectiveness. *Nursing Research, 36,* 303-308.

Fenton, M. V., Rounds, L. R., & Anderson, E. T. (1991). Combining the role of the nurse practitioner and the community health nurse: An educational model for implementing community-based primary health care. *Journal of the American Academy of Nurse Practitioners, 3,* 99-105.

Flexner, A. (1910). *Medical education in the United States and Canada: A report to the Carnegie Foundation for the advancement of teaching.* New York: Carnegie Foundation.

Fuchs, B. C. (1990). *Mandated employer provided health insurance* (IB87168). Washington, DC: Congressional Research Service, Library of Congress.

Graham, M. V., & Pierce, P. M. (1989). Assessing the need for family nurse practitioners: The Florida experience. *Journal of the American Academy of Nurse Practitioners, 1,* 63-68.

Gurwitz, J. H., Col, N. F., & Avorn, J. (1992). The exclusion of the elderly and women from clinical trials in acute myocardial infarction. *Journal of the American Medical Association, 268,* 1417-1422.

Harrison, M. (1982). *A woman in residence.* New York: Random House.

Harrison, M. (1989). *Premenstrual syndrome and the airplane.* Unpublished manuscript.

Harrison, M. (1990). Woman as other: The premise of medicine. *Journal of the American Medical Women's Association, 45,* 225-226.

Harrison, M. (1992). Women's health as a specialty: A deceptive solution. *Journal of Women's Health, 1,* 101-106.

Hawkins, J. E., & Rafson, J. (1991). ANA council merger creates council of nurses in advanced practice. *Clinical Nurse Specialist, 5,* 131-132.

Hillman, B. J., Olson, G. T., Griffith, P. E., Sunshine, J. H., Joseph, C. A., Kennedy, S. D., Nelson, W. R., & Bernhardt, L. B. (1992). Physicians' utilization and charges for outpatient diagnostic imaging in a medicare population. *Journal of the American Medical Association, 268,* 2050-2054.

Hudson, R. P. (1992). Abraham Flexner in historical perspective. In G. Barzansky & N. Gevitz (Eds.), *Beyond Flexner: Medical education in the twentieth century* (pp. 1-18). New York: Greenwood.

Igou, J. F., Hawkins, J. W., Johnson, E. E., & Utley, Q. E. (1989). Nurse-managed approach to care. *Geriatric Nursing, 10,* 32-34.

Johnson, K. (1992). Women's health: Developing a new interdisciplinary specialty. *Journal of Women's Health, 1,* 95-99.

Johnson, K., & Dawson, L. (1990). Women's health as a multidisciplinary specialty: An exploratory proposal. *Journal of the American Medical Women's Association, 45*, 222-224.

Kiesler, C. A. (1992). U.S. mental health policy: Doomed to fail. *American Psychologist, 47*, 1077-1082.

Krumholz, H. M., Douglass, P. S., Lauer, M. S., & Pasternak, R. C. (1992). Selection of patients for coronary angiography and coronary revascularization early after myocardial infarction: Is there evidence for a gender bias? *Annals of Internal Medicine, 116*, 785-790.

Lamper, L. C., Goetz, K. J., & Lake, R. (1983). Developing ambulatory care clinics: Nurse practitioners as primary providers. *Journal of Nursing Administration, 13*, 11-18.

Mahoney, D. F. (1992a). A comparative analysis of nurse practitioners with and without prescriptive authority. *Journal of the American Academy of Nurse Practitioners, 4*, 71-76.

Mahoney, D. F. (1992b). Nurse practitioners as prescribers: Past research trends and future study needs. *Nurse Practitioner, 17*, 44-51.

McElmurry, B. J., Swider, S. M., Bless, C., Murphy, D., Montgomery, A., Norr, K., et al. (1990, September). Community health advocacy: Primary health care nurse-advocate teams in urban communities. *NLN Publ.*, pp. 117-131.

Meigs, C. D. (1859). *Woman: Her diseases and remedies*. Philadelphia: Blanchard and Lea.

Mitchell, J. M., & Scott, E. (1992). Physician ownership of physical therapy services: Effects on charges, utilization, profits, and service characteristics. *Journal of the American Medical Association, 268*, 2055-2059.

Mulligan, J. E. (1983). Some effects of the women's health movement. *Topics in Clinical Nursing, 4*, 1-9.

Nagel, M. (1988). Nurse practitioners: Primary health care nursing for women. *Imprint, 35*, 115-118.

Olade, R. A. (1989). Perception of nurses in expanded role. *International Journal of Nursing Studies, 26*, 15-25.

Redman, S., Hennrikus, D. J., Bowman, J. A., & Sanson-Fisher, R. W. (1988). Assessing women's health needs. *Medical Journal of Australia, 148*, 123-127.

Reeves, J., Dan, A. J., Keys, E., & Hennein, S. (1989). Primary health care for women's health: Using a negotiated process approach in an urban setting. *Boletin de la Ofecina Sanitaria Pan Americana, 107*, 93-100.

Reid, R. A., Eberle, B. J., Gonzales, L., Quenk, N. L., & Oseasohn, R. (1975). Rural medical care: An experimental delivery system. *American Journal of Public Health, 65*, 266-271.

Spitzer, W. O., Sackett, D. L., Sibley, J. C., Roberts, R. S., Gent, M., Dergin, D. J., et al. (1974). The Burlington randomized trial of the nurse practitioner. *New England Journal of Medicine, 290*, 251-256.

Utley, Q. E., Hawkins, J. W., Igou, J. F., & Johnson, E. E. (1988). Giving and getting support at the wellness center. *Journal of Gerontological Nursing, 14*, 23-25.

Wallis, W. A. (1992). Women's health: A specialty? Pros and cons. *Journal of Women's Health, 1*, 107-108.

Wallis, L. A., & Klass, P. (1990). Toward improving women's health care. *Journal of the American Medical Women's Association, 45*, 219-221.

Walsh, M. R. (1992). Women in medicine since Flexner. In B. Barzansky & N. Gevitz (Eds.), *Beyond Flexner* (pp. 51-63, 211-214). New York: Greenwood.

Why women's health? Section for maternal and child health special report. (1990). Chicago: American Hospital Association.

PART II

Social and Political Issues

9

Building a New Specialization on Women's Health: An International Perspective

Carmen Barroso

I believe that, to be truly multidisciplinary, women's health has to be considered in the international context. Today, health is a global issue. From AIDS transmission to the effects of global warming, health issues cannot be considered as isolated within national boundaries. Even more closely linked are the effects of growing inequality and poverty, affecting the health of women both in this country and abroad.

Let us look at the international experience with women's health and see what lessons can be applied in reframing research and practice into a new specialization. But before I go into that, I have to present a word of caution: International experience is too vast a theme. I will be addressing mostly the experience of Third World women, which itself presents an enormous variety but with which I am more familiar.

1. The first lesson we can learn is the overarching importance of prevention. We need a new scholarship that includes the prevention and maintenance of health in all of its complex interrelationships. We need a conceptual framework in which prevention incorporates the social and cultural determinants of health. We need a multidisciplinary approach that fully explores the interaction of physical and mental health.

We all know that so-called health care services are just a small part of all the conditions and activities that affect our health. Our environment, our

AUTHOR'S NOTE: This chapter was originally a keynote address at the conference, "Reframing Women's Health: A Multidisciplinary Research and Practice," sponsored by the University of Illinois at Chicago, Center for Research on Women and Gender (October 17, 1992).

93

working conditions, our housing, our eating and exercise habits, and our lifestyles are all so important. A comprehensive approach to prevention is fundamental.

But in the technological society of the United States, so highly medicalized, prevention takes a backseat as people tend to naively believe that medical intervention can cure any and all ills.

This is not so in the Third World, where access to modern medical care is so restricted. It is a well-known irony that some people who cannot afford meat and other food rich in animal fat end up having healthier diets. More broadly, when medical resources are limited, an unexpected benefit may be greater emphasis on prevention and avoidance of overmedicalization.

Here I have to acknowledge that in the Third World resources for prevention are also scarce. I have no illusions about the overall health situation. Nevertheless, the relative emphasis given to prevention tends to be better than it is in this country.

One example is in the delivery of immunizations, which are offered free or at very low cost as part of the primary health care services provided by governments. With strong international support, Third World countries achieved the coverage of 80% of young children, according to UNICEF. In contrast, the median immunization rate across the United States is 57% of 2-year-olds (Morgan & Mutalik, 1992).

Obviously, prevention is much more than the provision of vaccines or even of primary health services. Also, the argument is not against research and practice of curative interventions. What we must do is to make a case for greater attention to the much neglected area of prevention.

I once wrote a paper in which I argued that women and Third World countries had a lot in common because both occupied a subordinate position in hierarchies of power. The metaphor is valid here too because women in this country seem to be pushing for a greater emphasis on prevention. But to promote this agenda it is important not only to bring it to public discussions but also to develop the scholarship that will bring weight and substance to a new approach to health.

2. *The second point is that a truly multidisciplinary approach will tie together macroeconomic policies and their effects on health.* Consider this description by Jodi Jacobson (1992):

> Two out of three women around the world presently suffer from the most debilitating disease known to humanity. Common symptoms of the fast spreading ailment include chronic anemia, malnutrition and severe fatigue. Sufferers exhibit an increased susceptibility to infections of the respiratory and reproductive tracts. And premature death is a frequent outcome. In the absence of direct interven-

tion, the disease is often communicated from mother to child, with marked higher transmission rates among females than males. Yet, while studies confirm the efficacy of numerous prevention and treatment strategies, to date few have been vigorously pursued. (p. 3)

The disease she is describing is poverty.

What is remarkable is that the same macroeconomic policies that increase inequality in the United States also generate a wider gap between the developed and the underdeveloped countries.

I do not need to describe the crisis in this country. But let me remind you of the worldwide crisis going on beyond our borders.

First (and it certainly will not come as a surprise to many), too many women are sick and dying unnecessarily from preventable causes. Hundreds of thousands of women are dying from lack of care during obstructed labor. Hundreds of thousands of women are dying from botched abortions. Hundreds of thousands of women are dying from undiagnosed cervical cancer. This is really a tragic situation when simple technology is available to prevent many of these deaths and when enormous resources can be quickly mobilized for destructive purposes—as we were made painfully aware with the Gulf War.

What makes this reality even more dramatic is that the 1980s brought sharp decay to an already dismal picture. The numbers of poor have increased in a more divided world. Conditions of health have deteriorated around the world and in the urban ghettos of this country. In some instances, the causes are very similar. In a recent study of the Bronx, Wallace (1990) studied the effects of misguided policies that resulted in cuts of much needed social services. The deteriorated housing forced out-migration, bringing what she called urban desertification: empty buildings and the flight from certain areas of the borough. She found a striking parallel between the health effects of urban desertification and the health consequences of disruption of social structure caused by forced migration and desertification of the Sahel and other agricultural lands of Africa. In both cases, the role played by improper policies has been crucial.

In many countries of the Third World, the World Bank and the IMF are playing major roles in the formulation of economic policies. To get loans, governments must devalue their currencies, freeze wages, raise food prices, and slash social services. The result has been particularly devastating for children and women.

The decade of the 1980s has been called the lost decade for most of the Third World. Per capita income has been drastically reduced and government's budgets also. *Today the average per capita income of the countries of the South is only about 6% of the countries in the industrial North.*

In this picture of human suffering and despair, the capital flow *from* the Third World to the First World has increased! Billions and billions of dollars are transferred each year from the Third World to the First World, mostly in the form of payment for foreign debts. The $42.6 billion transferred annually from the industrialized to the heavily indebted Third World countries in the early 1980s, mostly in the form of investments and loans, had by 1988 turned into a $32.5 billion transfer from the Third World to the industrialized countries (Speth, 1992).

Poverty is also linked to an international economic order that has perverse regressive effects. A variety of trade barriers in the industrial countries discourage Third World countries from expanding exports that would promote sustainable development patterns. Protectionism in industrial countries costs developing countries an estimated $100 billion annually (Speth, 1992). While many countries of the Third World are opening their markets, 20 of the 24 industrial countries are now more protectionist than they were a decade ago (Arias, 1992).

Gus Speth of the World Resources Institute argues that the United States must reorient its policies or risk political obsolescence. The United States's own interests call for a complete rethinking of its relations with the Third World countries. More than one third of U.S. exports now go to developing countries. Millions of U.S. jobs already depend on the economic health of the developing world, and the failure of heavily indebted countries to grow in the 1980s cost the United States an estimated 1.7 million jobs.

Also, the United States needs the cooperation of the developing world to protect its own environment. This cooperation will be difficult if large North-South disparities persist. Disparities among countries can diminish and jobs for unemployed Americans can be created by a new international program that includes access to capital and technology on favorable terms, reductions of external debt, and mutually advantageous trade reforms. In addition, those concerned with the environmental problems that loom over the quality of life of each and every U.S. citizen are becoming increasingly aware of the fact that the solution to those problems requires the collaboration of every country on this planet. Therefore they are arguing for an increase and a qualitative change in foreign assistance. Other industrialized countries have a much greater share of development assistance, if we take into account the relative size of their economies. If the United States doubles its contribution for development assistance, it will bring its contribution as a percentage of gross national product into the same league as Canada's, France's, and Germany's. Current economic assistance of the United States totals less than 1% of the federal budget, and half of it goes to Egypt and Israel.

In addition to the general economic crises, a decrease in resources allocated to health care has also contributed to the decline of women's health in many countries of the Third World. Women pay the heaviest price for the reduction in social services. They are the ones who take care of the sick when health services become unavailable.

The dire reality for health policymakers in the Third World is that their budgets are not only very low, they have been shrinking. The results of the transfer of resources from the poor to the rich can be seen in the health care system, which is being brought to a virtual collapse in many countries.

In Brazil, I have seen the best and the brightest occupying health policy positions—and having their hands tied, able to do very, very little. How can one implement policies to curb unnecessary cesarian sections, or to provide safe, legal abortions or quality sex education, when one has to spend half the time negotiating with health workers on strike? How can these workers offer quality care when they are pressed for survival and their salaries are being cut by half?

Since 1980 health spending per capita has declined in three quarters of the nations of Africa and Latin America, even as Third World countries' debt and interest payments reached three times as much as all the aid received from all industrialized countries in 1988 (UNICEF, 1990; World Bank World Debt Tables, 1988).

The truth of the matter is that public health as a whole is badly neglected. Much of modern medicine is driven by motives that have more to do with profits and prestige than with the well-being of the majority of human beings.

Research and interventions to address women's health are constrained by the resources available for public health as a whole. Women's health issues will be pitted against other health problems in difficult decisions. Therefore these are not merely technical problems, they are mostly political ones too.

The construction of a new specialization in women's health has to start from a full account of this broader political and economic context. It should combine theory building and a focus on policy. A multidisciplinary approach will make it possible to lay the firm foundation for effective strategies to change women's health in this country and abroad.

3. A third lesson that emerges from the international experience also rein-forces what has been learned in this country: A new discipline on women's health should be informed by a gender perspective. Everywhere we look, we can see how women's health problems are largely determined by women's subordination in gender power relationships.

When medical doctor Rani Bang tells us that, in the remote village of Gadchiroli in India, women never complain about the debilitating reproductive tract infections that seriously undermine their health and well-being, what is she talking about? She is describing women's powerlessness.

When the noted Harvard economist Amartya Sen estimates that 100 million women are missing from world statistics because they have died prematurely due to selective malnourishment of girls, lack of adequate health care, and various forms of violence, what is he talking about? He is describing a tragic picture of neglect and sex discrimination.

When the WHO reports that an estimated 200,000 or more Third World women die needlessly every year due to botched abortions, what does it tell us? There is an outrageous lack of recognition of women as autonomous human beings.

When research shows that the great majority of prostitutes in Zaire, who are at great risk of being infected by HIV, are not able to make men comply with their suggestion that they use condoms (Stein, 1990), what is the independent variable? Women's lack of power. (Which, incidentally, is not restricted to prostitutes. Monogamous married women whose husbands have multiple partners are usually in no better position to negotiate protective measures.)

When sexually transmitted diseases, including cervical cancer, are causing 750,000 deaths in women each year (far more than does AIDS—another STD—in men, women, and children combined; Germain, Holmes, Piot, & Wasserheit, 1992) and nevertheless the STD epidemic receives so little attention, what is the cause? Women's invisibility in public policy debates.

If we do research, our ultimate aim is intervention for changing unhealthy conditions. If our research does not take into account the power relations between the sexes, our understanding of health processes will be very limited. Change based on limited understanding will not go beyond the cosmetic level. Many of the problems of women's health arise from systems of relationships that deny access to information and resources to a large majority of women across the globe.

It is important to study the concrete mechanisms through which these systems work, but it is also important to keep in mind how each piece fits into the overall framework of power relationships. Otherwise, we may end up with specific descriptions, which, interesting as they might be, do not illuminate the underlying causalities.

So, what I am calling for is the development of a sound theoretical framework—one that takes into account not only gender hierarchies but also the linkages between different kinds of hierarchies of countries, classes, and ethnicities.

What could a framework like that do for research? It could stimulate the development of new areas for study and bring new approaches to old problems.

The area of adolescent fertility, for instance, could be seen in a new light if we took into consideration the social construction of the meaning of motherhood, and how that meaning is affected by the power relations in the family, in the labor market, and in the broader world.

What is the bargaining power that young women bring to the negotiation of sexual relationships? What are the mechanisms that reinforce or undermine self-esteem under culturally prescribed gender roles, and how are these related to the ability to construct a meaningful concept of the future? What sorts of conflicts do young women of different classes and ethnic groups face if they decide to write different scripts for their lives? What different meanings do love and intimacy have for young women and men, and what are the consequences for wanted and unwanted fertility, and the subsequent division of labor and responsibility for parenting? These and numerous other questions have far-reaching implications for policy. If we address them, we may loose our innocence and no longer be surprised when sex information is not sufficient to decrease teenage pregnancy rates.

Other areas of research would equally benefit from a gender perspective. The bottom line may well be that powerlessness is a very serious health hazard. But what do we make out of it? Perhaps not much, but perhaps a great deal. Power relations are not easy to change, of course. Gender relations, ethnic relations, class relations, and international relations are intertwined in systems that have very efficient self-perpetuating mechanisms. However, their "immune system" is not invulnerable. Recent history has shown remarkable changes. The modest contribution of research is to illuminate the linkages and, I hope, point out their vulnerabilities.

An important contribution brought by a gender perspective is that we will be dealing with a framework that allows for the consideration of men's roles as well.

In reproductive health, for instance, we shouldn't forget that reproduction usually involves the two sexes. The prospects opened by the new reproductive technology notwithstanding, we should keep in mind that both men and women are involved. Obviously, the quality of that involvement is widely different, but this is largely due to gender systems shaped by history, and as such amenable to change because historical forces may lead to different arrangements in the future.

A gender perspective may help us understand why men have been neglected by contraceptive research, for instance. And I suspect that will lead us directly to the current sexual division of labor of production and reproduction, *not* to the traditional explanations in terms of greater or lesser complexity of men's biological features. It will lead us into exploring the different meanings of sex for men and for women.

Bringing a gender perspective to reframing women's health will illuminate the social conditions that shape health and stimulate the creativity needed to solve old problems.

4. The fourth lesson from international experience is the need for close alliance between scholars and activists. I do not want to portray women as passive victims of gender power hierarchies. As social historians have shown repeatedly, women's resistance and creativity are boundless. And that is the picture you find throughout the Third World. To begin with, whatever health exists, it is mostly the result of women's labor. Women are the main producers of food; they are almost exclusively responsible for food processing and for the care of children. They are in charge of hygiene in their homes, and they are the main direct providers of health care in their homes or in health institutions.

In addition, organized women throughout the world are the most inventive in creating self-help initiatives, in criticizing distorted policies, in questioning the priorities in the choice of problems for research, in pushing for new values to guide health practices, in monitoring the implementation of governmental programs.

> Throughout Asia, Africa and Latin America, community based women's groups are bringing women together to share problems and find solutions on issues ranging from sexuality and reproductive tract infections to domestic violence and the availability of credit. And women in every region have begun to affect change by educating themselves and others, organizing to achieve common goals and lobbying to change discriminatory policies and practices. (Jacobson, 1992, p. 57)

> Third World non-governmental organizations are frequently the most visionary and creative groups in addressing the basic causes of ill-health. They regularly struggle, along with people at the grass-roots, to increase access to basic necessities of life. They have valuable experiences that need to be heard, and, where applicable, adapted to the efforts to widen space for community control and expand access to services among underserved groups in the United States. (Morgan & Mutalik, 1992)

The alliance between scholars and activists is fundamental for giving the specialization the social support it needs, for stimulating studies in neglected, important areas, for giving visibility to research findings, for implementing the policies derived from these findings, and for keeping us all true to our vision.

In conclusion, let me summarize by saying that the international experience points to the need for great attention to prevention, for a full account of the broader political and economic context, for a gender perspective, and for an alliance with activists.

As I said in the beginning, today health is a global issue. Major problems are shared across national boundaries. Fortunately, however, we can also benefit from ideas and solutions generated throughout the world.

References

Arias, O. S. (1992, September 9). Halting the reversal of democracy. *The Christian Science Monitor.*

Germain, A., Holmes, K. K., Piot, P., & Wasserheit, J. N. (Eds.). (1992). *Reproductive tract infections: Global impact and priorities for women's reproductive health.* New York: Plenum.

Jacobson, J. I. (1992). The health of women: A global perspective. In M. Koblinsky, J. Gay, & J. Timyan (Eds.), *Women's health: The price of poverty.* Boulder, CO: Westview.

Morgan, R., Jr., & Mutalik, G. (1992). *Bringing international health back home.* Presentation for the 19th Annual Conference of the National Council for International Health, Washington, DC.

Speth, J. G. (1992). A post-Rio compact. *Foreign Policy, 88,* 145-161.

Stein, Z. A. (1990). HIV prevention: The need for methods women can use. *American Journal of Public Health, 80,* 460-462.

United Nations Children's Fund (UNICEF). (1990). *State of the world's children 1990.* New York: Oxford University Press.

Wallace, D. (1990). Roots of increased health care inequality in New York. *Social Science Medicine, 31,* 1219-1227.

World Bank. (1988). *World debt tables.* Washington, DC: Author.

World Bank. (1993). *World development report: Investing in health.* New York: Oxford University Press.

10

Community-Based Research: The Case for Focus Groups

Sara Segal Loevy
Mary Utne O'Brien

Managers frequently develop new health care services without any input from the intended program participants. Then, when client satisfaction or client participation levels are low, managers must backpedal to discover the errors in planning or implementation. Even when the mistakes are identified, the obstacles encountered in changing the program and remarketing it to a disenchanted or disinterested community may be insurmountable.

Focus groups provide an effective means for including community women in program planning, thus avoiding the problem of installing the wrong set of services in the wrong place. Through focus groups, researchers and managers alike have the opportunity to present a program plan, often based on a series of demographically valid assumptions, and then adjust the plan to meet the specific local social, economic, or ethical needs expressed during the focus groups.

Background

We were trained as social scientists—the scientific sampling, quantifying sort. We cut our methodological teeth on multistage area probability samples, large-scale surveys containing hundreds of closed-ended questions, such as these: "Do you have a regular source of care?" and "What was the highest grade in school that you completed?" No matter how representative the sample, we prefaced all presentations with a series of methodological warnings and concluded them detailing the limitations of our findings.

We generally disregarded qualitative research, distanced by its frequent biases and lack of generalizability. That was until one of us called the other to say,

> The General Accounting Office wants to know why female drug addicts, particularly pregnant ones, are less likely to enroll in substance abuse programs than men. I have 8 weeks in which to gather the data and write the report, so there's no time for drawing probability samples and screening for drug use and pregnancy. I do have access to three AIDS risk reduction programs for female drug users—in Los Angeles, Chicago, and Boston—so do you want to try to do some focus groups with me?

We have discovered that focus groups provide rich research opportunities to develop hypotheses and to gather background information to learn how to ask the right questions. As program planners and evaluators, we learned that focus groups can serve as the voice of the community as participants talk about community strengths and weaknesses, needs and resources.

Findings

This section consists of our methodological findings on conducting focus groups and the key substantive findings from each of the focus group projects.

Methodology

We preface our findings with the following observation: We no longer ascribe to the myth that, to conduct a successful focus group or to do an interview, the researcher must be of the same sex and race/ethnicity as the participants. The success of the focus group depends on the circumstances, the topic, the style and the approach of the researcher.

1. Circumstances. Entrée to the community—who helps you organize the group—is an important element. When participants respect the person or organization convening the focus group, then the focus group leader is, by association, accorded that same respect. The focus group leader, viewed as acceptable in the critical opening minutes of the group session, thus speeds the process of earning trust.

Whenever possible, conduct the focus group in the participants' neighborhood. First, meeting in the community removes some of the barriers to attendance—travel time, travel costs, fear of unknown territory. Second, local, known settings remove some of the discomfort of unfamiliar experience. Third, entering the environment of the participants indicates respect, your willingness to try to walk in their shoes. This is particularly important if racial, ethnic, or socioeconomic differences exist between the focus group participants and the focus group leaders. Last of all, meeting in the community creates an opportunity for the researcher to understand even more about the participants through direct observation of their base of operation.

We always serve refreshments. They function as an icebreaker, lightening the mood and refreshing people's spirits. Fuss a bit over the refreshments to make them special, and make yourself part of the group by eating with the participant.

All groups involving women, and perhaps those with men only, should provide child care on site or through reimbursement. Participants should learn of this service during recruitment because providing child care removes a formidable barrier to participation for many focus group recruits. It avoids the difficulty of participants bringing children into the group, which is often distracting and disruptive. On-site care requires a small room and a locally recruited teenager or mother; often, the organization assisting in recruiting can also help you find a responsible person for child care.

Finally, we pay participants, and pay them fairly. By doing so, we acknowledge the worth of their time and participation. The notion of reciprocity encourages participants to give full value.

2. Topic. Few topics exist that cannot be approached in focus groups. If the topic is particularly sensitive, then it is helpful to broach it with a group that has had experience with it. When we discussed seeking treatment for substance abuse, for example, the women in several of the focus groups all came to a drop-in center for ex-users. For this group, the sensitive topic of substance abuse was an organizing characteristic of the group and an open topic of conversation.

In the case of traditionally taboo topics, such as incest, it may be that no amount of matching of group leader to respondents will allow full disclosure unless the group already exists around this issue. A very few topics may never lend themselves to focus group discussions among relative strangers.

There are very few topics about which the gender or race/ethnicity of the group leader preclude discussion. Race or gender matching, on the contrary, sometimes erects its own set of barriers or distortions in response. In discussing sexuality, for example, gender matching in a male group may create an atmosphere of muscle-flexing in which the discussion reflects expected behavior or group norms rather than actual behavior. Race or gender matching does affect the discussion. The effect, however, is as likely to be negative as positive. Each leader/group combination has consequences—there are biases built into matching as well as not matching—but a given combination should not *a priori* preclude proceeding on almost any topic.

3. Style. There is an inherent tension between researcher and respondent. The respondent knows something that the researcher also wants to know. When the researcher asks the question that permits the respondent to give the answer, then the information is shared. Quantitative research concentrates on how you ask the question. Qualitative research demands something quite different: Can you hear the answer?

Hearing the answer requires a different, but compatible, set of skills. First, leading a focus group is akin to being a good psychotherapist. It demands putting aside your ego so that you have removed any *a priori* investment in a given response. This may play out in very simple ways, such as vocabulary. During a focus group with Latinas who knew each other from the state penitentiary, one woman used the word *boosting* repeatedly while she recounted a particular important story. When she used the word for the second time, we realized that we needed to ask her to define the term so that we would understand the salience of the story. Asking did not label us as stupid or uninformed outsiders but as listeners who cared enough about accurate understanding to ask for a definition. Our willingness was clearly appreciated.

Hearing the answer means being open to the experiences of other people, and suspending all judgments, whether ethical or intellectual. It requires granting people their own time, their own place, their own experiences, their own views. You must assume that both you and your respondents are trustworthy, that you are genuine and honest.

And, finally, hearing the answer demands increasing the tempo of your own thinking, so that you can absorb and synthesize what you are hearing while you begin to frame the logical next question.

4. Approach. We begin each group with brief introductions of ourselves as well as the reason for conducting this group, including the sponsoring agency. Although we limit the information about ourselves to what we believe is of interest to the group, we do not always know what is most relevant. In one focus group with lesbian women led by one of us, I introduced myself and neglected to tell my sexual preference. Before the group moved forward one centimeter, I was asked if I were gay or straight. After I responded that I was straight, married, and the mother of a 17-year-old male, the rest of the evening proceeded smoothly. I clearly had omitted an important fact. While the response *per se* did not alter the group's attitude toward me, the absence of information was not comfortable for them.

Irrespective of the topic, we emphasize our interest in hearing about group members' opinions and experiences. We explain about the tape recorder, that we would like to tape the session so that we can review the discussion but will not tape it if anyone objects. Similarly, each participant is free to turn off the tape recorder if she feels inhibited in talking about a particular topic.

Then, we ask the participants to introduce themselves. These introductions serve two functions. First, each participant must speak in order to tell a bit about herself. In this way, the entire group loosens up. Second, it provides us with some basic background information about individuals and about the collective. These introductions often provide the first testing ground for our assumptions. Last year, for example, one of us convened a focus group to discuss breast and cervical cancer with a group of Latinas who spoke only Spanish. I assumed that because they spoke no English, they were newcomers to Chicago. Because I wanted to understand their contacts with the local health system, I asked the bilingual group leader to ask the respondents to tell their age, where they had come from and when, and, if they had any, the ages of their children. Much to my surprise, I found out that most of them had been living in the neighborhood for at least 15 years. Without this information, I would have assumed that their contacts with the system were much more limited in quantity and duration.

After the introductions, we begin the discussion by telling a simple story, a three-sentence narrative that allows them to focus on a stranger while drawing on their own experiences. In the study of breast and cervical cancer screening, I began with the following projective: "There is a woman named Angela, about age 50, and one day she notices a lump in her breast. What does she think, what does she feel?" Then, when they finish discussing Angela's immediate reaction, I continued with the following probes: "Will she talk about it with her friends? Or her mother and sisters? What will she say to them? What will they tell her?" Finally, I asked, "What will she do? Will she take any action?" Many of these questions were answered in the natural course of the discussion.

It is critical to keep the story simple. Do not make it too lavish or you will trip yourself up in the details, creating diversions that waste time. It is not important, for example, to explain just how Angela discovered the lump. If it is verboten in a given culture for women to touch themselves, then to say that Angela found the lump while doing breast self-examination or while bathing will be to introduce an element that will puzzle and sidetrack the discussion.

This fictitious character may befriend you, the researcher, in other ways. Angela becomes a convenient device for refocusing the conversation when personal narratives have ceased to move the discussion forward. It is wonderfully convenient, and indisputably polite, to return to the mythical guest of honor, to be able to say, "Well, let's get back to Angela." And, when the focus group ends, more often than not someone will come up to ask if everything worked out for Angela.

5. Quantifiable information. We often collect some demographic information during the introductions or at the end of the session. We use this data to help us understand the group—their ages, where they live, what provider they use—but tend not to report the numbers or percentages. If we report numbers, we run the risk of having the information treated as if it were generalizable, as in a random sample, rather than as explanatory information. We are more likely to report that "most of the women had never had a mammogram" rather than "80% of the participants had never had a mammogram."

Substantive Findings

In this section, we describe a research project that used focus groups and discuss some of the substantive findings that we believe would have been difficult to unearth and comprehend if we had been confined to a quantitative approach. We view these findings as illuminating albeit preliminary information, qualitative revelations that demand further exploration and quantified substantiation.

Women United Health Research and Policy Project. This research and policy project, sponsored by Women United for a Better Chicago and funded by the John D. and Catherine T. MacArthur Foundation, analyzed the systems of care that educate and screen publicly insured and uninsured women for sexually transmitted diseases, AIDS, and breast and cervical cancer. Through a combination of quantitative and qualitative research, we developed a series of recommendations for refocusing public health care into community-based health education, health outreach, and health care services.

One of us conducted eight focus groups around the city: four with women over the age of 25, concentrating on breast and cervical cancer screening, and four with adolescents, concentrating on AIDS and STDs. The groups included Latinas (one group spoke no English), African American women, and a multiracial gathering of lesbians.

One unexpected finding, which appeared when comparing the two age groups, seems elemental in hindsight. The barriers to care experienced by the two age groups are substantially different. The older women, at risk for breast and cervical cancer, have had considerable exposure to the medical care system. They have navigated the system through childbirth, childhood diseases, and the chronic needs of their elderly relatives and neighbors. For these women, key barriers to good health center on (a) lack of good health education that would enable them to reduce risk through self-care and screening and (b) staffing problems, which include language barriers and providers being unnecessarily rough during procedures.

The older women had sufficient experience to differentiate sensitive from insensitive care. As a woman in Austin said,

> When I went to get my first mammogram I was mad. They treat you like a sack of potatoes. They had me in tears. The first one, the nurse just told me it was going to be cold. Nobody told me it was going to hurt. It was like a bomb. I was upset. Like she was upset that my breast was so big. It made me not want to go back to get another one.

Teens, however, have had no experience using the health care system as autonomous adults. This lack of experience interacts with their difficulty acknowledging the implications of their sexual behavior, creating a nearly overwhelming obstacle to seeking care.

In addition to this distinction between access for adolescents and more mature women, two additional observations came to light that have enormous implications for education and outreach. In the projective, I said: "Yvonne had been seeing Kevin for awhile and was thinking about having sex with him." All four groups made it perfectly clear that many teens engage in sexual intercourse in the hopes of establishing a relationship, not to deepen an existing one. Safe sex education therefore must teach women how to use condoms in an encounter where trust has yet to be established.

The adolescents also noted that young women date boys who are several years older and who may not have been exposed to the same sex education. Cohort-based education will therefore miss the male partners until the 12-year-old boys become 17-year-old young men dating 12-year-old girls. Educational outreach therefore must aim for the entire community.

Finally, the young women equated the ability to be sexually responsible with the ability to envision and prepare for adulthood, with the ability to stay in school and to keep a job. From their perspective, teens who have a long-term plan—a future—are more likely to practice safe sex and use birth control. This implies that we must help all children to have a future. In the larger social context, until teens living in poverty are confident that they have access to a better future, preventive health measures may seem futile to them.

Conclusion

Focus groups provide a clear voice for women in differing communities. Their experiences, heard in group discussions, allow us to record coherent and compelling stories rather than string together a set of numbers. The discussions allow us to compare their reality with the reality of other groups. In the following two stories, one taken, undiluted, from a personal friendship, and the other pieced together from the stories of women using drugs who had sought help, we contrast the experiences of being affluent with being poor, with being a member of the majority versus a member of a minority, with being a man versus being a woman.

We know a young man in his early twenties, adopted at birth into an upper-middle-class family and raised in an affluent suburb. His mother owns a bookstore; his father is a senior partner in a prominent law firm. Paul has no particular interest in learning and does not have great intellectual capacity. As a result, he chose not to go to college but went through a 1-year auto mechanics course. Although he has had a series of jobs as a mechanic, his last employer went bankrupt and Paul returned to the state to live at home. Paul drinks too much and lost his Illinois driver's license for driving under the influence of alcohol. Last year, he went to meet his friends at a bar on Friday night. He drank a good deal, had a fight with his girlfriend, and left the bar in a rage. He jumped onto his motorcycle and immediately lost control of it, sideswiping three cars while driving 50 miles per hour.

Luckily, the paramedics carefully scraped Paul up from the pavement and took him to the nearest hospital, where he was stabilized. Then he was transferred by ambulance to one of the city's finest medical centers where orthopedic surgeons and neurosurgeons amputated one crushed leg at the knee, wired shut his broken jaw, set his fractured arms, and bound his broken ribs. He spent several weeks in the hospital, and then was discharged to a famous rehabilitation center to be fitted with a leg prosthesis and to have the physical therapy required by his broken and battered body. In addition, Paul was told by his family that he could recover at home if he would undergo intensive psychotherapy. He agreed to this and, in addition, the entire family participates in family therapy.

Consider Jackie, whom we got to know in the course of this study. She is 22, poor, and black. She quit high school and went to work as a cashier at McDonald's. Jackie had difficulty getting to work on time, so eventually she was fired. She lives in the ghetto, using crack cocaine. Her mother, with whom she has little contact, is also an addict, and she does not know her father. Although she had not menstruated for several months, she was not worried because she knows that crack interferes with the menstrual cycle.

One evening, Jackie hit the streets to turn a trick in anticipation of needing her next fix. Afterward, the man she had just had sex with beat her up to get his money back and left her lying in an alley. She got herself to an emergency room, where they discovered that her ribs were broken, and that she was pregnant and loaded. They bound her ribs, chastised her about what she was doing to the fetus, followed her into the hospital washroom to make sure she wasn't doing drugs in there, and sent her home with a bottle of codeine.

There are many differences. Paul is a white male from an affluent family. His employment opportunities provide health insurance coverage. He is addicted to alcohol, which many other people use in moderation. Jackie is an African American woman, poor, and uninsured; she has no family supports and lives in a tough neighborhood. She uses an illegal substance. The extent of the care and treatment they receive is profoundly different.

Paul's alcoholism, and the injuries that follow in its wake, are treated like a disease. Jackie's addiction, and the injuries that follow in its wake, are treated like a moral weakness. Until the commonalities of these addictions, and the common humanity of those afflicted and affected, are acknowledged, the insufficient treatment of pregnant addicts will not be remedied. It is not merely a matter of administrative barriers.

Resources

Loevy, S. S. (1993, March). *Women at risk, communities in need.* A report prepared for Women United for a Better Chicago.

Merton, R. K., Fiske, M., & Kendall, P. (1990). *The focused interview.* New York; Free Press. (Original work published 1956)

O'Brien, M. U., & Loevy, S. S. (1991, May). Critical barriers to drug treatment for pregnant women and mothers with young children. Appendix 2 in *ADMS Block Grant: Women's set-aside does not assure drug treatment for pregnant women* (GAO/HRD-91-80). Washington, DC: Government Accounting Office.

11

Women and National Health Care Reform: A Progressive Feminist Agenda

Judy Norsigian

Although hotly debated during the 1992 election, the topic of national health care reform usually left out the voices of women, although women use the health and medical care system far more frequently than men and constitute the vast majority of health workers (75% overall and 85% within institutions). More recently, however, organizations and coalitions such as the Campaign for Women's Health[1] have articulated an agenda for system reform that incorporates women's particular needs and concerns. As we move toward a national health system that guarantees access to care for everyone, we have a unique opportunity to reassess and improve the *quality* of that system as well. At the same time, we have to educate ourselves about health care financing, health care administration, quality of care, and ways of evaluating all of the above. Finally, women have to make our views known to legislators and other relevant policymakers.

Almost everyone now recognizes that the U.S. health and medical care system is in serious crisis. Here are just a few of the most obvious problems:

We are the only industrialized country except for South Africa that does not have a national health program.

We may not admit it, but we do ration medical and health care already—and on a most inequitable basis. And those who are uninsured appear to receive inferior care, even when they do receive medical care.[2] To be able to obtain coverage, we have to be employed at certain kinds of jobs and be financially

SOURCE: This chapter originally appeared in modified form in *Journal of Women's Health,* Vol. 2, No. 1, 1993, pp. 91-94; used by permission of Mary Ann Liebert, Inc., 1651 Third Ave., New York, NY 10128.

well-to-do or poor enough to qualify for Medicaid or other entitlement programs that frequently offer a substandard form of care. Even as older citizens qualifying for Medicare benefits, we find that Medicare covers on average only 40% of our medical expenses. There is now no basic legal right to health care recognized by our federal government.

Women are at significant risk for *overtreatment* when we have insurance (for example, unnecessary cesarean sections and unnecessary hysterectomies) and are under greater risk of *undertreatment* when we have no form of medical coverage. *Access to appropriate care* remains an unattained goal for many women regardless of their insurance status.

Women of color in general have poorer health status than white women. This is not surprising given that poverty has such a major impact on health, and women of color are disproportionately poorer than white women. But reduced access to needed medical care, and especially primary care, contributes substantially to this poorer health status.

The absence of long-term care coverage has placed a special burden on women, who constitute the majority of older persons (and thus are more likely to need care for chronic and disabling conditions) as well as the majority of caregivers—usually unpaid—who provide long-term care for others.

Several progressive feminist health organizations such as the National Black Women's Health Project, the National Women's Health Network, and the Boston Women's Health Book Collective have joined grassroots "health care for all" organizations across the country now calling for a single-payer system. They also go further in identifying those reforms particularly important to women. One synthesis of their principles and concerns would result in a national health program characterized by the following.

Comprehensive benefits. Of greatest concern to many women is *what services and programs* will be covered by any new national health program. This may well be the issue that draws most women into activism on the matter of health care reform. Women want to know the following:

Will mammography screening for older women and younger women at heightened risk of developing breast cancer be covered? Screening for cancers of the reproductive system, such as cervical cancer?

Will contraceptive services and supplies be covered? Voluntary surgical sterilization? Abortion? Routine gynecological care?

Will prenatal, intrapartum, and postpartum care be covered? Will a range of maternity options be included, including midwifery care (both nurse-midwifery and direct-entry midwifery), freestanding birth centers, and home-birth services?

Will a wide range of practitioners be covered, including homeopaths, midwives, acupuncturists, and chiropractors?

Will access to primary care providers be emphasized and encouraged?

Will midwives, family practice physicians, internists, nurse practitioners, and other qualified providers be classified as primary care providers for women?

Will occupational health services be covered?

Will long-term care be covered (e.g., nursing homes, hospice care, home services, and respite care)?

Will mental health services be covered?

Will dental services be covered?

Will prescription drugs be covered?

Quality of care and ongoing planning and evaluation. We certainly do not want "more of the same" in cases where the current provision of services does not offer an optimal approach. Proposals to guarantee good quality of care will have to include adequate technology assessment as a central component, consumer involvement in assessing quality, and the establishment of clinical practice standards, especially in areas of medical care where clinical practices vary significantly from one community to another. Ongoing research and evaluation are vital to effective planning and may help eliminate unnecessary costs as well as improve quality of care.

Disease prevention and health promotion. Without placing a greater emphasis on primary care, including greater use of family practice physicians, nurse practitioners, midwives, and other primary care providers, it is unlikely that we can achieve even modest goals in the area of disease prevention and health promotion. In addition, any new proposal for a national health program must acknowledge the importance of nonmedical factors on health status. General health education, occupational health and safety programs, and other public and community health measures that address the impact of the environment, for example, must be included.

Furthermore, we need more community-based primary care settings rather than tertiary care institutions or other settings devoted principally to specialty care. We can and should build upon our experience with community health centers, which currently provide comprehensive primary care services to several million people. Their expertise in providing ethnically, linguistically, and culturally appropriate care is an important resource to draw upon.

Finally, the government should fund additional research to investigate new approaches to disease prevention and health promotion. The NIH's Women's Health Initiative represents one such effort, but it does not adequately address the concerns of women from particular racial and ethnic backgrounds.

Training. National health care reform measures must address the issue of training. Currently, too many specialists and too few primary care providers have been trained. Federal funds and training opportunities should be redirected to alter this trend. (For example, many women's health advocates believe we need to be training more midwives and fewer obstetricians, so that we can establish a less interventionist, more primary care-oriented approach for childbearing women.)

Universal coverage. This is a system in which *no one* residing in the United States would be excluded from receiving health and medical benefits.

No financial barriers to care. At its best, this would involve having no co-payments, no deductibles, and no extra charges for covered services. (Out-of-pocket payments required at the health care visit often represent a major barrier for lower income people.)

Equitable distribution of services. This would especially include services to underserved groups and regions.

Equitable financing. How are we going to pay for a national health program? A progressive surtax on individuals and corporations is the fairest approach, but Republican administrations have been totally inhospitable to the idea of greater taxes for the rich. With a Democratic president in office during the coming years, this approach may at last be politically feasible.

Elimination of administrative waste. As has been so well documented (see, e.g., Himmelstein & Woolhandler, 1986), the insurance industry is responsible for considerable and unnecessary overhead waste (e.g., numerous and varied insurance forms, the ad nauseam billing of patients and clients, and the extensive machinery for collecting money from many different sources). Eliminating this waste means eliminating—or substantially curtailing—the enormous role of the insurance industry, an idea many have asserted to be politically unlikely, given the powerful lobby representing this industry in Congress. Surveys show, however, that the public is increasingly in support of a government-run system that would allow, at most, a minimal role for insurance companies.[3]

Sensible payment mechanisms. Global budgeting for provider institutions (as currently practiced in Canada) and payment to MDs on a capitation basis represent mechanisms (albeit imperfect ones) that already reduce the incidence of unnecessary surgery and other forms of overtreatment. Some women's health advocates have long cited the fee-for-service approach as a primary reason for women's inappropriate medical care, but elimination of "fee-for-service" has never been a very popular proposal in this country. Ironically, about half of all MDs in the United States are now salaried, but many institutions operate on a fee-for-service basis even when physicians are on salary.

The current political climate and economic realities make it more likely that sensible payment mechanisms will be incorporated into forthcoming health care reform proposals. These could encourage both appropriate treatment by providers as well as more appropriate use of services by consumers.[4]

Effective and responsive organization and administration. We now have some 1,200 insurance companies selling about $192 billion in health insurance each year. *A single-payer approach, similar to the Canadian model, will offer critical and essential cost savings as well as a significant reduction in frustrating "red tape" and other bureaucratic requirements.* Along with increasing numbers of national organizations, 70-80 members of Congress have endorsed the single-payer model, noting that it will offer far greater cost savings than any of the employer mandate proposals, whether "pay or play" or "play only."[5] Furthermore, tying coverage to employment is discriminatory toward women, because we are less likely to be employed full time and more likely to be employed by smaller businesses, which are exempted from requirements to provide coverage in many current legislative proposals.

It is critical that any national health program have publicly responsible mechanisms to assure responsiveness to our concerns. This requires some degree of community input into the nature and type of services. Furthermore, an adequate decision-making role for consumers needs to be addressed in any reform proposal. Almost two decades ago, Congressman Ronald Dellums offered an important step in this direction in his National Health Service Act, which incorporated directly elected community health boards (two third consumer and one third health workers) as well as indirectly elected regional and national health boards.

Many ethical issues loom large as we move toward national health care. For example, what about rights to refuse treatment or diagnostic testing or genetic screening? As the Human Genome Project (and similar research) progresses, will individuals be allowed to refuse genetic testing (or risk losing coverage)? Also, should a national health care program include procedures and treatments that have not undergone adequate technology assessment even though they are now available on a fairly widespread basis? IVF (and other assistive reproductive technologies) represents such a procedure—it continues to offer fairly low efficacy and entails risks that are still not well understood. Yet many women with severe tubal damage will insist that IVF remains their last chance for biological motherhood, one that a national health plan should recognize.

Women's health groups have been joined by disability rights advocates in emphasizing issues of consumer input and control:

Particular attention must be placed on the appropriateness of available services. It is of critical importance to the disability community that full involvement of the "consumer" is assured in all decisions affecting the selection of service, service provider, service timing, and service setting. CCD is concerned that certain forms of managed care create an incentive for under-serving persons with disabilities and often utilize gate-keepers who are not knowledgeable about the special health care needs of persons with disabilities.

The issue of consumer choice and participation has a particular importance for persons with disabilities. While the present acute-care oriented health care system has a tendency to relegate all "consumers" to a dependent status embodied in the "sick role," this indignity is particularly disempowering to persons with disabilities when their chronic health conditions are permanent. That is why the health related services for persons with disabilities must be delivered in a way that minimizes interference with normal activities, and that health care financing policies which govern access to health care for persons with chronic conditions must be sensitive to issues of locus and control. (Griss, 1992, congressional testimony)

Unfortunately, many of the most vocal advocates for "managed care" and "managed competition" would limit consumer/patient input even more than it is now. For women, this is an especially alarming trend, as we have had too many years of "experts" (primarily male) poorly defining what our problems are and how they ought to be solved. Policymakers solely focused on questions of access, administration, and financing must hear from women, people with disabilities, and other so-called minority constituencies, who care about the other equally important questions as well.

Notes

1. The Campaign for Women's Health is a project of the Older Women's League (OWL), 666 Eleventh St., NW, Suite 700, Washington, DC 20001 (202-783-6686). This broad coalition of over 70 national, state, and grassroots organizations works "to reform the health care system to meet the needs of women of all ages, races, income and lifestyles." To track general grassroots efforts across the country as well as the most recent legislative health care reform proposals, see *Action for Universal Health Care*, a newsletter published by the Northeast Ohio Coalition for National Health Care, 1800 Euclid Ave, Suite 318, Cleveland, OH 44115 (216-566-8100).

2. One recent study suggests that uninsured persons are at greater risk of suffering medical injury from substandard medical care. See Burstin, Lipsitz, and Troyan (1992).

3. See the section on "public opinion on health care reform" in *The National Health Program Chartbook*, by David U. Himmelstein and Steffie Woolhandler. Copies are available for $20.00 from the Center for National Health Program Studies, Harvard Medical School/Cambridge Hospital, 1493 Cambridge St., Cambridge, Ma 02139 (617-661-1064).

4. For a useful discussion of global budgeting and problems with fee-for-service, see Terris (1992).

5. One accounting firm (Milliman and Roberston) has gone even further in concluding that "pay or play" proposals face a significant danger of being actuarially unstable and consistently underfunded.

References

Burstin, H., Lipsitz, S. R., & Troyan, B. (1992). Socioeconomic status and risk for substandard medical care. *Journal of the American Medical Association, 268,* 2383-2387.

Griss, B. (1992, May 5). Testimony of the Co-chair of Health Task Force, Consortium for Citizens with Disabilities, Hearings, "Health Care Reform: How Do Women, Children and Teens Fare?" before the U.S. House Select Committee on Children, Youth and Families, Washington, DC.

Himmelstein, D. U., & Woolhandler, S. (1986). Cost without benefit: Administrative waste in U.S. health care. *New England Journal of Medicine, 314,* 441-445.

Terris, M. (1992, September). Global budgeting and the control of hospital costs. *Public Health Comments, 6*(9), 5-8. (Available from Public Health Information Services, 11661 Charter Oak Court, Reston, VA 22090-4533, 703-709-0020)

12

Institutionalizing Women's Oppression: The Inherent Risk in Health Policy Fostering Community Participation

Judith Wuest

Current Canadian health care policy emphasizes health promotion through self-care, mutual aid, and the promotion of healthy environments (Epp, 1986). Provincial health policy increasingly reflects a movement toward increasing community involvement and community-based services without putting in place the necessary social, physical, and economic supports essential for this changing focus. In the face of the shrinking health care dollar, Canada's forward-looking health promotion policy has become a justification for reducing institutionalized services and increasing individual and family responsibility under the guise of public participation (Laurence, 1992). The underlying assumption of many of these changes is that there is a woman willing, able, and morally obligated to provide care (Guberman, 1990). Currently, "the ideology of women as caretakers serves not only the interests of the family but also the society at large" (Anderson & Elfert, 1989, p. 741). Support structures for women as caregivers are minimal; thus the health of women receiving care and the health of women providing care are at risk (Laurence, 1992). Poland (1992) identified that, despite the changing trend in health promotion policy, traditional positivist research methods fail to uncover the social reality that influences health. An understanding of this social reality is essential for the development of health policy that is responsive to the health needs of women.

SOURCE: This chapter originally appeared in modified form in *Health Care for Women International,* Volume 14, 1993, pp. 407-417; used by permission of Taylor & Francis, Washington, D.C.

My purpose in writing this chapter is to explore through a feminist lens the assumptions underlying such partnership policy. Canadian women's health is examined within the environment of social control imposed by their position in society. The responsibilities and societal expectations of women as family caregivers are considered. Suggestions will be made for health promotion research and health policy implementation that acknowledges sociopolitical responsibility for health and responds to the complexity of women's health experience.

Social Inequity: The Context of Women's Health

Graham (1983) discussed caring as the major defining characteristic that distinguishes men from women in Western society. "Caring is 'given' to women: it becomes the defining characteristic of their self-identity and their life's work" (p. 18). Graham developed the distinction between women accomplishing their feminine reproductive roles simply by *being* and men fulfilling their public sector roles by *doing*. This difference is the foundation of the caring role, which is

> constructed through a network of social and economic relations, within both the home and the workplace, in which women take responsibility for meeting the emotional and material needs not only of husbands and children, but of the elderly, the handicapped, the sick and the unhappy. (Graham, 1983, p. 22)

The Ideology of Familism

The ideology of familism is the dominating principle of social organization in Western society (Dalley, 1990). The nuclear family is the primary structure for the organization of daily living and the functions of caring. This ideology fosters relationships of domination and subordination, patterns of domestic labor, altruistic caregiving for the children and the elderly, and patterns of dependency, all of which serve women poorly. "Caring-by-wives-and-mothers is seen as the mechanism by which families are reconstituted on a daily basis. It is the provision of high quality and unpaid care within the home which keep the family going" (Graham, 1983, p. 23).

These principles extend to the public sector and govern the field of social care. The position of women in society is reflected in the position of women in the Canadian health care system (Begin, 1989; Laurence, 1992). The hegemony of patriarchy continues despite the changing roles of women.

Men manage the public domain, which governs, legislates, sets policy and controls the allocation of resources (money, power, authority, services, opportunities). Women manage the private domain, which provides the male power (bearing and caring for children) and the support structures that maintain and nurture the public domain: the private domain does not set policy and has little say in the distribution of resources. (Laurence, 1992, p. 31)

This pattern is evident in the health care system, where male physicians and administrators wield the most power and women as nurses, social workers, aides, and volunteers have progressively less power. This ideology of familism nurtures the prevailing belief that care in the home is better than institutional care. The hegemony of familism is demonstrated in the fact that public policy for social care is increasingly based on this model when in reality the family is currently a changing structure that does not reflect the model revered by policymakers (Dalley, 1990).

Dependency and Poverty

The ideology of familism while liberating for men results in dependency for many women because family responsibilities limit their opportunities. "However, for women, the experience of dependency is . . . contradictory. Their dependent status—as housewives, mothers, dutiful daughters—is not absolute but is conditional upon their being simultaneously depended upon by others" (Graham, 1983, p. 24). Although they are in a dependent position in the family, their position is characterized by giving, not receiving, care, and the cost of caring is often economic dependency and poverty (Graham, 1983).

Single mothers and women living on their own are most vulnerable to poverty (Evans, 1991). Women have maintained a disproportionate share of the poverty (approximately 60% as compared with 40% for men) in all Statistics Canada figures from 1971 to 1988. Poverty is measured by household unit and Evans asserted that this practice masks female poverty because it assumes that women have access to the resources of the household, which is often not the case.

Many women work out of necessity but make less money for the same work than men do (Laurence, 1992). Women are concentrated in low-wage occupations and, even when employed in jobs of comparable skill and responsibility, women make only 80% of the salaries of men (Evans, 1991). Despite the gains women have made in entering nontraditional professions, redressing gender-based wage discrepancies, obtaining maternity benefits and leaves, and improving income security for the elderly, many groups such as elderly, young, visible minority, and immigrant women are vulnerable to poorly paid work and no job security (Canadian Mental Health Association [CMHA], 1987).

Visible poverty among elderly women is merely a continuation of lifelong poverty that may have been hidden by total family income. Elderly women have small pensions because they have spent their lives dealing with family responsibilities and often have only had part-time, low-wage work outside the home. Work interruptions are most commonly attributed to family responsibilities (Evans, 1991). Most elderly women can expect to live their later years in poverty, partially because they live longer than men and have minimal pension income (Harder, 1991). Single mothers are vulnerable to stress and social isolation but this is a result of economic circumstances rather than the absence of a partner. Evans found that almost half of single mothers are poor, and this can be attributed to low-paying jobs, limited child care and child support payments, and inadequate social assistance. "Women are tainted with economic dependency throughout their lives as a result of the domestic division of labour which accords a discounted value to women's paid work and no value to women's domestic labour" (Medjuck, O'Brien, & Tozer, 1992, p. 45).

Paltiel (1988) examined women's health in the context of poverty and noted that "the relationship between women's work and women's worth has profound consequences for their mental health" (p. 190). Summarizing the literature, she found that the poor are exposed to more environmental health hazards in their homes and in unrewarding, depersonalizing jobs. Paltiel further specified that poor Canadian women are more likely to demonstrate risk factors such as smoking, obesity, poor exercise habits, alcohol problems, poor nutrition, and drug use. Many of these habits are seen as responses to work roles, life conditions, and social status.

Dual Roles

When women are employed, they continue to assume responsibility for the domestic realm and thus carry a double load (Laurence, 1992). Ferguson (1990), using figures from Statistics Canada, identified that 58% of women with children under 3 and 65% of women whose youngest child was between 3 and 5 are working outside of their homes; 60% of women who are employed outside the home who care for the elderly also care for children who live at home (MacBride-King, 1990).

Since caring for children is considered women's work, the reality that women have at least two jobs is not acknowledged. For many women, child care is their "hidden" work while their paid occupation defines their public profile. In addition, this "invisible" work constitutes a very demanding twenty-four hour responsibility. (Ferguson, 1990, p. 82)

Women in dual roles face sexual harassment in their jobs, fatigue from double responsibilities, disruption to family life from shift work, and stressors of inadequate day care and limited benefits from part-time work (Ontario Advisory Council on Women's Issues [OACWI], 1990).

Medicalization of Women's Health

Waitzkin (1991) described medicalization as a form of social control. Problems originating in psychological, social, economic, and political realms are dealt with on a purely technical medical basis. This reification of social problems into medical labels is condemned in feminist analysis of women's health issues.

> Many of the typical female illnesses are the result of a highly coercive and highly effective labelling process exercised by the medical profession operating not only in its own self-interest . . . but in those of the state and other agents of control eager to restrict women's equal participation in society. (Pirie, 1988, p. 634)

Sociopolitical responsibility is diminished and individual ownership is emphasized. Thus health professionals reinforce dominant social ideology. Waitzkin stated that social control is not a conscious goal of most practitioners; however, the education and socialization of these professionals result in this behavior. Medicalization is especially evident in women's reproductive and mental health care (Clarke, 1990). Within these contexts, medicalization reinforces and intensifies the social inequity of women. Such diagnoses as Battered Woman Syndrome redefine the experience for the woman, deny social responsibility, and reinforce relationships of dominance.

Family Caregiving:
A Social Expectation of Women

> The provision of comfort and nurturing to children, an elderly mother, or a disabled member of a family is arduous work, but is usually undertaken in a network of relationships in which the emotions of affection are mixed with resentment, and norms of family responsibility and obligation are intertwined. (Baines, Evans, & Neysmith, 1991, p. 14)

Guardians of Family Health

In a study of the responsibilities and tasks of women in maintaining their own health and that of their families, Heller (1986) identified "the importance of the numberless daily, routine, preventive, monitoring, and promotional tasks which serve to maintain and build the health of the family, and by extension the health of the society at large" (p. 65). The major caregiving task in the nuclear family is the care of children. Dalley (1990) noted that the experts widely support the view that child care is best carried out in the home and that early separation from the mother is harmful. Ferguson (1990) recognized the controversiality of this position but suggested that it draws attention to the importance of the role of child care in women's lives: "Failure to acknowledge the significance of this work not only distorts the reality of many women's lives and vastly underestimates their working hours and conditions, but also undervalues the importance of the child-care component of their work" (p. 82). Most stay-at-home mothers perceive that their role lacks status and feel isolated and fearful of losing the ability to work outside the home (Kellerman, as cited in OACWI, 1990). Kellerman further noted that "women are ultimately damned if they do and damned if they don't when it comes to working inside or outside the home" (p. 16). Those who stay at home feel pressured to enter the workforce and not waste education or intelligence on child care. Those in the workforce are told their selfishness will result in damage to their children.

Caregiving for the Elderly and Disabled

Family caregiving is caregiving by women (Medjuck et al., 1992). Over 85% of care given to elderly Canadians is provided by family members (Chapell, Strain, & Blandford, 1986), especially women at midlife. "Society expects women to care for elderly family members in the same way it has traditionally expected women to care for children" (Medjuck et al., 1992). Laurence (1992) noted that, because this work in the home is invisible, the consequences of these demands are also invisible, and thus have little impact on the system. Burnout, stress, or inability to cope are viewed as personal failure.

Professionals and Policy:
Maintaining the Status Quo

Anderson and Elfert (1989) recognized that the ideology of the dominant health professionals reflects that of the society and serves "to sanction and legitimize the dominant ideology" (p. 736). In their study of women as caretakers of chronically ill children, they identified that professionals were powerful forces in maintaining women in their caretaking roles. Women who failed to meet professional expectations ran the risk of being judged incompetent and losing custody of the child. This promotes "the concept of 'homecare management' and the transfer of the economic costs of caring from the state to the family" (p. 736).

However, the focus of policymaking is "sustaining the present division of care rather than changing it or asking whether it is in women's best interests to be, effectively, pressed into caregiving" (Aronson, 1991, p. 143). "It is a social fact of life that women are responsible for families, and health professionals in their encounters with families collude to keep women in this field" (Anderson & Elfert, 1989, p. 741).

Long-term care for the elderly in Canada is increasingly community based in the form of home care programs. "Because research continues to confirm that women family caregivers provide the majority of support to their elderly kin, there is argument that community care public policy regards women caregivers as a resource which may be used (for free) in the success of community care programs" (Medjuck et al., 1992, p. 53). This community care public policy reinforces the traditional division of labor.

Impact of Caregiving on Women

Medjuck et al. (1992) reviewed the research on the cost of caregiving and summarized the effects under the dimensions of employment and earnings, expenditures, and physical and emotional impact. Employment opportunities may be curtailed by responsibilities that make it impossible to work longer hours, relocate, attend social functions, or take additional courses. Caregivers may have to reduce working hours or give up the job altogether or may be distracted by responsibilities during working hours.

> Women already vulnerable and usually caring for others as single mothers, delinquent girls, elderly or abused women are all too often revictimized through the underlying familial ideology of the welfare state, which emphasizes the importance of women providing care but limits their abilities to express their own needs for care. (Baines et al., 1991, p. 13)

A major consequence of a social policy that supports caregiving in the family is the increased demand on women and the isolation of women and those for whom they care in their homes. Dalley (1990) noted that, despite the rhetoric that suggests that professional services, voluntary organizations, and neighbors will provide support, research demonstrates that "most often, caregiving devolves on to those closest to the dependent person—and those deemed to be closest are generally wives, mothers and daughters—or the dependent person is left to cope alone" (p. 7). Society supports maternal child care and frowns on neglect (Ferguson, 1990).

> Financially, they derive little monetary reward, making women dependent and vulnerable to both men and the state. Dependent on men, they and their children risk physical and emotional abuse, and dependent on the state, they risk the stigma of charity or welfare. (p. 84)

Aronson (1991) found that, although women generally supported the view that daughters should care for their elderly parents, "they often find themselves in the midst of competing commitments, feeling over-extended and suppressed in terms of the pursuit of their own needs and objectives" (p. 153). Elderly women described the dual desire for security without being burdensome. Aronson found these women's lives reflected an ongoing tension between the normative expectations of society for caregiving and the lived reality of everyday experience. This internal struggle of self-enhancement versus self-sacrifice results in guilt for the caregiver, who constantly feels she is not doing enough. But elderly women also have a struggle between maintaining independence and self-sufficiency and voicing their needs for support.

Where Do We Go From Here?

The issues inherent in current public policy relate to the interpretation of health as a social responsibility and implementation of policies of public participation and partnership in a manner equitable for women. The issue of partnership in health promotion is critical. Partnership can only be based on equality between players. Yet it is clear that women have not been and are not equal partners in Western society, despite the gains that have been made. If partnership is truly intended, then representation of women at all levels within government, health departments, and health agencies is essential.

More significant, however, is partnership between these policymakers and the public. Policy invariably is based on research, research that often contains androcentric bias simply in the questions asked and in the theoretical perspective from which the findings are examined. Clarke (1992) urged that "it is important that preliminary exploratory research, which would distinguish between the health concerns of men and women in the language and the meaning and life-world relevancies which pertain to gender, be undertaken" (p. S57). Research to examine such differences cannot be conducted within a logical positivist paradigm but requires a more phenomenological approach that recognizes the primacy of lived experience. This approach values women's diversity and recognizes the complexity of women's lives. The findings of such research might ultimately form a base for more traditional survey research but the questions would be grounded in health needs identified by women. Kaufert (1988) suggested that a feminist epidemiology would be "rooted in the real experience of women, but would allow sharing on a larger scale than a local self-help group" (p. 13). She called for research approaches that take into account the social reality of women's lives and integrate women's perspectives. Findings from such research can provide support for changes within society and within the health care system.

> We can publicly legitimize and normalize the stifled and suppressed voices of women who feel the unfairness as they struggle to survive under their burden. We can publicly question the allocation of resources in a system that rewards the glorification of high tech medicalization of health care while embracing a model of care predicated on an outmoded definition of the place of women in society. (Laurence, 1992, p. 33)

Does this imply that caring should be maintained at an institutional level rather than within families and communities, that women should be freed of the caring role? Torjman (1988) offered this summary:

> This then is our reality: physical and mental stresses different from those experienced by men, a secondary economic role, and continued sublimation of our own needs. In order to change our reality, we need not give up nurturing, caring, and taking responsibility for others. But what we must do within the confines of our caregiving, is take greater control of our own needs. We must make society conform to *our* needs rather than continually molding, shaping, and accommodating our needs to meet the demands of society. (p. 2)

Health professionals can support this position by identifying what the needs of women are. "In the future, it will be crucial to foster the conditions in which women can speak about their experiences and make claims on their own behalf" (Aronson, 1991, p. 164).

We cannot operate on the assumption that care within the family unit is best or that care in the community means care by a family member.

> For instance, availability of a family member ought not to be a factor in determining the type and length of homecare made available to an elderly person. If the public policy of community care continues to be translated into care *by* the community, rather than care *for* the community, then women's economic vulnerability becomes reinforced by the state as women are entrenched in the caregiving role. (Medjuck et al., 1992, p. 54)

Much more emphasis must be placed on the community-based resources necessary to support and facilitate caregiving within the community setting.

Conclusion

It is clear that the issues surrounding the health of women are multifaceted and that inequities will not be addressed quickly. However, health care professionals have the power to effect change by developing a greater sensitivity to the social factors that influence women's health needs in today's society and by lobbying for social change. Professional behaviors that reinforce the prevailing social belief that women will be the caregivers and that any problems they have fulfilling their roles can be accounted for by individual failures must be identified and eliminated. Finally, research that centers on the social reality of women's experiences must be conducted and used for the development of health policy that acknowledges the contradictions and stressors in women's lives.

References

Anderson, J., & Elfert, H. (1989). Managing chronic illness in the family: Women as caregivers. *Journal of Advanced Nursing, 14*, 735-745.

Aronson, J. (1991). Dutiful daughters and undemanding mothers: Constraining images of giving and receiving care in middle and later life. In C. Baines, P. Evans, & S. Neysmith (Eds.), *Woman's caring: Feminist perspectives on social welfare* (pp. 138-168). Toronto: McClelland & Stewart.

Baines, C., Evans, P., & Neysmith, S. (1991). Caring: Its impact on the lives of women. In C. Baines, P. Evans, & S. Neysmith (Eds.), *Woman's caring: Feminist perspectives on social welfare* (pp. 11-35). Toronto: McClelland & Stewart.

Begin, M. (1989). *Redesigning health care for women*. Ottawa: Canadian Research Institute for the Advancement of Women.

Canadian Mental Health Association (CMHA). (1987). *Women and mental health in Canada*. Toronto: Author.

Chapell, N., Strain, L., & Blandford, A. (1986). *Aging and health care: A social perspective*. Toronto: Holt, Rinehart & Winston.

Clarke, J. (1990). *Health, illness and medicine in Canada*. Toronto: McClelland & Stewart.

Clarke, J. (1992). Feminist methods in health promotion research. *Canadian Journal of Public Health, 83*(Supp. 1), S54-S57.

Dalley, G. (1990). *Ideologies of caring: Rethinking community and collectivism*. London: Macmillan.

Epp, J. (1986). *Achieving health for all: A framework for health promotion*. Ottawa: Health Services and Health Promotion Branch, Health and Welfare Canada.

Evans, P. (1991). The sexual division of poverty: The consequences of gendered caring. In C. Baines, P. Evans, & S. Neysmith (Eds.), *Woman's caring: Feminist perspectives on social welfare* (pp. 169-203). Toronto: McClelland & Stewart.

Ferguson, E. (1990). The child-care crisis: Realities of women's caring. In C. Baines, P. Evans, & S. Neysmith (Eds.), *Woman's caring: Feminist perspectives on social welfare* (pp. 73-105). Toronto: McClelland & Stewart.

Graham, H. (1983). Caring: A labour of love. In J. Finch & D. Groves (Eds.), *A labour of love: Women, work, and caring* (pp. 13-30). London: Routledge & Kegan Paul.

Guberman, N. (1990). The family, women, and caregiving: Who cares for the caregivers. In V. Dhruvarajan (Ed.), *Women and well-being* (pp. 67-78). Montreal: McGill University Press.

Harder, S. (1991). *Women in Canada: Socioeconomic status and other contemporary issues.* Ottawa: Ministry of Supply and Services.

Heller, A. (1986). *Health and home: Women as health guardians.* Ottawa: Canadian Advisory Committee on the Status of Women.

Kaufert, P. (1988). Through women's eyes: The case for a feminist epidemiology. *Healthsharing, 10,* 10-13.

Laurence, M. (1992). Womancare—health care: Power and policy. *Canadian Woman Studies, 12,* 31-34.

MacBride-King, J. (1990). *Women and the family employment challenge of the 90's.* Ottawa: Conference Board of Canada.

Medjuck, S., O'Brien, M., & Tozer, C. (1992). From private responsibility to public policy: Women and the cost of caregiving to elderly kin. *Atlantis: A Women's Studies Journal, 17*(2), 44-58.

Ontario Advisory Council on Women's Issues (OACWI). (1990). *Women and mental health: A background paper.* Toronto: Author.

Paltiel, F. (1988). Is being poor a mental health hazard? *Women & Health, 12,* 189-211.

Pirie, M. (1988). Women and illness role: Rethinking feminist theory. *Canadian Review of Sociology and Anthropology, 25,* 628-648.

Poland, B. (1992). Learning to "walk our talk": The implications of sociological theory for research methodologies in health promotion. *Canadian Journal of Public Health, 83*(Supp. 1), S31-S46.

Torjman, S. (1988). *The reality gap: Closing the gap between women's needs and available programs and services.* Ottawa: Canadian Advisory Council on the Status of Women.

Waitzkin, H. (1991). *The politics of medical encounters.* New Haven, CT: Yale University Press.

13

My Mexican Friend Marta, Who Lost Her Womb on This Side of the Border

Ruth Behar

On a Sunday afternoon Marta phones to tell me she has just been offered a job at Meijer, the discount store. She had told me 2 weeks earlier that she had put in an application and I had asked her whether she hoped to get a job working the register. Oh, no, she was willing to do any kind of work, she said to me in Spanish, the language we always speak together; she'd even wash floors, she added, with a laugh.

We don't say much more about the job, because Marta is mainly calling to let me know they will be late; her brother Polo, who came from Mexico 2 years ago sponsored by Marta and her husband Saúl, is working until 3:00 at Farmer Jack's, and they have to pick him up before they can leave to come to our house. Am I sure I still want them to come? Do I really not have something more important to do? Of course, I still want them to come, I reply; I have no other plans but to see them.

On this occasion as on so many others, Marta reminds me that there is distance between us. We live a half hour away from each other, but there is

SOURCE: This chapter originally appeared in modified form in *Journal of Women's Health,* Vol. 2, No. 1, 1993, pp. 85-89; used by permission of Mary Ann Liebert, Inc., 1651 Third Ave., New York, NY 10128.

AUTHOR'S NOTE: All the names in this chapter are pseudonyms. I am grateful to my friend Marta for her willingness to speak openly to me and for her permission to let me write about her. The MacArthur Foundation has made it possible for me to take leave time to undertake my research, which I sincerely appreciate. I want to thank Alice Dan and Sarah Hemphill for inviting me to participate in the conference on women's health, in which this chapter was originally presented as a paper, and to Esther Parada for suggesting my name.

a gaping-wide border between her garden apartment on a shopping strip a few miles from Detroit and my two-story Victorian house in a quiet tree-lined neighborhood of Ann Arbor. Marta always addresses me in the formal you, as *usted*. She won't let me forget that I am 10 years her senior; that when we met in Mexico she was a young girl finishing high school and I was already a married woman embarking on a career as an anthropologist. After 7 years in the United States, and after knowing each other for 10 years, Marta insists on maintaining certain formalities that acknowledge the age, cultural, educational, and class differences between us.

We'll come for a little while, then, Marta tells me, so that Lisandra, her sister, can see my house. Lisandra, 17 and radiant, has just arrived from Mexico, with her papers in order, thanks to the efforts of Marta and Saúl. Like her brother Polo, she hopes to complete her last year of high school here and study in a community college. One of the sites Lisandra must see in the United States is my house. For Marta, my house is a museum. It is a house filled with books, embroidered cloths, and antique furniture; and there are clay pots, enameled trays, and bark paintings brought from Mexico. It is a house of many rooms, wood-framed windows, and a garden. Marta tells me she loves to come to my house; it is her dream house. She takes notice of anything new—a wicker chair, a used piano, a Turkish beaded good luck charm, new tiles in the bathroom, with whimsical nopal cactuses, also brought with us from Mexico. I have brought back folkloric, popular art things to remind me of my years in Mexico as an anthropologist. Marta, for whom Mexico is her grandparents, her seven siblings, and her mother and father, who were always working not to become poor, longs for none of these things; she dreams of packages filled with pretty white linens, edged in lace, that you order from catalogues, and she wants elegant, gold-trimmed porcelain dishes, the kind you can sometimes find on sale for $15, service for four, at Meijer.

The Cuban meal we always make when Marta visits is ready: black beans, white rice, picadillo, and a salad with slices of avocado; I even have an apple pie bought at the farmer's market and several bottles of beer ready for Saúl. I have also known Saúl for about as many years as I have known Marta. Born in the United States of Mexican parents, Saúl grew up in Michigan, working summers with his four brothers and their parents in the cherry, apple, and cucumber harvests. When I met Saúl, he was searching for his roots in the same Mexican town in which my husband and I were doing fieldwork. He'd usually visit around Christmas, hosting lively *posadas* at the house of his mother's cousin, where the tamales were plentiful and a big piñata bulging with sweets was never lacking. On one of his first visits, when I met him, he came with a girlfriend, a gringa with long curly blonde hair; and years before, he had come with a different girlfriend, also a gringa.

But during the Christmas season in 1983, he came alone. Marta, who had won a scholarship to attend a state boarding school, was home on a vacation from her job as a schoolteacher. Her hair was permed, she wore a pink knit blouse and fitted pants, and danced an entire night with Saúl at a fifteenth-birthday party, the quinceñera, of a cousin. Soon after, when he returned to the States, they wrote letters to each other every day. Two years later, they decided to get married, against the objections of Marta's father. He described Saúl, 13 years older than Marta, as a *gallo,* an old rooster, who wanted the hand of a *pollito,* a little chick.

Marta and Saúl were married in a big church wedding in Mexico in December 1985 and moved to East Lansing, where Saúl worked in the personnel department of Michigan State University. In the university setting, Marta met other women from Latin America and studied English. Saúl, who realized he'd taken Marta away from her job, hoped she'd prepare to become a teacher of bilingual education. But Marta soon decided she wanted to have a child and, without letting Saúl know, let him get her pregnant. What she hadn't expected was that it would happen so quickly. Their son Eduardo was born in 1988, when Marta was 23, and in 1989 they moved to the Detroit area, where Saúl found a better paying job in a state government office. For the next 3 years they lived in a garden apartment in Romulus, under the flight paths of the Detroit Metro airport, where few families lived and Marta felt unsafe. She stayed indoors all the time, shut within the four walls of their apartment, with her baby and the television as her only companions. Marta says she has learned English from watching soap operas. When she was asked at Meijer whether she'd work in their television and video department, she said she would not; I've spent almost all of my years in the United States inside a room with a television, she told her interviewer. Saúl told her she wouldn't get the job because she had said that, but fortunately he turned out to be wrong. Recently, they have moved to another apartment in Westland, where there are more families and children and the stores are within walking distance. It's not yet Marta's dream house, but at least she doesn't feel so isolated anymore.

The doorbell rings and I run to answer it. Marta, Saúl, Lisandra, and little Eduardo come in. I'm used to kissing hello, Cuban style, and they politely do the same. Polo, I learn from Marta, has stayed home to study. I bring out the tortilla chips, the pistachio nuts, the cashews, the beer for Saúl, and the Coke for Marta and Lisandra, pulling out the Mexican inlaid wood nesting tables to set everything on. "One table's enough," Saúl says, moving the bowls around. "No, here, let me get the other one," I say. "Oh, you just want to show off your little tables," Saúl says, good-naturedly, but I start to feel self-conscious. After a while, Marta announces that she will be working in the picture frame department, near the jewelry exhibition cases, at Meijer. She won't be washing floors, after all, she says. Will they offer her any benefits or health insurance, I ask. She shrugs; she hadn't asked, but she thinks they offer you those things after you've been working for some time.

Just before dinner I ask Lisandra if she'd like to have a tour of the town. She would, she says, and Marta suggests that the three women go off together. The three of us get in the car, Marta in back, Lisandra and me in front. I am conscious of being in the driver's seat because Marta has just said that she doesn't feel ready to start driving and that Saúl will have to take her back and forth from her job at Meijer. We drive to the university, circling around the bookstores, the campus buildings, the coffee shops, the T-shirt shops, the silver jewelry shops, the overpriced clothes shops, the law quad glistening with ivy, the orange brick building where I point out the anthropology department is housed. On Main street we get out of the car. Marta says it reminds her a little bit of Mexico, where there are places to just walk. Let's go see the stores, she says, but on a Sunday in Ann Arbor, at dinnertime, only the bookstores are open. We wander into Falling Water, a New Age bookstore, looking at amber and crystals and self-help books, which Marta examines intently, and then we go to Afterwords, a remaindered books bookstore, where Marta and Lisandra admire the books on lace and embroidery. "There's a book for everything, isn't there?" Marta remarks. And she adds, "You probably have this many books in your house."

After the Cuban dinner and a few minutes spent watching the presidential debate, Marta says it's time for them to go. Lisandra has to get ready for school the next day. We are saying good-bye when Marta says to me, "I didn't bring what I promised. I've only written one page. I'll mail it to you." I tell her I need it right away and that I'll visit her in 2 days, so we can talk.

*   *   *

A few days before her visit to my house, I had finally told Marta on the phone that I wanted to write about her. With some hesitation, I also told her I wanted to write about her *operación*. From the time she had her hysterectomy in May, I had known I would write about her, but I had been afraid to tell her. My worries about her denying me permission turned out to be unfounded; she told me she'd be happy if I wrote about her. Knowing that she likes to write long letters, I asked her if she'd write something down for me about her life, maybe in the form of a letter. She said she would. When I asked her if she'd ever written anything about her experience giving birth, which I remembered had been by cesarian section, she started to cry. "You know what, Ruth," she said to me after a pause, "I just threw away a few pages I wrote about that." I realized I had opened the floodgates and I felt scared. Then Marta added, "And when they did the operation, they cut along the same scar where they had cut before." She was crying again.

Maybe in a way I was wishing Marta would deny me permission to write about her, because what I feared most was having to tell her what I haven't been able to tell her. I have not been able to tell her that I feel distressed and guilty about her hysterectomy. I don't think it should have happened. I feel I ought to have stopped it from happening. Marta and Saúl seemed so certain they had come to a wise decision; moreover, they had not asked me for my opinion. And yet I have a debt to Marta. Her family in Mexico was always kind to us. I have not forgotten that her father asked me to watch over her, that her grandmother, when I said good-bye, cried for her Martita, and also asked me to look out for her. I feel I have failed my friend.

Marta came from Mexico with all the illusions of youth, seeking nothing more than to be a good wife to her husband and to live a decent life here in America, where everything is supposed to be better; at the age of 26, she should not have had her womb thrown into a garbage can.

*   *   *

I am sitting with Marta on her bed with the white lace coverlet. A mirror is behind Marta and I try not to look at my face in it. Little Eddy is in the living room playing with my husband David, who has accompanied me on this trip because I always get lost driving into the Detroit area. The tape recorder is on the bed and I hold up the microphone toward Marta. We don't know that the tape recorder is not recording anything; only later, when I get home, will I learn that David forgot to put the batteries in the microphone. I will get angry at him for his carelessness and angry at myself for depending on him to do what I should have done.

On three sheets of lined loose-leaf paper, Marta has begun to write her life story in a few broad strokes. I read her handwritten words and notice how careful she has been to leave out anything painful; but her sense of solitude is profound and it surfaces, unwillingly, several times in her brief text, which ends in midsentence, with the words, "I have tried not to be an abnegated wife, but a . . ." She has held within herself all the pain of social and cultural displacement, all the tension of her rite of passage from virgin to wife, and all the anxieties of losing her womb so soon after becoming a mother.

Women think back through their mothers, and, indeed, an important goal for Marta was to become a mother totally unlike her own mother. As I sit holding the microphone toward her, Marta tells me that her adult self comprehends that her mother had to work hard, first as a peddler and then as a

schoolteacher, to care for her eight children; but even so, she says with
anguish, she can't forget how as a child she felt neglected and wished she
could be wrapped inside her mother's arms, those arms that were always busy
working. In the United States, Marta imagined she could become the mother
she didn't have, the mother who would plan her pregnancy and be exclusively
devoted to her child. And so she has chosen to have one child and to stay at
home with him during the early years of his childhood. She has taken the job
at Meijer only because the hours are 6 to 11 in the evening, when she will
be able to count on Saúl, Polo, and Lisandra to care for little Eddy. As she
admits, they need the additional money now that Polo and Lisandra are living
with them. They are like two more children, who need to be fed and clothed.
Having taken them away from home, Marta wants to support her younger
brother and sister properly. Her brother had two pairs of pants in Mexico;
he'd be washing one pair when he was wearing the other. If nothing else, she
wants him to have enough pants to be able to wear a clean pair each day.

Knowing that she planned to have only one, or maybe two, children of her
own, Marta tells me she tried to enjoy every moment of her pregnancy. It was a
special time that she remembers with joy. But giving birth was a nightmare
for her. At the hospital, when she became fully dilated, the doctors told her
that the baby's head was too big and that they needed to perform a C-section.
They had given her a spinal block for pain relief and later they put her under
total anaesthesia to perform the C-section. Saúl was not allowed to be present
at the birth and the staff delayed bringing the baby to her. Apparently the
anesthesiologist was sloppy, because after giving birth Marta suffered from
terrible spinal headaches and body pains for 4 months. She cries remember-
ing how she could barely take care of Eddy at first. Was the C-section really
necessary, she asks herself now. And then she adds, "The operation wasn't
so bad. In a week I was perfectly fine. I felt better than after giving birth." It
has always seemed to me that the rate of C-sections and the rate of hysterectomies are intimately related. For Marta, having a C-section, especially one
that was botched and alienating, opened the way for her feeling that her
womb wasn't worth much; and sure enough, for the doctor who took out her
uterus, it must have been easy to cut along the dotted line of her C-section
scar.

Marta found the doctor who performed her hysterectomy, a board-certified
OB-GYN, in the phone book. She had already gone to two other doctors,
both women, before seeing him. The two previous doctors, she felt, were
unscrupulous in their desire for money; after learning what a good health
insurance plan she had through her husband's job, they had immediately
wanted to perform hysterectomies without even running a single test or
analysis. As a rule, she prefers women doctors, she says, because she's Latina
and finds it shameful to be examined by a man. But the doctor she found in

the phone book impressed her enough that she put her trust in him. He's Cuban, she tells me, which I already know, cringing at the horrible thought that Marta, in a subliminal way, may have put her trust in him because she's learned from me that Cubans are OK. I am holding the microphone that is taping nothing as she tells me that she wanted to have tests done and the Cuban doctor did them. She wanted to be sure she needed this operation and he convinced her she did. Her heavy menstrual bleeding had worried her since she was a young girl but, after giving birth, it had gotten worse. She had to rest during her periods and take iron; during those days, she fell behind on the cooking and cleaning and she didn't like that, because if the house was going to be her only responsibility, she wanted to do it well. The doctor told her if she went on bleeding so heavily, one day she'd have a hemorrhage. He also told her that she had a tumor in her uterus, but, after removing it, he told her there was no tumor at all, that it was her uterus itself that was abnormally enlarged, that it had not shrunk back to its proper size after pregnancy.

Marta is beginning to question her doctor's advice and motives. She's not so sure anymore that he wasn't out for the money too. And she recognizes that he's not so honest, perhaps, as she thought at first. When she tells him she's been gaining weight after the operation, he pretends it's her eating habits that are responsible—you know, too many tortillas. But later she finds out that it's very common for women who lose their uterus to put on weight. But what matters is her health, she says. It's nice not to be worried about her periods anymore or about getting pregnant. She couldn't have gone on taking iron pills forever. And if she's not going to have any more children anyway, then she really doesn't need her uterus. She's lucky, she tells me, that Saúl is educated and accepts her in her new wombless state. In Mexico, she says, there are men who won't have a woman who's had a hysterectomy; they claim those women aren't women anymore.

I realize that she needs to affirm to herself that her decision was a wise one. She thought about it for a year and she feels she explored her options by getting several medical opinions. She has to believe that her health has improved, that she is really better, much better. But the loss of her uterus has made her aware of all her losses—of everything she has given up, everything she is giving up, to make a new life for herself and her family on this side of the border.

You know, Marta says to me, the last time she was in Mexico she and her mother were joking around and her mother called her a good-for-nothing. Those words—*no sirves para nada*—stung, and the pain was compounded when Saúl recently said the same thing to her, also as a joke. As she recounts this, Marta's eyes fill with tears. Marta was the second daughter; it was her sister, the eldest, who was always the smart one, always the favorite of her father. When she was in Mexico, her father told her how proud he was of her older unmarried sister for having gotten so far in her studies and achieving degrees in two fields. But he didn't say anything to Marta about being proud of her. She longs for greater affirmation from her parents, and yet her deepest wish is to bring them both to the United States someday and be able to provide for them in their old age.

Marta left everything behind to come to the States with Saúl, but she didn't receive a very warm welcome from his family. When her mother-in-law suddenly developed an inexplicable illness, her father-in-law accused Marta of having used witchcraft to cause the illness; later he told Marta that Saúl didn't love her and that she was lucky he had paid any attention to her. One brother-in-law called her an Indian from the rancho because she refused to drink beer; another brother-in-law told her she was *un perro entrenado* (trained dog) because she was so concerned to keep Saúl happy, having dinner on the table when he returned from work and setting his clothes out for him, neatly ironed, each morning. She doesn't do those things for Saúl anymore, Marta says, because he never thanked her, never showed any appreciation. If Saúl thought he was bringing back a young and innocent Mexican wife to do all his housework for him, those days are over, she says, wiping her last tears, her face recomposing itself into a hard cast.

                              *   *   *

What happened to Marta can happen to any woman. In 1991 nearly 1 million hysterectomies were performed in the United States. Nine out of ten of those procedures were carried out as elective surgery. By the age of 65, three fourths of American women can count on losing their uterus for no justifiable medical reason. In recent years, both a female OB-GYN and a male OB-GYN have spoken out on the subject, showing that at least half of all hysterectomies carried out in a year are unnecessary. The procedure is sold to women by male physicians who use the operation as a major source of income, finding it easier to remove a woman's uterus than to explore complicated, and often lengthier and less lucrative, alternative therapies. It has also been shown that the rate of hysterectomy varies greatly among doctors, regions, and hospitals and that it often correlates with the practice of other common surgical procedures such as tonsillectomy. While right-wing political pressure has succeeded in reducing the number of hospital training programs that teach doctors how to perform abortions, women have not yet mounted a strong enough campaign to train doctors to curtail the excessive number of hysterectomies (Blum, 1992; Gittelsohn & Wennberg, 1976; Hufnagel, with Golant, 1989; McPherson, Wennberg, Hovind, & Clifford, 1982; Smith, 1992; Wennberg, 1979). We cannot keep waiting, as in Jan Clausen's

(1992) brilliant sardonic tale, for our discarded wombs to rise up for us in all their fury, "like a sticky organic glacier, leaving a trail a mile and a half wide of a shiny material that reminded some viewers of banana slug slime" (p. 423).

Indeed, what happened to Marta can happen to any woman, yet the point I want to make here is that nothing that happens to a woman ever happens to another woman in exactly the same way. Each of us needs to be listened to, one at a time. We are not cases. We are not statistics.

The Algerian writer Marie Cardinal describes how her menstrual blood once "flowed in such large clots that it might have been said I was producing slices of liver," making the doctor want "to make a long incision in the skin, in the muscles, in the veins, open up the flesh of the belly, the viscera, and take hold of that hot, pinkish organ, cut it away and eliminate it." When the tests showed nothing was seriously wrong with her, Cardinal bundled herself in cotton pads and, in a last desperate move, went to an analyst, under whose guidance the bleeding stopped completely as she found the words to tell her life story (Cardinal, 1983, pp. 31, 34).[1] What I regret deeply is that Marta wasn't given the chance to do that; instead, she sacrificed her womb. Her bleeding has stopped, but her tears are flowing.

In learning about Marta's medical history, I came to see just how deeply enmeshed that history is in the whole of her life history. With Marta, I have come to realize that, until you know the whole of a woman's life story, you cannot know anything about her health, let alone what to tell her to do for her own good. When doctors will sit with us in our homes and listen to our life stories, learning about the old hurts we've carried around since childhood and the new hurts of our adulthood, then we will be able to say that we have achieved a field truly concerned with women's health.

Note

1. Although I feel that an opportunity to have told her life story to a receptive medical practitioner might have helped Marta to find an alternative to hysterectomy, I want to stress that telling her life story after the hysterectomy offers important and necessary healing. I have written about the need for women to tell their life stories after a hysterectomy in my essay, "The Body in the Woman, the Story in the Woman: A Book Review and Personal Essay" (1990).

References

Behar, R. (1990). The body in the woman, the story in the woman: A book review and personal essay. *Michigan Quarterly Review, 29*(4), 694-738. (Reprinted in L. Goldstein, Ed., *The female body: Figures, styles, speculations*, pp. 267-231, Ann Arbor: University of Michigan Press, 1991)

Blum, D. E. (1992, May 6). Fewer programs found to teach future doctors how to perform abortions. *The Chronicle of Higher Education*, p. A39.

Cardinal, E. M. (1983). *The words to say it.* Cambridge, MA: Van Vactor & Goodheart.

Clausen, J. (1992). The end of history. *Feminist Studies, 18*(2), 421-429.

Gittelsohn, A. M., & Wennberg, J. (1976). On the risk of organ loss. *Journal of Chronic Diseases, 29,* 527-535.

Hufnagel, V., with Golant, S. K. (1989). *No more hysterectomies.* New York: New American Library.

McPherson, K., Wennberg, J. E., Hovind, O. B., & Clifford, P. (1982, November 18). Small-area variations in the use of common surgical procedures: An international comparison of New England, England, and Norway. *The New England Journal of Medicine,* pp. 1310-1314.

Smith, J. (1992). *Women and doctors.* New York: Atlantic Monthly Press.

Wennberg, J. (1979). Factors governing utilization of hospital services. *Hospital Practice, 14*(9), 115-127.

PART III

Reproductive Health and Sexuality

14

Contraception and Abortion: Challenges Now and for the Next Century

Nada L. Stotland

It seemed that the development of relatively safe, inexpensive, and effective methods of contraception for women should have ended the era, dating from the origins of humankind, in which women's lives and deaths were largely dominated by the exigencies of childbearing. Many researchers and health care providers, and political leaders in some societies, themselves ardent subscribers to technical advances and careful planners of the courses of their lives, have little patience with the failure of individuals and of whole social subgroups to take rational control of their reproductive lives. The timing and number of births, they believe, should be determined by factors such as economics, population size, and the provision of family circumstances suitable for child nurturance.

For most people, however, that is not how it works. Large numbers of young women who have not completed their educations, and without mates to share the financial and psychological burdens of parenthood, become mothers. Overcrowded countries strive to feed their populations. Many or most well-educated, comfortably off, mature individuals, married and unmarried, with access to contraceptive techniques and medical care, conceive pregnancies without conscious intention and go on to become parents.

Is this carelessness, or the result of biological forces that supersede economic and social contingencies? Are there psychological factors between the biological and the social that we and our political leaders have failed to take into account? Contraceptives must be effective not only in vitro, but in vivo,

AUTHOR'S NOTE: I gratefully acknowledge the editorial contributions of Bevanne Bean-Mayberry.

in situations in which the application of cognitive knowledge is complicated by power imbalance and abuse, exhaustion, conscious and unconscious attempts to bind the relationship between the partners, haste, and embarrassment, not to mention lust. In fact, none of cognitive knowledge, contraceptive effectiveness, or access to abortion can be taken for granted. Ignorance about reproductive anatomy and physiology is rampant and not limited to the lower socioeconomic classes. Contraceptives fail and cause unacceptable side effects. Many women face realistically formidable obstacles to obtaining abortions.

Very little is known about the motivation for parenthood. Some would argue that the biological drive for heterosexual intercourse is what perpetuates the species, and that conception is only an unconsidered by-product of that activity. The large number of induced abortions supports that view. On the other hand, most pregnancies are carried to term. Is there a drive for parenthood as well as for sex? Our challenges in contraception and abortion must be viewed from technical, social, and psychological perspectives.

Historical and Anthropological Perspectives

These issues have been with us since the beginning of recorded time. Repeated conceptions dominated the lives, and often caused the deaths, of women until very recently in human history. Diaries of women through the centuries reveal that, after marriage, they were nearly always either pregnant or breast-feeding. Breast-feeding, if used as the infant's only source of not only nourishment but also sucking and soothing, suppresses ovulation fairly effectively. Prolonged breast-feeding may explain the spacing of childbirth in some so-called primitive societies, although other sociobiological factors may play significant roles as well. The birth of many children in succession is more common under circumstances of high infant mortality, and may contribute to it.

On the other hand, in every society there are circumstances in which pregnancy is regarded as a liability. Efforts to prevent or end pregnancy have been documented at least as early as ancient Greece, and in all cultures studied around the world. Given that one form of abortion is specifically mentioned in the Hippocratic oath, and given that abortion was illegal in most Western countries until recent decades, many people believe that it has been officially prohibited throughout history. In fact, for most of history, abortion was ignored or considered acceptable under certain circumstances.

For example, the Roman Catholic church via canon law permitted abortions early in pregnancy until "formation" of an embryo. It was believed that the female embryo did not have a soul until the 80th day, and the male until the 40th day, of pregnancy (Luker, 1984). Abortion services, like other women's reproductive health care, were provided by lay women in the community. It was only as medicine became increasingly professionalized and systematized, and incorporated midwifery, that abortion came to be officially deplored and then outlawed, late in the last century (Luker, 1984).

In nonindustrialized societies, the termination of pregnancy is universally practiced, though official attitudes range from disapproval to requirement. Methods include pharmacological abortifacients, primitive surgical interventions, and gross external abdominal pressure. Anthropologists reported one society in which the aborted fetus is fed to its would-have-been siblings. For most of history, in most places, pregnancy and abortion have been associated with a high rate of morbidity and mortality. It was the care of women following septic abortions that prompted Margaret Sanger to campaign for the provision of contraceptives. Before abortion was legalized by the U.S. Supreme Court in the 1973 *Roe v. Wade* decision, approximately 20% of maternal deaths were attributable to the complications of illegal abortions. Their number was estimated at 1 million per year.

The Current Situation

The generation of health care providers currently being trained has had no such direct exposure to the real-life consequences of bans and limitations on abortion. In the United States, only a minority of residents in obstetrics and gynecology learn to perform abortions (Westoff, Marks, & Rosenfield, 1993). Efficiently and safely carried out in freestanding outpatient clinics, outside the mainstream of training, the performance of abortions is seen as just a service, without intellectual, technical, social, or financial rewards. Abortion is legal in Canada and in most European countries. Current U.S. incidence is about 1½ million per year. Most are performed on young white women. The vast majority take place in the first trimester.

It might seem that the control of human reproduction has been achieved. We have effective contraceptives and legalized abortion. The U.S. Supreme Court was said to have upheld the *Roe v. Wade* (1973) decision in the 1991 *Casey* case (*Planned Parenthood v. Casey*, 1992). However, it was not until the plague of HIV infection threatened the middle classes that sexual practices and the use of condoms became acceptable topics of private conversation and public discourse. Ronald Reagan's surgeon general, chosen for his antiabortion stance, shocked and enraged the administration with his insistence upon educating the public about the transmission of HIV and educating himself about abortion. Despite his courageous efforts, despite our prosperity, enlightenment, and advanced technology, pregnancies continue to be conceived "accidentally" and terminated deliberately, sometimes not until the second trimester. Why should this be?

Contraceptives and the human behaviors required are far from infallible. A new wrinkle in a long history of reproduction, they have been introduced without sufficient knowledge of the realities of human reproductive psychology and behavior. Barrier methods require premeditation and/or interruption of an act characterized by powerful instinctual urges and emotions that sweep thoughts of consequences from awareness. Diaphragms slip; condoms leak and break. Hormonal contraceptives are tainted by our fascination with the manipulation of women's reproductive anatomy and physiology, often before we consider the long-term consequences, a fascination that has given us diethylstilbestrol; intrauterine devices that caused infection, sterility, and death; a 25% Cesarean section rate; and a 50% hysterectomy rate. Paradoxically, surgical interventions and hormonal manipulations are rewarded with generous monetary fees, prestige, and public and institutional attention, while providers of abortion services, and members of their families, can expect harassment, physical danger, and, in one recent tragic incident, assassination.

The most effective forms of contraception for women are available only by physician's prescription, requiring an office appointment and submission to a pelvic examination. This is a major psychological barrier, especially for young, nulliparous women, who find the examination embarrassing and uncomfortable and fear that their sexual behavior, as well as their sexual organs, will be probed and judged in the health care setting (Zabin, Stark, & Emerson, 1991). It is a social barrier for women who must bring children or find child care, travel long distances, endure long waits, and/or obtain leave from their jobs for doctor visits. The male condom must be purchased and requires advance planning, interruption, and the consent and cooperation of the male partner. While it is appropriate for sexual partners to share the contraceptive burden, the medical consequences of unprotected sexual intercourse fall on the woman only.

What we know about the psychology and sociology of family planning highlights the clash between our narrow biomedical thinking and the realities of the challenge. Aside from the unconscious biological drive for parenthood, conception is driven by the wish to prove one's fertility, to cement a relationship, to be loved by the partner and the child, to receive financial support. In certain subcultures, not only sexual intercourse, but the impregnation of a woman, is required to prove a man's virility and manhood. Many women consider intercourse outside of marriage more or less immoral or at least improper. Somehow the idea of being overcome by romance and passion is a mitigating factor. Because all contraception requires advance planning of one kind or another, contraception is associated with precisely the deliberate preparations for sex that would make one a "bad girl." Some women who engage in prostitution to support their drug addiction (i.e., heroin) reserve contraception for their paying customers and regard it as an inappropriate barrier between them and the men they genuinely love (Kane, 1991). Moreover, women who exchange sex for money or drugs (e.g., crack, cocaine) are less likely to use contraception and are more apt to be at risk for STDs (Fullilove & Fullilove, 1989; Schwarz et al., 1992). Recent data on women attending family planning clinics indicates women are less likely to use condoms with their regular partners (Soskolne, Aral, Magder, Reed, & Bowen, 1991).

The provision of contraceptive health care, and general health care to women with contraceptive needs, must be informed by an appreciation of these realistic factors and empathy for the women influenced by them. The challenge is not only that we health care providers are biomedically oriented; it is also that we are accustomed to valuing and striving for what we consider to be a highly "rational" approach to our lives and our practice. With its extremely competitive, long, and demanding training, the field of medicine selects for those obsessionals best able to implement and tolerate the delay of gratification, and specifically of reproductive gratification. Families had better be planned, or at least postponed. Because this style is adaptive in the professional setting, providers may mistakenly confuse it with moral superiority. This attitude has no useful place in the provision of care to patients with other styles.

Politics also plays a major role in family planning. Under the Reagan and Bush administrations in the United States, there was active government resistance not only to the provision of family planning services at home and abroad but also to the development of new contraceptive techniques and the education of the population about currently available methods. Fear of hormonal contraceptives, inspired by reports in the media and by past experience, as with diethylstilbestrol, expose many young women to the probably greater dangers of unwanted pregnancy (Zabin et al., 1991). Aside from refinements in oral contraception and the creation of a cumbersome so-called female condom and Norplant, there have been no significant additions to the contraceptive armamentarium in several decades. Increasingly stringent requirements for the informed consent of research subjects, and immense, escalating liability awards, have also contributed to the narrowing of options for family planning (Kaeser, 1990). Intrauterine devices disappeared almost completely from the market after the revelation of the dangers of the Dalkon Shield. The enormously inflated price of the remaining product is due to the cost of liability insurance for the manufacturer.

It would seem that the medical community, and society as a whole, is far more willing to experiment and interfere with female reproductive capacities than with males'. This disparity is reflected not only in the paucity of male contraceptives but also in the relative rates of sterilization among men and

women. Though vasectomies are far less expensive and medically complicated than tubal ligations, the latter greatly outnumber the former. Perhaps
the difference also reflects the fact that it is women who become pregnant
and who have few other reliable means of establishing control over that
vulnerability.

When political, psychological, sociological, and/or biological factors impede the effectiveness of contraception, and pregnancy occurs, the next
possible intervention is abortion. Again, it is vital to recognize the distinction
between theoretical and actual access. Abortion has been legalized in much
of the Western world, but legality is not equivalent to availability. In North
America, there are vast stretches of territory where abortion services are so
scattered as to be virtually inaccessible (Henshaw, 1991; Henshaw & Van Vort,
1990). Antiabortion forces, driven by powerful convictions, have succeeded
in establishing a variety of restrictions that appear harmless or even sensible
but that in fact have a major dampening effect on women's reproductive
choices. This effect falls disproportionately on rural, uneducated, and/or poor
women, women below the age of majority, women of color, and women lacking
English language skills and knowledge of the health care and judicial systems.

Laws vary from state to state and from week to week as legislators respond
to strong political pressures and the findings of the courts. Typical restrictions include requirements of parental notification or consent for young
women (laws requiring notification and consent of the woman's husband or
male partner have been passed, but overturned), prohibitions on the discussion of abortion in public family planning clinics, mandated delays between
the woman's presentation for care and the performance of abortion, and
scripted lectures describing fetal development and the alternatives to abortion. Those not immediately involved may not be fully aware of the realities
for many women most at risk of unwanted pregnancy.

Adolescents from chaotic, incestuous, and abusive families are at highest
risk of unplanned pregnancy (Boyer & Fine, 1992). A teenage girl from an
abusive family may have to obtain both parents' permission, risking violence
and exclusion from the family, unless she is sophisticated enough to know
that she can bypass this requirement by getting permission from a judge. To
obtain a judicial bypass, she must find the courthouse and the correct courtroom.
She must manage to absent herself from her usual workday activities. She
may have to make more than one trip; in many areas, the courts are not in
session every day. She is likely to be overawed by courts and judges.
Guarantees of confidentiality have little meaning; courthouse personnel may
know her family, friends, teachers.

Once before the judge, her chances of being granted permission for the
abortion depend largely on the state. Though they may have nearly identical
laws, one state grants, and another denies, nearly all such petitions. After

obtaining a bypass, she still must obtain the abortion. U.S. federal law forbids the use of national funds to pay for abortions. This procedure appears to protect children and their parents' prerogatives in helping them to make major life decisions. However, no such regulations pertain when it comes to continuing a young woman's pregnancy. She is free to undergo 9 months of pregnancy, labor, and delivery, and to assume total responsibility for a newborn child, without any participation by her parents.

As it is quite clear that the provision of legal, safe abortions results in less medical morbidity and mortality than either illegal abortions or childbirth (Henshaw, 1990), antiabortion proponents have often focused on the psychological effects of abortion. They allege that women are permanently emotionally scarred, unable to form normal maternal attachments. They speak to the public of an "abortion trauma syndrome" that the psychiatric community deliberately covers up. There have been several exhaustive reviews of the literature on the psychosocial sequelae of abortion, including one by Paul Dagg (M.D.) (1991) at the University of Ottawa.

The methodological challenges attendant on the study of abortion are formidable. Abortion is probably most often performed on women in stressful, if not traumatic, situations. Either some psychosocial barrier has interfered with their use of contraception, or their contraceptive method has failed them. Some have persistent or recurrent psychiatric illnesses. For some, the male partner with whom the pregnancy was conceived may have forced the sexual act, fled when it was over or when the pregnancy was conceived, or demanded a pregnancy—or an abortion—as a condition of continuing the relationship. Family or religious mores may condemn both sex outside of marriage and abortion. Family finances may demand a choice between the welfare of existing dependents and the continuation of a pregnancy.

It is difficult indeed to dissect the effects of such circumstances from the effects of the abortion itself. The logistics of obtaining the abortion may involve illegality, secrecy, desperate attempts to find a provider and the money to pay for the abortion, judgmental and rejecting significant others, and protesters blocking the entry to the abortion clinic, chanting: "Don't kill your baby." An appropriate control group must consist of women who carried pregnancies—optimally, pregnancies conceived under similar circumstances—to term; delivery is the only other option available to a woman considering abortion.

No study yet performed or planned meets all these criteria. Nevertheless, there is a good deal of information about the psychiatric sequelae of abortion. Studies from Scandinavia and Czechoslovakia have compared the outcomes of pregnancies carried to term after the mothers were refused abortions with matched control pregnancies. A U.S. study followed a group of adolescent women who sought pregnancy tests in a clinic (Zabin, Hirsch, & Emerson,

1989). The young women who chose abortions fared best, even better than those who had not been pregnant at all, while those who chose to deliver children fared worst.

Most studies concern groups of women who chose abortions, and some compare them with published studies of women who delivered. The incidence of adverse psychiatric outcomes is many multiples higher among the latter than the former. Risk factors include previous and/or ongoing psychiatric illness, paralyzing ambivalence, a decision made under pressure from others, and particularly stressful life circumstances. Women who had desired the pregnancy, but chose abortion after learning that the fetus was abnormal, have more emotional difficulty. Most women who undergo abortions report a sense of relief and brief, self-limited sadness. The best predictor of postabortion adjustment is the woman's psychological condition before the abortion. There is no scientific evidence of any discrete psychiatric syndrome. There are self-selected groups of women, affiliated with groups opposed to abortion, who feel strongly that abortions played a significant role in their ongoing psychosocial difficulties.

Another risk factor for adverse psychiatric outcome is abortion in the second trimester of pregnancy. Delays in arranging abortion are caused by the same array of factors that lead to unintended pregnancy (Henshaw, 1991). Some women experience extraordinary difficulties in making a decision about the pregnancy; they are not psychologically able to acknowledge the fact of the pregnancy for psychodynamic reasons or are subject to confounding external pressures. The wait for the results of prenatal testing delays some abortions. By far the most common reason for second trimester abortions in the United States at this time is difficulty finding funds and/or a provider in the first trimester.

Implications for Women's Health and Health Care

A short generation ago, all medical students were exposed to hospital wards filled with patients dying or recovering from septic abortions. But today many physicians not directly involved in the provision of gynecological care doubt that they should be concerned about contraception and abortion. Control over their reproductive lives has, however, been critical to women's general health, life expectancy, and participation in society. Counseling about reproductive choices is essential to the care of women who have suffered adverse consequences following previous pregnancies, to others at high risk, and to women who require or are inadvertently given pharmacological agents, exposure to radiation, and other potentially teratogenic interventions in early pregnancy. Limitations on contraceptive and abortion services produce an intolerable situation, in which our rich and sophisticated patients obtain appropriate care that our disadvantaged patients are denied. Many of the restrictions imposed have entailed intrusions into the trust, collaboration, and confidentiality of the doctor-patient relationship. Finally, without control over conception, women of reproductive age have been excluded from medical research studies vital to diagnosis and treatment.

Research Directions

In one sense, there is little use trying to determine whether contraception and abortion are "good for" women. Women have consistently demonstrated that they will risk their lives to obtain them. It is shameful that we have so few techniques to offer and so little basic reproductive education for young people. We will follow the outcomes of RU 486 abortions with interest. Certainly we need to know how we can help women to achieve more sense of control over their own reproductive lives. We need to know why the techniques effective in vitro do not work in vivo. It would be helpful to be able to identify women at risk of adverse outcomes following either abortion or delivery and to study the effectiveness of monitoring and preventive interventions. Very little is known about the attitudes of men toward contraception as well as their response when their partners, or other women important in their lives, undergo abortion. It is also vital to foster a medical and social climate in which these critical issues can be studied without fear of their misapplication to further limit women's reproductive choices and health.

Resources

Stotland, N. L. (Ed.). (1991). *Psychiatric aspects of abortion.* Washington, DC: American Psychiatric Press.
Tribe, L. H. (1990). *Abortion, the clash of absolutes.* New York: Norton.

References

Boyer, D., & Fine, D. (1992). Sexual abuse as a factor in adolescent pregnancy and child maltreatment. *Family Planning Perspectives, 24,* 4-11, 19.
Dagg, P. K. B. (1991). The psychological sequelae of therapeutic abortion—denied and completed. *American Journal of Psychiatry, 148,* 578-585.

Devereux, G. (1976). *A study of abortion in primitive societies* (rev. ed.). New York: International Universities Press.

Fullilove, M. T., & Fullilove, R. E. (1989). Intersecting epidemics: Black teen crack use and sexually transmitted disease. *Journal of the American Medical Women's Association, 44,* 146-153.

Henshaw, S. K. (1990). Induced abortion: A world review, 1990. *Family Planning Perspectives, 22,* 76-89.

Henshaw, S. K. (1991). The accessibility of abortion services in the United States. *Family Planning Perspectives, 23,* 246-252.

Henshaw, S. K., & Van Vort, J. (1990). Abortion services in the United States, 1987 and 1988. *Family Planning Perspectives, 22,* 102-108, 142.

Jones, E. F., & Forrest, J. D. (1992). Contraceptive failure rates based on the 1988 NSFG. *Family Planning Perspectives, 24,* 12-19.

Kaeser, L. (1990). Contraceptive development: Why the snail's pace? *Family Planning Perspectives, 22,* 131-133.

Kane, S. (1991). HIV, heroin and heterosexual relations. *Social Science Medicine, 32,* 1037-1050.

Klitsch, M. (1991). How well do women comply with oral contraceptive regimens? *Family Planning Perspectives, 23,* 134-136.

Luker, K. (1984). *Abortion and the politics of motherhood.* Berkeley: University of California Press.

Planned Parenthood of Southeastern Pennsylvania v. Casey (1992) 112 5 cf 2791, 120 LiEd 2d 674, 60 U.S.L.W. 4795.

Roe v. Wade (1973) 410 U.S. 113.

Schwarz, S. K., Bolan, G. A., Fullilove, M., McCright, J., Fullilove, R., Kohn, R., et al. (1992). Crack cocaine and the exchange of sex for money or drugs. *Sexually Transmitted Diseases, 19,* 7-13.

Soskolne, V., Aral, S. O., Magder, L. S., Reed, D. S., & Bowen, G. S. (1991). Condom use with regular and casual partners among women attending family planning clinics. *Family Planning Perspectives, 23,* 222-225.

Speert, H. (1980). *Obstetrics and gynecology in America: A history.* Baltimore: American College of Obstetricians and Gynecologists, Waverly.

Tavris, C. (1992). *The mismeasure of woman.* New York: Simon & Schuster.

Westhoff, C., Marks, F., & Rosenfield, A. (1993). Residency training in contraception, sterilization, and abortion. *Obstetrics and Gynecology, 81,* 311-314.

Zabin, L. S., Hirsch, M. B., & Emerson, M. R. (1989). When urban adolescents choose abortion: Effects on education, psychological status and subsequent pregnancy. *Family Planning Perspectives, 21,* 248-255.

Zabin, L. S., Stark, H. A., & Emerson, M. A. (1991). Reasons for delay in contraceptive clinic utilization: Adolescent clinic and nonclinic populations compared. *Journal of Adolescent Health, 12,* 225.

15

Women's Sexuality:
Not a Matter of Health

Leonore Tiefer

The Power of Naming

This chapter will consider the advantages and disadvantages of locating women's sexuality under the rubric of health issues. Perhaps unexpectedly, or even counterintuitively, I want to argue that considering women's sexuality a matter of health is premature at this point for two main reasons. First, there are assumptions hidden in a health model that seem to me disadvantageous for a liberated view of women's sexuality. And, second, adopting a health model for women's sexuality would support even greater institutionalization of the dominant paradigms in medical sexology, a situation I also feel is not in women's best interests. Instead, I will argue that there are some short-term "health-oriented" clinical and research goals we can advocate while at the same time working outside the medical model to shift the prevailing sexology paradigm to a more woman-friendly (even woman-centered) one.

This approach is based on the premise that designating an area of human behavior and experience such as sexuality a matter of "health" is a choice, with important ramifications in terms of appropriate authorities, institutional control, and so on (Conrad & Kern, 1981; Featherstone, Hepworth, & Turner, 1991). "Health" is not dictated by biology any more than "sexuality" is dictated by biology (Scott & Morgan, 1993). They are both matters of language and culture, using a set of biological potentials that are expressed and constructed very differently in different sociohistorical situations.

This perspective derives from the larger political recognition that language doesn't just name reality, it organizes reality, and gives names to that organization (Potter & Wetherell, 1987). Naming takes on fundamental importance in areas such as health, mental health, or sexuality, which are subject to repeated redefinition, often moralistically, and "the categories, taxonomies, or units of analysis used in the investigation of a certain problem tend to influence the findings and also the conclusion" (Edwards, 1981, p. 4). Because sexuality is contested political terrain where various ideological forces constantly struggle for legitimacy and cultural authority (Weeks, 1981), all discourse about sexuality, including the scientific and clinical, represents some worldview and political agenda. The informed discussant accepts that there is no neutral ground, no apolitical ground of technical expertise where one can coolly and objectively discuss the facts and leave politics at the door.

Thus feminists and women's health activists construing sexuality as a matter of health (to be covered in health training programs and by health policies) should be seen as an important decision with wide-ranging consequences, undertaken only after a review of the covert as well as the overt implications of such jurisdictional allocation.[1] This chapter will first examine some of the appeals of a health model of sexuality, then turn to an examination of the hidden assumptions of such a model. It continues with a worrisome examination of how men's sexuality has been dealt with in the world of medicine and health and with an analysis of how the field of sexology is currently dominated by a male-centered model of sexuality. Finally, I will recommend some limited, short-term research on women's sexuality that might be conducted while longer-term transformations of the fundamental sexological paradigm are under way.

Appeals of the Health Model

Feminists are attracted to a health model for sexuality in large part because of its legitimacy and moral neutrality, its confident reliance on the objective facts of biological nature.[2] Feminists celebrated the publication of Masters and Johnson's (1966) physiological measures of people engaged in masturbation and coitus, for example, because they seemed to provide objective "proof" that women's sexual capacities not only existed but equaled those of men (e.g., Ehrenreich, Hess, & Jacobs, 1986). Feminists felt that finally they had ammunition against the tyranny of the Freudian vaginal orgasm (see Koedt, 1973), not to mention against the earlier claims of women's passionlessness and frigidity (see Sahli, 1990, for a summary of the prefeminist literature about women's sexuality). As Masters and Johnson (1966) themselves boasted, "With orgasmic physiology established, the human female now has an undeniable opportunity to develop realistically her own sexual response levels" (p. 138).

The legitimacy offered by the moral neutrality and authority of the medical/health model of sex extended beyond descriptions of women's sexual capacities to the implicit assumption that sexuality, at least the medically approved "normal" sort, was actually a component of health, that is, that sexuality itself was healthy. Because *healthy* has become the premiere adjective for goodness, it can be used to endorse everything from behaviors to products and services (Barsky, 1988). The importance of such an imprimatur for sexuality cannot be underestimated in a culture where sexuality has been for centuries a moral football, a religious and political weapon used to challenge social and personal virtue and decency (Freedman & D'Emilio, 1988).

The legitimacy and entitlement offered for women's sexuality by the medical model seems to derive directly from "nature," without the intervention of culture or cultural standards of right and wrong. I have elsewhere discussed how the discourse of "naturalism," or the reliance on "laws of nature," is rhetorically tempting not only for individuals but for sex researchers and activists (Tiefer, 1990). Once having opted for biological justification, supporters of women's sexuality can even recruit evolutionary theory, that replacer of (or, depending on region, competitor of) divine law, as the ultimate and inarguable source of authority (Caporael & Brewer, 1991).

Were women's sexuality, then, to be located under the rubric of health, it would appear to acquire there a strong, secure, and eminently respectable home that feminists could use as a base to press for improved sex education, protection against sexual violence, reproductive rights, elimination of the sexual double standard, and all the other components of the sexuality plank in the contemporary women's rights platform.

Hidden Assumptions of the Health Model

But, alas, all is not so simple. There are hidden assumptions that go along with the health model that make it deeply worrisome when applied to women's sexuality (Mishler, 1981). Let me briefly discuss the four medical model assumptions of norms and deviance, universality, individualism, and biological reductionism.

Norms and Deviance

First and most important is the fundamentally normative structure of the health and medicine model—the assumption that there is such a thing as healthy sexuality that can be distinguished from nonhealthy (diseased, abnormal, sick, disordered, pathological) sexuality. The normative basis of the health model is absolutely inescapable—the only way we can talk about "signs and symptoms" or "treatments and cures" or "diagnosis and classification" is with regard to norms and deviations from norms. But, where shall we get the norms for women's sexuality? What are the legitimate and compelling sources and what do they say?

At the present time, sexual norms are far better understood by sociologists than by health specialists. That is, sociologists have analyzed sexual category making as part of the social discourse of sexual normalcy versus sexual deviance in many texts on women's deviant sexualities such as promiscuity, prostitution, masturbation, nymphomania, frigidity, and so on (Sahli, 1984; Schur, 1984). Can health specialists demonstrate that their "sexual health" norms derive from more "scientific" sources than simply cultural values (Tiefer, 1986a)?

It is my opinion that there are no valid clinical norms for sexuality. There are diverse cultural and legal standards, and they have been selectively appropriated by the health and medicine domain. But, just as playing canasta 10 hours a day may be a sign of emotional malfunction, that doesn't mean there is a disease of "hypercanasta"![3] That is, without being facetious, there's just too much lifestyle, historical, and cultural variability in sexual behavior standards for us be able to establish clinical norms in lifestyle patterns of sexual activity performance, choices, frequencies, partners, subjectivities, and so on. One of my biggest worries about locating sexuality discourse within the domain of health is the potential abuse of norms. Sociologists point out that norms are the principal mode of social control over sexual behavior because the norms become internalized and even unconscious and are "policing" people 24 hours a day (e.g., DeLamater, 1981). What we don't need in a society with a history of women's sexual disenfranchisement are additional sources of repression.

Universality

Variability and diverse standards bring us to the second assumption of the health model: universality. The difference between clinical norms and cultural standards is, presumably, that health is based on pan-cultural standards of biological function and malfunction. The only such standards for sexuality currently derive from the physiological research of Masters and Johnson (1966), and I have written at length about how that research is based on a flawed and self-fulfilling design (Tiefer, 1991a). Masters and Johnson did not demonstrate a universal "human sexual response cycle" of arousal and orgasm because they only took measurements on subjects who were able to exhibit masturbatory and coital arousal and orgasm in their laboratory. I don't doubt that (many? most? all?) human bodies can produce genital vasocongestion and orgasm. But, should those physical performance capacities constitute the features of human sexuality that are enshrined as universal medical norms? In other words, does it make sense from a health point of view that absence of these features constitutes a universalizable condition of sexual disorder?

Individualism

Although family medicine comes close sometimes, I know of no medical specialty that does not consider as the appropriate unit of analysis the individual person (or something smaller, such as the individual organ or organ system) (Stein, 1987). Yet, should we follow the medical model and situate sexuality in the individual person's physiology/psychology? Is sexuality better understood as an enduring or even essential quality of the self or as a phenomenon that emerges in a deeply contextualized interaction? Given the abundant usefulness of systems perspectives in therapy for sexual problems, sexuality as a concept may have more in common with friendship than intelligence (Verhulst & Heiman, 1988). One can take a history of a person's lifetime experiences with friendship (or sexuality), but each experience will only be understood when issues such as scripting, choreography, expectations, and negotiations are analyzed.

Moreover, women's sexual lives are embedded in—we might say "constructed by"—sociohistorical contexts that feminists have identified as overwhelmingly patriarchal. Focusing on women's sexuality as individual capacity and expression, as occurs within the biomedical framework, not only ignores the relationship context but ignores the larger political and ideological framework. This introduces the danger of mistaking something socially constructed and internalized for some transhistorical essence, an error that many feminists believe has happened and continues to happen in our understanding of sexuality (e.g., MacKinnon, 1987).

The individual focus of the health model "privatizes" sexual worries and difficulties, making them the result of some malfunction of a "natural" and "normal" capacity. The individual is often blamed for causing or contributing to the problem (Crawford, 1977). This contributes to shame and perpetuates ignorance about the way sexuality is socially constructed. Any sense of entitlement to sexuality given by the health model is negated, it seems to me, when the same model implies sexuality is some individual and private birthright rather than a learned and deeply socialized phenomenon.

Biological Reductionism

Finally, a health model of sexuality is inevitably focused on the biology of sexuality and on establishing biological standards for normal and abnormal function. When sexuality is seen primarily as a matter of health, research focusing on biology predominates and is considered more central and definitive than research focusing on what are seen as sociocultural "influences." This contrasts with what feminist historians have seen as the more progressive trend—an ever-widening scope of awareness of the sociocultural factors that determine women's sexual opportunities and experiences (Duggan, 1990). "Social actors possess genitals rather than the other way around," as one feminist essay put it (Schneider & Gould, 1987, p. 123).

Biological reductionism is not only antifeminist because it precludes awareness of sociohistorical factors but because it is far less likely to result in policies that limit or reverse negative social elements. Caporael and Brewer (1991), for example, note that, "in the current Western milieu, people tend to feel a lesser responsibility to redress inequities attributed to biology than inequities that arise from defects in policy, law or social structure" (p. 2). If far more research is conducted showing the influence of hormones or neurotransmitters on women's sexual responsiveness, this will have a different impact on policy than research on the influences of gender socialization or contraceptive availability.

The Medicalization of Men's
Sexuality: An Object Lesson

These hidden assumptions of the health model are not just abstract worries—they have actually come to pass in the medicalization of men's sexuality (Tiefer, 1986b, 1993, in press-a, in press-b). To make a long story short, sexual health for men has been reduced to the erectile functioning of the penis. There's a new and highly successful medical subspecialty for urologists ("impotence") along with a growth industry of diagnostic and treatment technology, all focusing on a specific physical organ with universalized standards of function and malfunction. There's no real interest in the sexuality of a person, not to mention that of a couple with a particular culture and relationship. There's just universalized biological organ norms—as for the heart or the kidney.

This medical juggernaut has resulted from the collusion of a number of social actors: men's interests in a face-saving explanation for poor "performance," societal perpetuation of a phallocentric script for sexual relations, economic incentives for physicians and manufacturers, the media appeal of medicalized sexuality topics, the absence of a strong alternative metaphor for sexuality that would stress variability, and so on. These are powerful social forces, and in the presence of continuing social pressure for sexual adequacy as defined by intercourse performance, they have created an explosive new medical development.

The clinical developments around "impotence" are supported by a tremendous quantity of basic cellular research on the penis, assuring a long life to the hunt for biological variables that might affect erectile function and that might therefore be a source for new diagnostic or treatment interventions. This past year, the first National Institutes of Health Consensus Conference on a sexuality topic was held (these conferences, several a year, go back to 1977!), and it further confirms these trends—the topic: "impotence"; the participants: overwhelmingly urologists; the outcome: a lengthy document essentially ignoring culture, the partner, lifestyle, or lifetime differences and a document reifying "erection" as the essence of men's sexuality and the medical model as the proper frame of reference for understanding and intervention.

I foresee the same outcome for women's sexuality, should some new physiological discovery about the genitalia emerge that could be developed into an industry and a clinical practice. For example, *The New York Times,* covering the 1993 American Urological Association, quoted one urologist as speculating that vascular abnormalities of the clitoris might play the same role in women's sexual problems as the extensively researched vascular penile abnormalities (Blakeslee, 1993). Discussing women's sexuality in terms of health leads directly, it seems to me, to a biologically reductionist, compartmentalized, economically driven system that will ignore far more than it will include of what women's sexuality is all about.

A Man-Centered Sexology

It is not difficult to demonstrate that sexology is man centered (Tiefer, 1991b). Despite the incorrect impression that sexology is friendly to women's interests (sex therapy seems to include a lot about communication and whole body pleasure, lesbianism is considered a normal sexual orientation alternative, and so on), there is actually active resistance to feminist analysis within the field (research dominated by biological variables, almost complete neglect of cultural variables, the perpetuation of a phallocentric, that is, coitus centered, design for heterosexual relations).

The most dramatic example of this comes from a careful examination of the nomenclature for sexual dysfunction (Boyle, 1993; Tiefer, 1988). There seems to be scrupulous gender equality in the numbers of sexual dysfunctions, and there is remarkable similarity in the types of dysfunctions listed. Yet, women's complaints as they are reported in their own voices are absent (Frank, Anderson, & Rubinstein, 1978; Hite, 1976). Women's official dysfunctions almost all are directly related to performing coitus—proper vaginal lubrication, orgasm, absence of vaginal constriction, desire, no aversions. There's nothing about love, gentleness, kissing, passion, body freedom, freedom from fear, lack of coercion, communication, emotional involvement, manual skills, cooperative contraception and infection avoidance, and so on. Despite numerous letters directed to the revisers of the official diagnostic nomenclature, there are no expected changes in the upcoming revisions.

Thus sexology, in its current phase of tunnel vision, continues to neglect many variables important to women. Popular authors and feminist activists fill the bookstores with discussions addressing women's issues and presenting diverse women's voices, but you will not see these in the professional texts, training programs, and licensing requirements or in the insurance-reimbursable complaints, sex education curricula, or government conference topics. Until the schism between the feminist literature and sexology is reduced, the male-centered paradigm of sexology is dangerous for women.

Short-Term Recommendations
for Women's "Sexual Health"

There are some short-term suggestions I can make, however, for constructive clinical and research approaches to women's sexuality even within the current paradigm.

More Clinical Concern for the Sexuality
Implications of Chronic Disease in Women

Patients and doctors alike will tell you that asking questions about sexual practices and problems is not a common part of patient-doctor interactions, whether we are talking about primary care providers or specialists. Sexual practices and concerns are usually omitted from preliminary complaint checklists in the office and from conversation during physical examination. When the medical provider is younger than the patient or when there are pressing medical concerns for the consultation, there is even more complete silence about sexual matters.

I can tell you from working in a urology department for 10 years that sexual issues are only briefly or obliquely brought up even when the consultation is about urinary tract infections or genital pain. The extent of the current discussion might be to advise women to urinate before and after intercourse, with advice given in a formulaic way. There's never a detailed discussion of sexual practices and values to understand the impact of a condition on individual or couple sexual patterns and preferences.

There is very little training currently in medical schools on sexual topics outside of genital anatomy, physiological functioning, and venereal diseases. This represents a drastic rollback from the liberal 1970s when medical education included a week or more devoted to lectures by a diverse group of visiting speakers, dozens of explicit films, and small group discussions about sexual practices and concerns of different social groups. During that brief period, a genuine consciousness-raising about sexuality as it is lived in real people's lives was part of medical training, but even with that education, studies show that doctors were still hesitant to bring sexual topics into their consultations. So clearly there is room for improvement.

More Research on the Sexuality Implications
of Disease and Medications on Women

Part of the reason for practitioner silence is that there has been very little research on how diseases affect women's sexuality (Schover & Jensen, 1988). We have every reason to suspect that diseases that affect sensory, motor, or circulatory function, or that cause fatigue, pain, or depression are likely to have an impact on sexual life, yet there is very little research on effects on women. There must be 10 studies on diabetic men, for example, for every study on diabetic women; 20 studies on effects of antihypertensive medication in men for every 1 on women; and so on.

"Lifestyle Variables" and Women's Sexuality

In a similar vein, we know next to nothing about the impact of such variables as cigarette smoking, alcohol intake, recreational drugs, exercise, diet, and the like on women's sexuality. We have looked at the impact of these variables on fertility, pregnancy, menstrual function, and infant health, but not on women's sexuality, as these factors affect interest in sex and ability to experience desire, pleasure, or become physically aroused or have orgasms.

Fourth, and Finally, Some
Sexual Research on "Taboo" Subjects

A completely neglected subject is the experience and physiology of sex during menstruation. And while we are looking at the realities of women's lives, I'd like a little research on sex and uterine fibroids. And I would really like some more basic anatomical work on the never-answered questions about clitoral anatomy and physiology raised in "A New View of the Clitoris" (in Federation of Feminist Women's Health Centers, 1981).

Long Term:
Women-Centered Sex Research

My experiences with men's medicalized sexuality and my experiences with the unyielding male-centered sexology paradigm frighten me about the future of women's "sexual health." Sexuality is so poorly understood by ordinary people that they are especially vulnerable to mystification and exploitation. As feminists, our efforts on behalf of women's sexuality should be in terms of providing and financially supporting education and conscious-ness-raising rather than health care at the present time. Sex research should raise up women's diverse voices rather than imposing a preexisting paradigm through questionnaires or measurements. And, of course, promoting women's political and economic power will have the most beneficial effect of all on women's sexuality.

Notes

1. Just to consider alternative "jurisdictions" briefly, we could consider sexuality not a matter of health but a relational issue, primarily a matter of consensual intimacy and cooperation. Or we might construe sexuality as similar to dancing, a cultural expression of human physical capacities, with many (though not all) members of a culture interested (though not necessarily participating), in very different styles and settings. It was to make this point that I considered titling this chapter, "Is Sex More Like Dancing or Digestion?"

2. This sentence, of course, could also read ". . . in large part because of its 'legitimacy' and 'moral neutrality,' its confident reliance on the 'objective facts' of 'biological nature'."

3. And, as always with behavior, it could turn out that "the patient" was a tournament canasta champion and earned her living that way!

References

Barsky, A. J. (1988). *Worried sick: Our troubled quest for wellness.* Boston: Little, Brown.

Blakeslee, S. (1993, June 2). New therapies are helping men to overcome impotence. *The New York Times,* p. C7.

Boyle, M. (1993). Sexual dysfunction or heterosexual dysfunction? *Feminism and Psychology, 3,* 73-88.

Caporael, L. R., & Brewer, M. B. (1991). The quest for human nature: Social and scientific issues in evolutionary psychology. *Journal of Social Issues, 47,* 1-9.

Conrad, P., & Kern, R. (Eds.). (1981). *The sociology of health and illness: Critical perspectives.* New York: St. Martin's.

Crawford, R. (1977). You are dangerous to your health: The ideology and politics of victim blaming. *International Journal of Health Services, 7,* 663-680.

DeLamater, J. (1981). The social control of sexuality. *Annual Review of Sociology, 7,* 263-290.

Duggan, L. (1990). Review essay: From instincts to politics: Writing the history of sexuality in the U.S. *Journal of Sex Research, 27,* 95-109.

Edwards, S. (1981). *Female sexuality and the law: A study of constructs of female sexuality as they inform statute and legal proceedings.* Oxford: Martin Robertson.

Ehrenreich, B., Hess, E., & Jacobs, G. (1986). *Re-making love: The feminization of sex.* Garden City, NY: Anchor, Doubleday.

Featherstone, M., Hepworth, M., & Turner, B. S. (Eds.). (1991). *The body: Social process and cultural theory.* Newbury Park, CA: Sage.

Federation of Feminist Women's Health Centers. (1981). *A new view of a woman's body.* New York: Simon & Schuster.

Frank, E., Anderson, C., & Rubinstein, D. (1978). Frequency of sexual dysfunction in "normal" couples. *New England Journal of Medicine, 299,* 111-115.

Freedman, E. B., & D'Emilio, J. (1988). *Intimate matters: A history of sexuality in America.* New York: Harper & Row.

Hite, S. (1976). *The Hite report.* New York: Macmillan.

Koedt, A. (1973). The myth of the vaginal orgasm. In A. Koedt, E. Levine, & A. Rapone (Eds.), *Radical feminism.* New York: Quadrangle.

MacKinnon, C. A. (1987). A feminist/political approach: "Pleasure under patriarchy." In J. H. Geer & W. T. O'Donohue (Eds.), *Theories of human sexuality* (pp. 65-90). New York: Plenum.

Masters, W. H., & Johnson, V. E. (1966). *Human sexual response.* Boston: Little, Brown.

Mishler, E. G. (1981). Viewpoint: Critical perspectives on the biomedical model. In E. G. Mishler, L. R. AmaraSingham, S. T. Hauser, R. Liem, S. D. Osherson, & N. E. Waxler, *Social contexts of health, illness and patient care* (pp. 1-23). Cambridge, MA: Cambridge University Press.

Potter, J., & Wetherell, M. (1987). *Discourse and social psychology: Beyond attitudes and behavior.* Sage: London.

Sahli, N. (1984). *Women and sexuality in America: A bibliography.* Boston: G. K. Hall.

Sahli, N. (1990). Sexuality and women's sexual nature. In R. D. Apple (Ed.), *Women, health, and medicine in America: A historical handbook* (pp. 81-100). New York: Garland.

Schneider, B. E., & Gould, M. (1987). Female sexuality: Looking back into the future. In B. B. Hess & M. M. Ferree (Eds.), *Analyzing gender: A handbook of social science research* (pp. 120-153). Newbury Park, CA: Sage.

Schover, L. R., & Jensen, S. B. (1988). *Sexuality and chronic illness.* New York: Guilford.

Schur, E. M. (1984). *Labeling women deviant: Gender, stigma, and social control.* New York: Random House.

Scott, S., & Morgan, D. (Eds.). (1993). *Body matters: Essays on the sociology of the body.* London: Falmer.

Stein, H. F. (1987). Polarities in the identity of family medicine: A psychocultural analysis. In W. J. Doherty, C. E. Christianson, & M. B. Sussman (Eds.), *Family medicine: The maturing of a discipline.* New York: Haworth.

Tiefer, L. (1986a). "Am I normal?": The question of sex. In C. Tavris (Ed.), *Everywoman's emotional well-being* (pp. 54-71). New York: Doubleday.

Tiefer, L. (1986b). In pursuit of the perfect penis: The medicalization of male sexuality. *American Behavioral Scientist, 29,* 579-599.

Tiefer, L. (1987). Social constructionism and the study of human sexuality. In P. Shaver & C. Hendrick (Eds.), *Review of personality and social psychology: Vol. 7. Sex and gender* (pp. 70-94). Newbury Park, CA: Sage.

Tiefer, L. (1988). A feminist critique of the sexual dysfunction nomenclature. *Women and Therapy, 7,* 5-21.

Tiefer, L. (1990). *Sexual biology and the symbolism of the natural.* Paper presented at the International Academy of Sex Research, Sigtuna, Sweden, and subsequently published (in German translation) in *Zeitschrift für Sexualforschung, 2,* 97-108 (1991).

Tiefer, L. (1991a). Historical, scientific, clinical and feminist criticisms of "the human sexual response cycle" model. *Annual Review of Sexuality, 2,* 1-23.

Tiefer, L. (1991b). Commentary on the status of sex research: Feminism, sexuality and sexology. *Journal of Psychology and Human Sexuality, 4,* 5-42.

Tiefer, L. (1993). A progress report on the medicalization of male sexuality. *Zeitschrift für Sexualforschung, 6,* 119-131.

Tiefer, L. (in press-a). The medicalization of "impotence": Normalizing phallocentrism. *Gender & Society.*

Tiefer, L. (in press-b). Three crises facing sexology. *Archives of Sexual Behavior.*

Verhulst, J., & Heiman, J. R. (1988). A systems perspective on sexual desire. In S. R. Leiblum & R. C Rosen (Eds.), *Sexual desire disorders.* New York: Guilford.

Weeks, J. (1981). *Sex, politics and society: The regulation of sexuality since 1800.* London: Longman.

16

Problems and Prospects of Contemporary Abortion Provision

Jean Hunt
Carole Joffe

Legal abortion—albeit with restrictions—seems assured for the foreseeable future in the United States, due both to the Supreme Court *Casey* decision of 1992, which reaffirmed the essential finding of *Roe v. Wade*, and the election, also that year, of Bill Clinton, a "prochoice" president. Nonetheless, access to abortion services for many women in this country is in serious jeopardy. In starkest terms, there are not enough abortion facilities in this country, and there are not enough providers willing to perform abortions. At present, some 83% of all U.S. counties do not have any abortion services (Henshaw & Van Vort, 1992, p. 38). It is estimated that only about one third of all currently active obstetricians/gynecologists are trained to do abortions, and the number of hospital residencies that train in this procedure has been steadily decreasing, with only 12% now routinely offering training in first trimester abortion procedures to their residents and 6.7% of residencies offering training in second trimester techniques (Grimes, 1992; McKay, 1992). This chapter will discuss some of the factors accounting for this shortage of abortion providers and some of the strategies now under way to address this problem.

Historical Background

It is tempting of course to attribute the present crisis in abortion provision directly to the activities of the contemporary antiabortion movement. An organized antiabortion movement, which began to mobilize in this country immediately after the *Roe* decision in 1973, entered a particularly militant—

often violent—stage starting around 1988, with the formation of Operation Rescue and similar groups, and this violence has only intensified since the election of Clinton. Clinic blockades and "invasions" have become common-place (National Abortion Federation [NAF], 1993) as have such tactics as introducing butyric acid and other nausea-inducing gases into abortion-providing facilities. A number of clinics have been firebombed and otherwise destroyed. Most pertinent, for our purposes, *abortion providers and other clinic staff* have, in the 1990s, become particular targets of antiabortion militants. Though long subject to picketing in front of their workplaces, abortion personnel have recently been the targets of a campaign of escalating violence and intimidation. "Nowhere to hide campaigns" have brought antiabortion-ists to individual providers' homes, churches, and even favorite restaurants. Providers have been the subjects of "wanted posters" displayed prominently in their communities. Children of abortion staff have been singled out for harassment at schools and at their homes. Medical students have been targeted by antiabortionists, as, for example, in a recent mailing to first-year students across the country that contained vulgar jokes directed at abortion providers. This wave of intimidation culminated in spring 1993 with the murder of David Gunn, an abortion-providing physician, in front of a clinic in Pensa-cola, Florida. Gunn's murder, while denounced by some antiabortion groups, was seemingly condoned by others, and in any event does not appear to have weakened the resolve of antiabortion militants to target individual abortion providers for terrorist campaigns.

No doubt, such activity does have a chilling effect on abortion provision—leading some already in this field to retreat and others, at earlier stages of their careers, to shy away from this work. Yet, it would be a mistake to attribute the shortage of abortion providers wholly to the phenomenon of contemporary antiabortion activity. Rather, physicians' reluctance to provide abortions has far deeper roots, dating back to conflicts within U.S. medicine in the nineteenth century.

As a significant body of recent scholarship has demonstrated (Luker, 1984; Mohr, 1978; Petchesky, 1990; Smith-Rosenberg, 1985), the abortion issue played a key role in the mid-nineteenth century struggle of "regular" or "elite" physicians (that is, those who were university trained) to attain professional dominance over the wide range of "irregular" medical practitioners—heal-ers, homeopaths, midwives, and the like—who had flourished throughout the first part of the nineteenth century. The American Medical Association (AMA), founded by the "regulars" in 1847, made the criminalization of abortion—until then largely unregulated in American society—one of the highest priorities of the new organization. The argument of these physicians, in brief, was that abortion was both an "immoral" act and a medically dangerous one, given the incompetence of many of the practitioners then providing abortion. Abortion was a particularly fruitful territory over which to stake the regulars' claims of professional monopoly, both because so much of the irregulars' activity apparently was abortion based and because much abortion work was being done by lay people with no claims whatsoever to medical credentials.

The AMA campaign to criminalize abortion, which included other allies as well, was highly successful, and by 1880 all states had statutes regulating abortion. The objective of these regular physicians, however, was not simply to abolish all abortions. Rather, the AMA argument, which ultimately prevailed, was that physicians should control the terms under which "approved" abortions were performed—that is, "legal" abortions were now to be confined to those performed in a hospital, for "medically indicated" reasons. As is well known, one result of this "century of criminalization," which lasted until the *Roe v. Wade* decision in 1973, was a flourishing market in illegal abortion; in the period immediately before *Roe*, some estimates put the number of illegal abortions as high as 1.2 million a year. Those providing the illegal abortions were a combination of lay abortionists, women attempting self-abortion, and physicians, with one observer estimating that the latter accounted for about one third of all illegal abortions (Callahan, 1970, p. 131).

These earlier struggles over abortion, entwined as they were with professionalization efforts, have created a complex legacy for late twentieth-century abortion practice. For even though a substantial majority of contemporary physicians now see *abortion* as a valid choice for a woman to make, the figure of the "abortionist" is still received far more ambivalently. This ambivalence, we argue, stems from still salient images of the abortion climate of the pre-*Roe* era. From the nineteenth century, the prevailing image of the abortionist is the "quack," the ill-trained practitioner who scarcely merits the title of "physician." From the twentieth-century period up till *Roe*, the dominant image of the illegal abortionist is the "butcher," the physician who is both incompetent and exploitative and who presumably is engaged in abortion work because he cannot make a living in mainstream medicine. Indeed, in interviews one of us has done with a group of dedicated prochoice physicians, who were involved, as a matter of conscience, in abortion activity before *Roe*, it is striking how even this group had to struggle to overcome earlier negative messages about illegal abortionists. As one of these physicians, who was a third-generation obstetrician-gynecologist, remarked, "In my family, the worst thing that could be said about anybody was that he was an abortionist." Another, speaking of the climate of the 1950s, said, "*Abortionist* was such a dirty word then, it was one step above a pervert" (Joffe, 1991, p. 53).

In a related manner, the present crisis in abortion provision can also be traced to the lukewarm response of the medical establishment to the question of abortion services in the period immediately after *Roe*. The story of abortion after legalization is one of marginalization and isolation from most sectors of the medical community. As indicated, abortion training has not become a routine part of the education of obstetrician/gynecologists. Most hospitals have not established abortion services. Individual physicians who offer abortions often find themselves subject to various sanctions by medical colleagues (Imber, 1986).

Obviously, this marginalization of abortion services has been caused by a number of factors. Beyond the controversy and stigma that often accompany abortion, certainly one reason for the low status of abortion within mainstream obstetrics/gynecology is simply the technically unchallenging nature of the abortion procedure—especially the first trimester abortions performed by vacuum suction, which account for 89% of all abortions performed in the United States (Henshaw & Van Vort, 1992, p. 38). Numerous providers, in our encounters with them, have acknowledged that the actual performance of abortions—especially when this work is not mixed with other duties—can become tedious and, especially for those interested in advancing in academic medicine, devoid of the intellectual challenges found in other areas of obstetrics and gynecology.

An additional disincentive for abortion provision is the low rate of remuneration for this work. In marked contrast to most other medical procedures, the cost of abortion in most localities has stayed well below inflation. David Grimes, a leading student of abortion services, has pointed out the average cost of a first trimester abortion in 1991—below $300—is, in 1991 dollars, about half that of the cost of such a procedure at the time of legalization (Grimes, 1992).

Ironically, one of the key achievements in the *Roe* era of prochoice physicians and their allies—the development of the freestanding abortion clinic—has also contributed to the present marginalization (and low cost) of abortion services. The freestanding model, developed in the early 1970s in states that had already liberalized their abortion laws, offered a way to deliver outpatient abortion, under local anesthesia, with personnel—including a specially trained "abortion counselor"—with a particular commitment to this work. This freestanding model of abortion service was an attractive alternative to the more expensive, more cumbersome hospital-based abortion, which involved general anesthesia and, quite often, staff who might be themselves opposed to abortion, and thus hostile to abortion recipients. The clinic model continued to flourish after *Roe* and currently accounts for about 86% of all abortions performed in the United States (Henshaw & Van Vort, 1992, p. 45).

In retrospect, however, the very success of the clinic model seemingly has contributed to the avoidance of abortion services on the part of mainstream medical institutions. The original vision of the pioneers of the freestanding clinic—that the clinic would have a strong link to teaching hospitals and other medical institutions (Hodgson & Ward, 1981)—did not materialize in most communities. Rather, the existence of the clinics facilitated a situation in which most individual OB/GYNs could maintain a prochoice position and yet not perform abortions, in which OB/GYN residencies could decreasingly require abortion training as a matter of course, in which hospitals could readily yield to antiabortion pressure to abolish abortion services—all on the premise that "the clinics" would take care of those women needing abortions and would accommodate those physicians who sought abortion training.

In sum, the present situation of abortion provision in this country is one in which a relatively small number of providers are performing most procedures and in which these procedures are increasingly concentrated only in certain metropolitan areas. Many of those now performing abortions, moreover, are "graying" physicians, with memories of the medical horrors of the pre-*Roe* era, and current obstetrical/gynecological residencies are not doing an adequate job of training a new generation to replace the considerable number of currently active providers who are nearing retirement.

This physician shortage translates itself into situations of extreme difficulty for clinics. A clinic in Philadelphia took the following steps, between 1989 and 1992, to find new abortion providers willing to work with them. The executive director met with the chairs of three local OB/GYN departments in an attempt to identify interested attending physicians or residents or to promote a training program at her clinic. One chair told her, "Abortion is a dirty job but someone has to do it." This chair had recently closed his hospital's abortion clinic and was referring everyone seen in their OB/GYN clinics who wanted abortions to freestanding clinics. Letters were mailed to every graduating OB/GYN resident and fellow in the area seeking interested physicians. Mailing lists of progressive physician organizations were used for mailings that explained the problem and asked for help. Ads were run in local and national papers and in journals. There was not one positive response to any of these attempts. One national ad did elicit an inquiry from a physician in New York, who when he discovered there was a credentialing and reference process involved hung up the phone. It was clear he thought that the clinic had no standards for physicians doing abortions and would be willing to take anybody. A clinic director in Atlanta, Georgia, was even more aggressive, and mailed out inquiries to every single graduating OB/GYN resident in the nation. She also received no replies.

In addition to the historical problems that have kept physicians from performing abortions, and the current attack on abortion providers from the right wing, the final blow to the teaching of abortion services has come through the struggle over insurance funding. When the Hyde Amendment was first passed in 1977, it eliminated the use of federal funds for the provision of abortion services. This had a dramatic effect on the availability of services to women insured by the Medical Assistance (Medicaid) program, but it additionally had a hidden and in many ways more deadly effect on the training of abortion providers.

Most physicians learn to do procedures in clinics of teaching hospitals where there is a group of patients needing services. For example, residents in OB/GYN learn to do births, hysterectomies, and tubal ligations on clinic patients, insured by Medical Assistance, who come for care to the OB/GYN clinic. When Medical Assistance funds are not available for a procedure, that procedure ceases to be available in the teaching hospital setting. A poor woman would have to pay upward of $800 out of pocket for a hospital-based abortion, as opposed to a procedure in an outpatient clinic costing between $225 and $400. Therefore there is no way to build the routine teaching of abortion procedures into OB/GYN residencies without sending residents off site for training. This option is cumbersome, time-consuming, and not ideal for already overworked residents. Unless a resident is strongly personally motivated to receive training in abortion procedures, this training will not be routinely available during the course of training.

Solutions

Various solutions to this provider shortage are now under discussion in the medical community and within the prochoice and health reform movements. One of the most significant initiatives has been undertaken by the National Abortion Federation (NAF), an organization of abortion providers. In 1990 NAF and the American College of Obstetrics and Gynecology jointly sponsored a symposium on the crisis in abortion provision (NAF, 1991). The recommendations resulting from the symposium fall into three general areas: pressuring relevant medical organizations to develop firmer standards for the routine integration of abortion training within medical education, especially within obstetrics/gynecology residencies; training physicians other than obstetricians/gynecologists, such as family practitioners and "midlevel" practitioners (e.g., nurse midwives, nurse practitioners, and physicians' assistants) to perform abortions; and devising strategies to build stronger public support—both within medicine and in the general community—for the abortion provider.

RU 486

The development of RU 486 as an alternative method of providing abortions in the first trimester of pregnancy also presents the possibility of increasing access to abortion. RU 486 holds the promise of providing a way for women to get abortion services at a wide range of primary care settings, in privacy, without the kind of public attention to them and to their providers currently focused on clinics. Should RU 486 become widely available in the United States—and, as of fall 1993, such a prospect appears several years off, at best—OB/GYNs and family practice physicians would be able to provide abortions for their patients in the privacy of their offices.

Even if the availability of RU 486 is achieved, however, there would still remain some problems. One is that private practitioners will have to learn to do more extensive counseling and listening to women who arrive in their offices uncertain about a pregnancy. Historically, the freestanding clinics have developed counseling protocols that are designed to assist a woman in making the correct choice for her and guaranteeing that she is not seeking an abortion because of coercion from a partner or parent. Private physicians have not necessarily received training in these kinds of counseling services, and they will need to learn how to do this effectively and sensitively.

The second problem is that RU 486 will not be able to be used for every woman seeking an abortion, thereby requiring the maintenance of a skilled group of clinicians able to perform surgical abortion. We fear that this group might become even more visible and vulnerable in a system where there is even less incentive for physicians to learn the techniques involved in vacuum aspiration abortions and to maintain their skill level. Medical procedures are performed effectively and skillfully by those who do them frequently and regularly. Therefore the health care system is obligated to develop ways to teach surgical abortion techniques and sustain that technique in the clinicians who will be required to provide these services for women. One potential solution to this problem is that physicians who provide RU 486 be required to provide backup abortion procedures when they are needed for women in their practices. Another would be a grouping of physicians agreeing to support, defend, and refer to a practice or clinic that will continue to provide surgical abortion procedures post-RU 486.

The Prochoice Movement and Health Care Reform

Finally, we will address the possible roles in the immediate future of the prochoice movement and the health reform movement in increasing access to abortion. We stress that in the following pages we speak both as observers and as participants in these overlapping movements.

It has taken the prochoice movement a long time to overcome a historical antipathy to abortion providers. Until recently, the prochoice movement has poured almost all of its energy into the struggle for preservation of the legal right to abortion in both legislative and judicial settings. The providers of the medical service have been invisible to the movement and, in some cases, unwanted guests at the table. This has grown to some extent out of the historical conditions described above and out of a climate in which abortion is seen as a necessary evil (raising questions about who performs this necessary evil) rather than as a legitimate piece of medical care historically required and needed by women.

A simple example of the different approach to the medical service between the prochoice and antiabortion movements has been the extent to which these movements have attached their own personal medical care to their principles. One of us worked at a maternity hospital in Philadelphia during the 1980s and was aware that we routinely received calls from women inquiring about whether our obstetricians and nurse midwives performed or referred people for abortion services. These calls were from women in the antiabortion movement who were prepared to boycott the hospital if any providers were involved with the provision of abortion, even though those services were not provided on site. There has never been a corresponding move by prochoice women to question their OB/GYNs about a willingness to provide abortions. When women are asked if they have ever inquired about their doctors' position on abortions, they are often stunned and amazed that this has not occurred to them. Thus a scenario has emerged in which OB/GYNs routinely hear from the antiabortion movement as potential consumers but never hear from prochoice people. It is clear to the physicians that they have more to lose by providing abortion services than by refraining. This has encouraged the strange development by which a large number of OB/GYNs count themselves as personally prochoice but do not perform the service in their own practice (Imber, 1986).

The obvious solution to this problem is a widespread campaign that encourages prochoice women of all ages to question their OB/GYNs and family practitioners about abortion services. If a physician does not provide services and is not willing to provide them, women ought to be prepared to see physicians who are.

Many clinics that have sustained the provision of abortion for the past 20 years also provide high-quality well woman gynecological care. Prochoice women ought to consider switching their routine care to these clinics, bringing their health care dollars to the clinics as the most tangible sign of their support.

Abortion providers, who have an understanding of the abortion experience, which is deeper and more complex than the understanding of many other segments of the prochoice movement, need to be invited to the prochoice table, invited to educate the rest of the movement about the reality of the lives of those seeking services. They need to be listened to in terms of the development of legislative and judicial strategies as well as organizing drives to extend support for reproductive rights in communities. Many women working in clinics are African American, Latina, and Asian and are often working class. Their experience and knowledge have not been used by the prochoice movement, and their perspective is critical. This coalition between providers and activists provides a much stronger base for future reproductive rights work and is pivotal to our long-term success.

Rachel Atkins, a physician's assistant who has provided abortions and taught the procedure to OB/GYN residents at the Vermont Women's Health Center, has observed,

> As a provider of women's health care for over 15 years, it is absolutely clear to me that there are not two groups of women—women who have abortions and women who have babies. We are the same group of women at different times in our lives. This polarized thinking that allows women and their health care providers to be targeted, disrespected and marginalized has got to stop. (personal communication)

This observation reinforces our understanding that the fight for abortion must be placed in the context of a fight to provide high-quality health care services for all women, regardless of their reproductive status. One cannot provide one piece of reproductive rights without providing the whole pie. Much of the women's health movement in this country has suffered from a narrow focus on abortion rights, as if the securing of these rights would be adequate to assure women healthy lives throughout our life cycle. To this end, the abortion rights movement must join forces with a movement for structural health care reform that extends comprehensive health care services to all women, increases funding for women's services and research, and improves the quality of primary care services currently available to women and children.

As of fall 1993, the prospects of abortion coverage within the Clinton administration's health reform package are highly uncertain. As a possible harbinger of battles to come, prochoice forces within both the House of Representatives and the Senate have recently received a major setback in their attempts to lift the Hyde Amendment from the budget process. This setback appears to indicate that we will have great difficulty in getting abortion services funded under national health care reform. Additionally, as states embark on reform, they too have the power to restrict the allocation of state monies to the coverage of abortion services. In fact, states can restrict family planning monies as well, if they are inclined.

These realities mean that the prochoice movement has to be much more active and visible in the movement for health care reform, and has to state such a strong case for the coverage of abortion services that we can overcome this most difficult obstacle. The right wing has promoted a very effective argument against coverage of abortion services by posing it as a tax issue and by stimulating racist and anti-poor people and antiwoman rhetoric to isolate support for Medical Assistance coverage.

We can answer the Right by making clear that, under national health care reform, a restriction on coverage for abortion services would potentially effect every single woman in the United States. No one would have funding for an abortion procedure unless she paid extra for this benefit in her insurance package. The strategy to oppose such restrictions ought to be broad based, linked with unions, health care activists, community organizations, college students, high school students, public health workers and administrators, consumer advocates, and legislators. In all these settings, several simple arguments can be made.

1. It is immoral to force women to have children they do not want and cannot raise.

2. Abortion will always be a required part of medical care, but we can decrease its incidence by promoting broad-based women's health care services.

3. Abortion is the most common surgical procedure performed on women of reproductive age, and one cannot build a health care payment plan that excludes the single most common procedure.

4. Without coverage for abortion services, infant mortality and maternal mortality increase. The health care system cannot afford to pay these increased costs, which are totally unnecessary. And individual women should not be forced to undergo unnecessary suffering.

5. The devastation in human and family life that results from a policy of enforced childbearing presents public health and safety questions that cannot be ignored. There is more than adequate data to document this devastation and we must begin to design policies to reduce rather than increase its incidence.

If we can positively affect the direction of health care reform, it will have an immediate impact on the training of future abortion providers. Hospital clinics will have little rationale for not providing abortions within the clinic setting. If funding is available, activists will be more successful in forcing hospitals to provide the procedure, and thus the necessary training. This would have an immediate impact in rural areas and areas in which there are few freestanding clinics.

A victory in the national health care reform arena would also confirm that abortion is a legitimate part of women's health care, not separate and different than everything else that women need to maintain healthy bodies and lives.

A strategy that sees building a broader based movement, which allies itself with health care reform and actively reaches out to abortion providers, can only help solidify the position of providers within the medical system and will help to defend and protect them within their communities. For physicians currently wanting to provide services, but afraid, such developments would help encourage them to step forward.

A climate in which abortion is not stigmatized is one in which the provider is not stigmatized. A climate in which abortion is seen as a routine but, we hope, not frequent part of health care is a climate in which it becomes more available. A climate that recognizes the unique health care needs of women and that is responsive to those needs is one in which abortion providers will be seen as good rather than as sinister people. If the majority of the public could see the real providers, see their intense commitment to women and women's health, see their courage and humor and persistence in the face of unbelievable attacks, then much of the current belief system that sustains a negative image of providers would erode.

References

Callahan, D. (1970). *Abortion: Law, choice, and morality.* New York: Macmillan.

Grimes, D. A. (1992). Clinicians who provide abortions: The thinning ranks. *Obstetrics and Gynecology, 80*(4), 719-723.

Henshaw, S., & Van Vort, J. (1992). *Abortion factbook: Readings, trends and state and local data to 1988.* New York: Alan Guttmacher Institute.

Hodgson, J., & Ward, R. (1981). The provision and organization of abortion and sterilization services in the United States. In J. Hodgson (Ed.), *Abortion and sterilization: Medical and social aspects* (pp. 519-541). New York: Academic Press.

Imber, J. (1986). *Abortion and the private practice of medicine.* New Haven, CT: Yale University Press.

Joffe, C. (1991). Portraits of three "physicians of conscience": Abortion before legalization in the United States. *Journal of the History of Sexuality, 2*(1), 46-67.

Luker, K. (1984). *Abortion and the politics of motherhood.* Berkeley: University of California Press.

McKay, H. T. (1992). *Abortion training in U.S. obstetrics and gynecology residency programs: A follow-up study.* Paper delivered at annual meetings of the National Abortion Federation, San Diego.

Mohr, J. (1978). *Abortion in America: The origins and evolution of national policy, 1800-1900.* New York: Oxford University Press.

National Abortion Federation. (1991). *Who will provide abortion? Results of a symposium.* Washington, DC: Author.

National Abortion Federation. (1993). *Incidents of violence and disruption against abortion providers in 1992.* Washington, DC: Author.

Petchesky, R. (1990). *Abortion and woman's choice: The state, sexuality and reproductive freedom.* Boston: Northeastern University Press.

Smith-Rosenberg, C. (1985). The abortion movement and the AMA, 1850-1880. In C. Smith-Rosenberg, *Disorderly conduct: Visions of gender in Victorian America* (pp. 217-244). New York: Knopf.

17

Women and HIV

Mary Driscoll
Mardge Cohen
Patricia Kelly
Deane Taylor
Mildred Williamson
Gigi Nicks

Worldwide, a stage has been set for the relationship of women and HIV. The acted upon are women. The actors are poverty, racism, gender inequality, and violence, plus homelessness, chemical dependency, or simply the inability to refuse unprotected sex from fear of personal or economic instability or both. As long as the condition of the majority of women is one of powerlessness and dependency, the HIV epidemic will not be contained.

This chapter discusses the epidemiology of women and HIV, explores areas of social and biomedical research agendas, briefly looks at service delivery needs, and addresses HIV as a public health problem. There is much more to be said about women and HIV than these brief pages will allow, and by necessity some issues have been highlighted over others. The authors of this section are advocates of women and children's health and believe that to work with women with HIV is to work for human rights and social justice.

Epidemiology and Transmission

As of 1992, estimates by the World Health Organization cite 12.6 million people with HIV infection, 36% of whom are women (CDC, 1992a). Women represent the fastest growing group of new cases of AIDS in the United States, Latin America, and other large urban areas where there are high rates of other sexually transmitted diseases, IV drug use, or both (CDC, 1992b;

Schietinger, 1990). In 1992 in the United States, women accounted for 13.4% of persons diagnosed with AIDS as compared with 6% of cases in 1985 (CDC, 1992a). In New York City and major cities in Sub-Saharan Africa, AIDS is the leading cause of death among women 12 to 44 years of age (CDC, 1990). These global statistics show HIV as a growing public health epidemic, particularly in women and especially in women of reproductive age. To a greater degree than in men, the effect of HIV disease in women affects whole families. In the United States alone, the Centers for Disease Control projects that, by the year 2000, the number of children and adolescents orphaned by HIV will exceed 82,000 (CDC, 1993). In African countries, where the epidemic is more far reaching, effects on families will be even more devastating. The HIV epidemic raises issues of family policy, such as long-term care of infected children, guardianship, and medical care and subsidies for undocumented families as sickness and death of parents and siblings occur.

Little statistical data exist about the course of HIV disease in women and its impact on their lives. To date, there are no published natural history studies of women with HIV infection. (The first national natural history study received funding and began the planning phase in October 1993.) Most current data about women relate to pregnancy and maternal fetal transmission. These data tend to conceptualize women as vectors of HIV transmission (Hankins & Handley, 1992). However, the two longitudinal studies of women and HIV contradict the above impression. The studies are conducted in Rwanda, Africa, and Providence, Rhode Island. They show similar demographic information about women with HIV infection. The cohort participants were poor and young and had several children. Most had only one lifetime partner and their risk factor for HIV transmission was heterosexual contact. The mortality rate for women in these studies is 7% every 2 years (Carpenter, Mayer, Fisher, Desai, & Durand, 1989).

Homelessness and domestic violence have been strongly correlated with HIV infection in women (Chavkin & Paone, 1991; Torres, Lefkowitz, Kales, & Brickner, 1990; Worth, Drucker, Eric, & Pivnick, 1990; Zolpa et al., 1991). Estimates of HIV seroprevalence among homeless persons vary geographically, but overall are much higher than in the general population. One Chicago study of the social service needs of HIV-infected women stated that 27% of the women needed long-term housing assistance (over 1 month) and 15% needed emergency housing assistance (under 1 month) (Carr, 1991). Several studies have found high prevalence rates of domestic violence among women at risk for HIV infection (Chavkin & Paone, 1991; Fullilove, Fullilove, Gasch, & Smith, 1992; Worth et al., 1990). A pilot study of 60 HIV-positive women conducted in the Women and Children's HIV Program at Cook County Hospital found that there was an 83% prevalence rate of domestic violence.

Both domestic violence and homelessness affect women's general health and compliance with health programs (Elvy, 1985). More studies are needed that look at these factors in relation to the progression of HIV disease. Also needed are strong and forceful public policies promoting low-income housing and gender equality.

Women of color are disproportionately represented in the HIV-infected population. In the United States, women made up 13.4% of reported AIDS cases (CDC, 1992a). African Americans make up 12% of the U.S. population, but African American women are 62% of the women reported to have AIDS. Latinos make up 7% of the U.S. population but Latinas make up 20% of women reported to have AIDS (CDC, 1992a).

This disproportionate burden is caused by the same social, economic, and racist reasons that cause women of color to have higher infant mortality and morbidity rates (David & Collins, 1991), higher incidence of violence and greater use of drugs in their communities, and in general higher incidence and rates of most public health hazards and many life-threatening diseases. Specifically, because HIV is transmitted through blood and body fluids, it is the high incidence of IV and other drug use and lack of awareness of sexual transmission of HIV from men to women that is asymmetrically assigning the burden of HIV disease to communities of color (Flaskerud & Nyamathi, 1990). Programs that effectively combat substance abuse and provide preventive education and positive behavior change cannot be undertaken on a widespread basis in the current societal climate of victim blaming and false morality.

In most urban areas in the United States, the number of drug users seeking treatment far outnumbers the available treatment program openings (NIDA, 1991-1992). While studies show that it is possible to decrease HIV transmission between people who use injectable drugs, such as with needle exchange programs (Kirp, 1993), our society continues to taboo these methods as so-called contributors to moral decay.

In the United States, 57% of women report IV drug use as the primary source of infection. Globally, however, it is heterosexual contact that is clearly the major vehicle for transmission (World Health Organization, 1990), and here in the United States heterosexual transmission is increasing (Johnson & Laga, 1990). HIV appears to be transmitted sexually more efficiently from men to women. The reasons for this are multifactorial (Johnson & Laga, 1990), but the importance of sexual behavior change regarding use of condoms by men and a full speed ahead approach toward a female-controlled viricide can be appreciated in light of this information. Unfortunately, like the current societal approach to drug issues, open discussions of sexuality are discouraged or prohibited.

Research Issues

Sexism and Biomedical Research

Women historically are underrepresented in all biomedical research cohorts and clinical trials. Recently this gender bias was widely publicized in the all-male study of aspirin prophylaxis in coronary artery disease (Ridher, Manson, Buring, Goldraber, & Hennekens, 1991). The research community maintains this gender imbalance in AIDS-HIV studies. Men have been the focus of epidemiological and natural history studies as well as of clinical drug trials for the treatment of HIV and associated opportunistic infections. Until recently, most published research has focused on women only as vectors of infection to children and sexual partners (Levine, 1991). Even as the percentage of U.S. AIDS cases has increased steadily, from 6% in 1985 to 13.4% in 1992 (CDC, 1992a; Ellerbrock, Bush, Chamberland, & Optoby, 1991)—and in addition AIDS is now the leading cause of death in women of childbearing age in the New York metropolitan area (Chu, Buehler, & Berhelman, 1990)—few women with AIDS or at risk of acquiring HIV infection have been enrolled in HIV/AIDS research studies (Levine, 1991; Murphy, 1991). For instance, in the original trial documenting AZT efficacy, only 13 of the 282 subjects were women (Fischl et al., 1987).

In addition, a traditional bias against medical research exists within low-income and minority communities, where the majority of HIV-infected women live. The perception that all research is racist and concerns about being used as guinea pigs are primarily the legacy of the Tuskegee syphilis study (Jones, 1981) in which treatment for syphilis was withheld from a cohort of African American men. The clinical trials of oral contraceptives on Puerto Rican women (Potts, Feldblum, Chi, Liao, & Fuertes, 1982) and the sterilization without knowledge or informed consent of African American women by physicians are examples of the real vulnerability of minority women at the hands of health care providers with nonclinical agendas.

Just as in other areas of research, it is misleading to assume that the research findings from all (or even predominantly) male cohorts will be valid for women. Women must be the subject of epidemiological and clinical drug trials. Women's physiology relative to drug metabolism is frequently affected by factors such as age and weight; it is dangerous to assume no such impact from hormones, percentage of body fat, menstrual cycle changes, or other less tangible female-specific factors. The specific questions that exist can only be answered by involving large numbers of women in biomedical research trials. Questions include the following:

- Does the natural history of HIV disease differ in women?

- Are there any unique manifestations of HIV disease in women?
- What are the gynecological manifestations of HIV disease?
- Are the effects of the various drugs the same in women?
- What are the side effects of the various drugs in women?
- How does access to care affect clinical outcomes for women?
- How do social forces, such as poverty, race, ethnicity, and gender, interact with one another and affect the psychological and biomedical outcomes of women with HIV?

Ethical Issues of Women and HIV Research

Participation in clinical trials of women with HIV may result in material as well as clinical gains. The most obvious benefit for someone who has a potentially fatal illness with no cure is the chance to access the latest medical treatments. Also, trials offer concrete psychological advantages as participants feel they maximize their involvement in control over the disease processes. They may gain a sense of personal contribution in assisting the discovery of an effective treatment or cure for the disease. Participants in clinical trials often receive extra attention, education, and support from research staff, who are generally responsible for fewer patients than clinical staff.

The use of incentives as enticement into studies has tangible implications for women. Patient-focused research staff argue that study participation should result in direct benefit to individual women. The use of cash or material incentives or enhanced clinical care has been seen both to facilitate recruitment efforts by making it easier for a woman to agree to study participation (C. Booth, Research R.N., ACTG Clinical Trials, Cook County Hospital, personal communication, 1993) and also to provide study participants with a small but concrete return for their time. Meal vouchers, baby supplies, or a $10 transportation stipend (which can be used for cab fare or put away for unaffordable necessities) will make it easier for a woman to attend a study visit than the minimal bus or subway token. But are women agreeing to study enrollment only to get the $10? Is real informed consent possible in such a situation? And at what point do these incentives become coercive to poor women? In retrospect, there is agreement that paid funeral expenses for long-term Tuskegee study participants and the misplaced sense of being cared for by study organizers moved these incentives into the coercive realm (Jones, 1981). Is it a misuse of the trust component of a long-term clinician-patient relationship to suggest a research trial to a patient? Does it depend on the personality of the patient—that is, the desperate need to please ("I'll do anything you say") patient or the patient who questions and makes her own decisions? What about clinical services that are not available except in the context of a research study? Is it pressuring women to participate in a study by offering gynecological services, when these services are not easily available to HIV-positive women? There are not simple answers to these questions. But these are issues that must be raised in a thoughtful, meaningful context as we enter into women's HIV research trials.

Necessary Services

Many families affected by HIV have previously experienced negative interactions with health care institutions and social service agencies. These institutions may create obstacles to accessing their limited resources such as long waiting periods or difficult application procedures. Service organizations may be unfamiliar with meeting the needs of poor women and their families, such as providing needed child care, transportation, or food vouchers. Sometimes the agencies are insensitive to the health beliefs, cultural concerns, or language of the families and therefore are personally inaccessible to many people with HIV. Agencies may intentionally discourage those who use drugs or even have a history of drug use from participating in their programs. Personnel may display a punitive approach, blaming the women and families for HIV infection and the situation in which they find themselves. To engage families in ongoing care at HIV sites, all agencies and institutions involved in the delivery of such care must make a concerted effort to acknowledge clients' previous experiences, to be sensitive to behavior resulting in negative client interactions. The creation of care settings where there is appreciation and respect for HIV-infected families and their concerns presents a creative challenge to health workers. Attitudes of caregivers and the establishment of a caring and respectful environment are as important as any service provided.

Women and their families affected by HIV have multiple health, psychosocial, and economic needs in addition to their HIV infection. Because of their multiple problems, care for these families must be intended to be as comprehensive as possible. A primary care model that includes HIV-specific care as well as all aspects of health maintenance, general medical (including gynecological), and psychosocial care is best suited for HIV-affected families (Starfield, 1992). Counseling for all reproductive choices, as well as the existence of perinatal and abortion services, must be available on site or through referral.

For women, HIV is a family disease. If more than one family member is infected or sick with HIV, negotiation of the different medical providers and institutions each family member must visit is complicated and customarily a woman's responsibility. When children are sick or require special services, women make the child's health a priority, often at the expense of their own health. Scheduling appointments for children and mothers to receive all care at a single health care visit relieves the family of the stress of multiple visits. This provides the rationale for providing HIV services for women and their children in the same setting.

The necessary services for complete HIV care for women are best provided by a multidisciplinary team. These services include chemical dependency treatment, nutrition, mental health counseling, case management, child care, pastoral care, legal services, ongoing health education, and support groups. The following paragraphs focus on women's support groups and will high-light a peer approach to education and counseling. More important, this approach begins to develop a definition of women's empowerment in the context of HIV.

Support Groups: The Evolution of Dignity

The evolution of dignity is a process experienced and named by women attending weekly support group sessions at the Women and Children's HIV Program at Cook County Hospital. Prior to participating in the group, many of the women had literally no support systems. Concretely, this means the women had no one to talk to about their illness, their feelings, and their issues of self-esteem.

Through group discussions, women were able to identify barriers to care for HIV-infected women and discuss their own feelings relative to these barriers. Listed below are some of the women's support group concerns:

- There is a lack of women-focused substance abuse programs.
- There is a need for affordable, accessible child care.
- There is a dearth of culturally relevant AIDS services located in the African American and Latino communities.
- Immediate needs for food, clothing, shelter, and freedom from violence for themselves and their families prevent women from complying with medical treatment and making long-term behavior changes.

Members of the group share personal experiences and thoughts with an emphasis on confidentiality, women-to-women expertise, and personal shar-ing. Women discuss survival strategies, child care experiences, and "manipu-lating the system" stories. Participants learn from each other's experiences and begin to develop their own problem-solving strategies.

As women interact with each other, recognition of similarities in the patterns of their lives that led to contracting HIV can become a source of liberation. If they can go a step further to correlate their similar life experiences with poverty, racism, and sexism in their communities, HIV becomes a shared human problem with a social and political activist agenda. Paradoxically, HIV becomes a means for "transformation and hope" (Boudin, 1993). Through participation in the support group, each woman has experienced growth of self-esteem and pride manifesting in greater openness with family and friends, successful enrollment in drug treatment, partnership in medical treatment, development of future plans for themselves and their children, and a desire to educate people in their communities about preventing HIV/AIDS.

Peer Education

Peer education is an extension of the Women and Children's HIV Program women's support group. This model is the most innovative, energetic, and successful method of educating communities about HIV/AIDS (Taylor, Irvin, Rodriguez, Cohen, & Williamson, 1990). In addition, it satisfies the need of empowered HIV-positive women for more information about HIV/AIDS and helps them to share their experiences with their communities, thereby contributing to the prevention of the virus. This model of prevention and risk reduction information, delivered by someone who is living with HIV, is very powerful. In the Women and Children's HIV Program, peer educators work in a variety of settings, both clinical and community. For example, many women are paid stipends or given honoraria, which assist them to provide for their families. Peer educators have become nationally recognized as leading advocates for women and children with HIV, from speaking at conferences to serving on boards and advisory boards of governmental agencies that provide resources for HIV care. The intelligence and skills that these women have used for daily survival are now unleashed in service to their communities. The results are staggering.

Public Health Model

HIV/AIDS is a public health epidemic and demands a public health solution. A public health approach to HIV disease will provide the triad of treatment resources, disease prevention, and health promotion (an increase in the standard of living) on an individual and communitywide basis. A public health approach provides a living standard compatible with health—meaning decent shelter, food, clothing, freedom from violence, education, employment, and so on. This strategy employs effective disease prevention programs. It also provides comprehensive primary medical treatment as necessary (Editorial, 1990). Nationally, there has been little leadership in this arena. A public health solution to the HIV epidemic would by definition have to address issues of poverty, racism, and allocation of health dollars away from special medical interests. To date, almost the exact opposite has been happening. Currently, the U.S. standard of living continues to decline for all but the most wealthy. The wealthiest 1% of the population now owns 37% of the wealth, while the bottom 90% owns only 31% of wealth in this country, and the standard of living for four out of five American families went down during the 1980s (Sanders, 1993); only 3% of all funds allocated to health are spent on prevention (CDC, 1992c); and medical treatment is fragmented and specialized.

The lessons for health workers are simple but powerful. First, a personal lesson—compassion: Stop victim blaming, stop viewing HIV-infected women as the "other." If some women are infected, all are affected. As Jonathan Mann of the Harvard School of Public Health aptly stated, "Male supremacy is a public health danger" (Mann, 1991). Second, health workers must join with communities to advocate for more services that are comprehensive, woman and family centered, and therefore accessible. Finally, it is essential to recognize health prevention and promotion as the only real weapons against HIV. Health providers are then obligated to advocate for increasing dollars spent on prevention education programs that are culturally sensitive to the issues of particular communities and for a universal public health approach to HIV.

Food for Thought

In closing, pressing issues present themselves for intervention before the spread of HIV in women can be halted, and so that women and families can receive necessary services. Questions must be addressed by public policies that promote attitudinal change and allocate dollars for programs that will educate, implement, and enforce such innovation.

1. Health dollars must be reallocated for STD/HIV prevention, education, counseling, and testing to be integrated into women's health and social service programs, such as family planning, gynecological and prenatal, abortion, domestic violence, or housing programs, and, conversely, so the above services can be provided for HIV-infected families.

2. Research dollars must be allocated to develop a woman-controlled barrier viricide that effectively prevents HIV and STDs.

3. Substance abuse is a cofactor with HIV disease and a complex health problem that causes harm to the abuser and those around her. Substance use is neither a moral nor a criminal issue. Research must begin to address the multiple causes of chemical dependency as well as the relation of drug

addiction to socioeconomic and political factors. Successful models of treatment can be evaluated and replicated.

4. Honest discussion of sex and sexuality must began in institutional settings, such as schools, teen centers, or health centers, before sexual activity starts. Open discussion of sexism and homophobia can be initiated so as to change behavior regarding safe sexual practice.

5. A moral standard forbidding violence against women must be put forward in community and institutional settings, so that violence against women can be eradicated.

6. Comprehensive treatment services, with support groups and peer education components, must be replicated in HIV-affected communities.

7. Dollars must be reallocated from the current societal approach of "just say no" to sex and drugs, and punishment and blame for HIV-infected persons, to a real public health solution developed jointly with affected communities, taking into account standard of living issues.

Unless sexuality and drug abuse become societally viewed as part of the human condition and a health problem, respectively, and until the problems of poverty, racism, and violence are considered not as individual failures or attitudes but as our greatest national priority, HIV-infected people will continue to be discriminated against and blamed for the disease. These outlooks also continue to inhibit efforts to provide adequate prevention and treatment programs for women with and at risk for HIV.

The challenge of HIV in women calls upon national and local leadership to develop a broader understanding of HIV/AIDS and to look beyond medical models and understand the social and economic nature of HIV disease. Infected persons and affected communities will become copartners in treatment, program planning, and the creation of a prevention strategy powerful enough to affect everyone's daily behaviors. Only then will we see an impact on this worldwide epidemic that knows no borders, no gender, but can be prevented.

References

Boudin, K. (1993). Teaching and practice. *Harvard Educational Review, 65,* 207-232.

Carpenter, C. C., Mayer, K. H., Fisher, A., Desai, M. B., & Durand, L. (1989). Natural history of acquired immunodeficiency syndrome in women in Rhode Island. *American Journal of Medicine, 86,* 771-775.

Carr, A. (1991). *Changes in the health care and social services needs of HIV+ women and children in metropolitan Chicago.* Chicago: Visiting Nurse Association of Chicago.

Centers for Disease Control and Prevention. (1990). Risk for cervical disease in HIV infected women—New York City. *MMWR, 39,* 846-849.

Centers for Disease Control and Prevention. (1992a, October). *HIV/AIDS surveillance report, third quarter.* Atlanta, GA: Author.

Centers for Disease Control and Prevention. (1992b). Mortality patterns—United States: 1989. *MMWR, 41,* 121-125.

Centers for Disease Control and Prevention. (1992c). Estimated national spending on prevention—U.S. 1988. *MMWR, 41*(29), 529-531.

Centers for Disease Control and Prevention. (1993). Update projections of persons with AIDS in the U.S.—1992-1994. *MMWR, 41*(no. RR-18), 1-29.

Chavkin, W., & Paone, D. (1991). *Drug treatment for women with sexual abuse histories* (Abstract No. WC3260). Paper presented at the VII International Conference on AIDS, Florence, Italy.

Chu, S. Y., Buehler, J. W., & Berhelman, R. L. (1990). Impact of immune deficiency virus epidemic on mortality in women of reproductive age. *Journal of the American Medical Association, 264,* 225-229.

David, R. J., & Collins, J. W. (1991). Bad outcomes in black babies: Race or racism? *Ethnicity and Disease, 1,* 236-244.

Editorial: Confusion worse confounded: Health promotion and prevention. (1990, Summer). *Journal of Public Health Policy, 2,* 144-145.

Ellerbrock, T. V., Bush, T. J., Chamberland, M. E., & Optoby, M. J. (1991). Epidemiology of women with AIDS in the U.S. 1981-1990. *Journal of the American Medical Association, 265,* 2971-2975.

Elvy, A. (1985). Access to care. In P. W. Brickner, L. K. Scharer, B. Conanan, A. Elvy, & M. Saverese (Eds.), *Health care of homeless people* (pp. 223-236). New York: Springer.

Fischl, M., et al. (1987). Efficiency of azidothymidine (AZT) in the treatment of patients in AIDS and AIDS related complex. *New England Journal of Medicine, 317*(4), 185-191.

Flaskerud, J. H., & Nyamathi, A. N. (1990). Effects of an AIDS education program on the knowledge, attitudes and practices of low income black and Latina women. *Journal of Community Health, 15*(6), 343-355.

Fullilove, R. E., Fullilove, M., Gasch, H., & Smith, M. (1992). *Violent trauma and HIV risk* (Abstract PoC4252). Paper presented at the VIII International Conference on AIDS, Amsterdam, the Netherlands.

Hankins, C. A., & Handley, M. A. (1992). HIV disease and AIDS in women: Current knowledge and a research agenda. *Journal of Acquired Immune Deficiency Syndromes, 5,* 957-968.

Johnson, A. M., & Laga, M. (1990). Heterosexual transmission of HIV. In N. J. Alexander, H. L. Gabelnick, J. M. Spieler, & R. Alan (Eds.), *Heterosexual transmission of AIDS* (pp. 9-24). New York: Liss.

Jones, J. (1981). *Bad blood: The Tuskegee Syphilis Experiment: A tragedy of race and medicine.* New York: Free Press.

Kirp, D. L. (1993). Fighting AIDS in the streets: Needle exchange comes of age. *Nation, 256,* 559-560.

Levine, C. (1991, January-April). Women and HIV/AIDS research: The barriers to equity. *IRB,* pp. 18-22.

Mann, J. (1991, April). *Women and AIDS conference.* Boston: Fenway Clinic.

Murphy, T. F. (1991, January). Women drug users: The changing face of AIDS clinical drug trials. *QRB,* pp. 26-32.

NIDA. (1991-1992, Winter). Researches, clinicians, practitioners discuss emerging drug abuse treatment needs. *NIDA Notes.*

Potts, M., Feldblum, P. J., Chi, I., Liao, W., & Fuertes, A. d. (1982). The Puerto Rican contraceptive study: An evaluation of method and results of a feasibility study. *British Journal of Family Planning, 7,* 99.

Ridher, T. M., Manson, J. E., Buring, J. E., Goldraber, S. Z., & Hennekens, C. H. (1991). Effect of chronic platelet inhibition with low dose aspirin on atherosclerotic progression and acute thrombosis: Clinical evidence from health study. *American Heart Journal, 122,* 61588-61592.

Sanders, B. (1993). Clinton must go to the people. *The Nation, 256,* 265-267.

Schietinger, H. (1990). A global view of women and HIV. *Focus, 6,* 3.

Starfield, B. (1992). *Primary care: Concept, evaluation, and policy.* New York: Oxford.

Taylor, D., Irvin, Y., Rodriquez, A., Cohen, M., & Williamson, M. (1990). *The evolution of dignity: The role of support groups for HIV infected women.* Presentation at the VI International Conference on AIDS, San Francisco.

Torres, R. A., Lefkowitz, P., Kales, C., & Brickner, P. W. (1987). Homelessness among hospitalized patients with the acquired immunodeficiency syndrome in New York City [letter]. *Journal of the American Medical Association, 258,* 779-780.

World Health Organization. (1990). *Current and future dimensions of the HIV/AIDS pandemic: A capsule summary* (WHO/GPA Rev. 1). Geneva: Author.

Worth, D., Drucker, E., Eric, K., & Pivnick, A. (1990). *Sexual and physical abuse as factors in continued risk behavior of women IV drug users in a South Bronx methadone clinic* (Abstract ThD786). Paper presented at the VI International Conference on AIDS, San Francisco.

Zolpa, A., Gorter, R., Meakin, R., Keffelew, A., Wolfe, H., & Moss, A. (1991). *Homelessness and HIV infection: A population based study* (Abstract MC3244). Paper presented at the VII International Conference on AIDS, Florence, Italy.

PART IV

Violence, Abuse,
and Women's Health

18

The Negative Impact of Crime
Victimization on Women's Health
and Medical Use

Mary P. Koss

The frequency of crime in the United States is staggering: National Crime Victimization Survey (NCVS) estimates suggest that Americans sustained almost 19 million violent crime victimizations in 1990 (Bureau of Justice Statistics, 1992). Victimization is a diagnosis that physicians are increasingly expected to make as frontline health care providers (American College of Obstetrics and Gynecologists, 1989; Council on Scientific Affairs, 1992; U.S. Department of Health and Human Services, 1986; U.S. Department of Justice, 1984). Because of their high level of public contact and the decreased stigma compared with mental health providers, primary care physicians are an important resource for women victimized by crimes including rape and domestic violence (Steinwachs et al., 1986). Until recently, the medical literature had focused exclusively on forensic issues and acute treatment (Goldberg & Tomlanovich, 1984; Hicks, 1988, 1990; Hochbaum, 1987; Martin, Warfield, & Braen, 1983). Consideration of somatic consequences that extended beyond the emergency period was limited to the psychological aftereffects. Now, a rapidly growing body of research associates victimization by violence to chronic illnesses (Koss & Heslet, 1992). Unfortunately, examination of changes in medical use subsequent to victimization has been limited by the reliance on subjective documentation of health including self-reported

SOURCE: This chapter originally appeared in modified form in *Journal of Women's Health*, Vol. 2, No. 1, 1993, pp. 67-72; used by permission of Mary Ann Liebert, Inc., 1651 Third Ave., New York, NY 10128.

physician visits and medical expenses (Leymann, 1985; Sorenson, 1988; Waigandt & Miller, 1986). In the present study, crime's long-term effects on health were documented with objective health service use data. Women were chosen for the focus because the scope of criminal violence against them is of stunning magnitude when crimes by both intimate and stranger perpetrators are considered: One in five women has been the victim of completed rape and one in four women has been physically battered, according to the results of recent community-based studies (American College of Obstetrics and Gynecologists, 1989; Koss, 1993). The burden of sexual violence, in particular, falls heavily on women, who represent more than 90% of the rape victims identified in the NCVS (Koss & Heslet, 1992). Also, women are more likely to report illnesses and to seek medical care, although much of the increased medical use can be accounted for by reproductive health care needs (Verbrugge, 1985; Waldron, 1983). Nevertheless, risk factors such as interpersonal violence, which have a disproportionate impact on women, could also increase their requirements for health care (American College of Obstetrics and Gynecologists, 1989; Strickland, 1989; U.S. Department of Health and Human Services, 1985).

Methods

The site of the present study was an urban, work site-based health maintenance organization. Numerous crime victims have been identified among primary care patients (Koss, Woodruff, & Koss, 1991). Specifically, the lifetime prevalence of crime victimization was 57% among a sample of 5,086 women health plan members who received a mailed survey (45% response rate). New victimizations by violent crimes, including robbery with force, assault, and rape, occurred during a 12-month period at an estimated rate of 77 per 1,000 women patients. Many of these crimes occurred in highly intimate contexts. For example, 29% of the assaults and 39% of the rapes were perpetrated by husbands, partners, or relatives of the victims. Only 17% of the rapes and 41% of the assaults were perpetrated by strangers.

Participant Characteristics

The sample in the present study was a diverse group of urban, working women with an average age of 36, of whom nearly half were married or living with a partner, slightly more than one third (37%) were African American, and just one quarter had a high school education or less.

Interview Procedures

All data were collected by interviews held at the work site, which raises special human subjects considerations that have been elaborated upon elsewhere (Koss, Koss, & Woodruff, 1991). Medical records were accessed only upon the signed consent of participants. Participants were recruited from names generated by sampling every 10th person on the female patient register. The number of victimized women was then augmented by recruitment, which was accomplished by mailing a crime screening survey to the members of the health plan. Together the two sampling methods generated 413 participants. Demographic comparisons of recruited crime victims and the randomly selected women indicated no significant differences in age, marital status, ethnicity, income, or education.

Measurement of Crime Victimization

All participants were screened for severity of crime victimization with questions taken verbatim from the NCVS including those that focus on purse snatching, home burglary, attempted robbery, robbery with force, threatened assault, and assault (Koss & Heslet, 1992). Typical of these items is this one: "Did anyone take something directly from you by using force such as a stickup, mugging, or threat?" The NCVS procedure for identifying rape or attempted rape consists only of a single item, which reads: "Did someone attack you in some other way?" (The NCVS procedure for measuring rape was revised after the present study was completed.) This item was not used because it fails to provide the detailed cues typical of the nonsexual crime screen items and has been heavily criticized in the literature. Instead, five screening questions for rape and attempted rape were written to parallel the style of NCVS. Rape was defined according to reformed state statutes as penetration, no matter how slight, including vaginal, oral, or anal intercourse; against consent; and through force, threat of force, or when the victim was incapacitated. Typical of these items is this one: "Has a man made you have sex by using force or threatening to harm you? When we use the word 'sex' we mean a man putting his penis in your vagina even if he didn't ejaculate (come)." Participants also designated their most significant crime incident, if any, and provided the date of occurrence. A summary measure of crime severity was used in these analyses. The measure included responses to all 12 sexual and nonsexual crime screening items and scored each woman according to the most severe crime she had experienced. The rationale for the scores was the empirically derived *Wolfgang Crime Severity Index* (Wolfgang, Figlio, Tracey, & Singer, 1985). Among a national sample of adults who rated the seriousness of various crime descriptions, the second highest severity weight was applied to crimes that involved rape (the highest was for murder), and the next highest weight was applied to situations where bodily harm was present. Crime severity was scored as follows: A score of 1 was nonvictimization. This level applied to women who responded no to all of the crime screening items (19% of participants). A score of 2 was mild victimization and reflected experiences with noncontact crimes or crime attempts including illegal entry of the home, purse snatching, attempted robbery by threat or force, or threats to harm with a weapon but without exposure to any completed contact crimes (13% of participants). A score of 3 was moderate victimization. It was applied to women who had experienced crimes with bodily harm but without attempts to commit sexual acts such as being robbed with force, beaten up or attacked, or attacked with a weapon (23% of participants). A score of 4 represented serious victimization and was applied to women who had experienced crimes in which they were forced to engage in unwanted oral, anal, or vaginal intercourse (24% of participants). The score of 5 represented multiple assaults. It was assigned to the 21% of participants who both had experienced a completed forcible rape and had experienced physical assault separate from the rape.

Measures of Service Use

The measures of health service use, in accordance with common practice in the literature, were the number of physician visits and the outpatient costs. Visits focused on physician services and excluded psychotherapy, podiatry, physical therapy, dietetics, optometry, and dentistry. Outpatient costs focused on charges for treatments by physicians and excluded charges for psychological testing, laboratory, and X-rays. Childbirth services are the primary cause of female medical service usage, yet they are unlikely to be influenced by crime exposure. Therefore childbirth-related visits and charges were also excluded. Use indices were calculated for each woman for the calendar year 1986 (the latest for which complete data were available), which is hereafter referred to as the index year. Medical charges for earlier years were converted to 1986 dollars using actual price increases provided by the institution.

Results

Service Use

Criminal victimization severity influenced the number of physician visits made in the index year: $F(4,377) = 5.57$, $P = .001$. All the levels of victim-

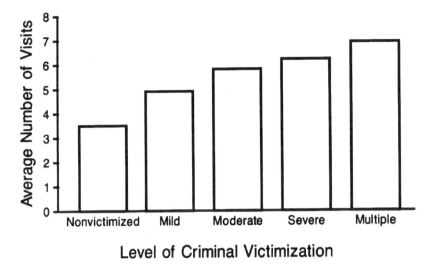

Figure 18.1. Mean Outpatient Visits in Index Year by Criminal Victimization Severity

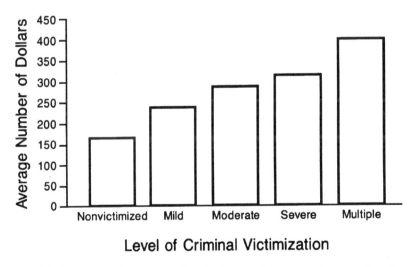

Figure 18.2. Mean Outpatient Expenses in Index Year by Criminal Victimization Severity

ization severity differed significantly from the others. For example, multiply victimized women visited their physician 6.9 times per year, which was twice as often as nonvictimized women, who made an average of 3.5 visits. The mean number of visits made in the index year according to the severity of victimization are illustrated in Figure 18.1.

Crime victimization severity also affected outpatient medical costs and all the levels of severity differed from each other: $F(4,375) = 8.29$, $P = .001$. The cost of treating a multiply victimized woman was \$401, which was 2½ times higher than the cost of treating a nonvictim (\$161). The mean expenses according to severity of victimization are illustrated in Figure 18.2.

Although these effects appear to be sizable, hierarchial multiple regression analysis was used to determine the power added to the prediction of medical use by knowledge of a woman's victimization status. Two multiple regression equations were developed: to predict visits in the index year and to predict outpatient costs in the index year. The 14 predictor variables comprised five demographic variables (age, marital status, ethnicity, income, and education), four health status assessments (which have not been described here due to space limitations; they were standard assessments taken from the Rand Health Insurance experiment covering self-reported symptoms, emotional well-being, functional status, and health hazards; Brook et al., 1979, p. 7), and five trauma and stress measures (12-month life change, lifetime exposure to divorce, deaths, and major illness, and criminal victimization severity). The variables were entered in blocks in the following order: demographic variables, health status assessments, and stress measures. Thereby the predictive power of criminal victimization severity is examined only after accounting for the contributions of all other variables. All of the predictors entered the equations and accounted for 19% of the variance in physician visits and 18% of the variance in outpatient costs. These analyses are summarized in Table 18.1.

Each increment in criminal victimization severity was associated with increases of 33% in physician visits and 56% in outpatient expenses above the use figures that characterized the former level of severity. Criminal victimization severity was the single most important contributor to the predictive power for both use criteria. In the case of physician visits, the variables that were the prominent predictors included marital status, age, health hazards, and criminal victimization severity. The size of the beta weights indicates that a 1 standard deviation increase in criminal victimization severity would have an effect on health service use approximately equal to a 3 standard deviation increase in age or a 2 standard deviation increase in health hazards. The women most likely to have high numbers of physician visits and medical expenses were those who were older, living alone, had more injurious health practices, and had suffered severe criminal victimization.

This analysis is not proof of a casual relationship between victimization and increased medical use, however. It is possible that a third variable, such as alcohol abuse, could both increase vulnerability to victimization and independently cause higher medical use. To address the causal relationship, prospective data were necessary.

TABLE 18.1 Prediction of Index Year Medical Use by Demographic Variables, Health Status, and Life Stressors

Block and Predictor	Beta	R	Multiple R^2	F	df	P
Visits:						
Demographic variables		.247	.061	4.10	5316	.0005
age	.09					
marital status	−.13					
education	−.03					
income	−.01					
ethnicity	−.02					
Health status		.335	.111	4.37	9312	.0005
total symptoms	.01					
health hazards	.14					
General Health Index	−.08					
Mental Health Index	.06					
Life stressors		.436	.192	5.18	14307	.0005
life changes	−.08					
family illness	.08					
divorce	.01					
family deaths	.08					
criminal victimization	.27					
Outpatient Costs:						
Demographic variables		.254	.064	4.36	5316	.0005
age	.11					
marital status	−.12					
education	−.04					
income	−.02					
ethnicity	−.06					
Health status		.340	.116	4.53	9312	.0005
total symptoms	−.01					
health hazards	.17					
General Health Index	−.07					
Mental Health Index	.06					
Life stressors		.423	.179	4.78	14307	.0005
life changes	−.09					
family illness	.06					
divorce	.01					
family deaths	.09					
criminal victimization	.24					

Temporal Links

To demonstrate that any elevated health service usage followed crime rather than preceded it, a subsample of participants was selected whose health service use for 5 years surrounding a discrete crime incident could be reconstructed from their longitudinal care records. Excluded were cases where more than one crime occurred during the 5-year period itself or for 2 years prior to it. A total of 68 crime victims met these criteria, including 15 completed rape victims, 26 assault victims, and 27 noncontact crime victims. A comparison sample of 26 nonvictims was selected who had 5 years of continuous medical data available. A sad comment on this sample is that it was the nonvictimized group rather than the victimized that was more scarce.

Crime victims were compared with nonvictims on demographic variables to address potential alternate explanations for any use differences that might be found. No significant differences were present in age, education, or income and the groups were equivalent in ethnic composition (46% of nonvictims were African American compared with 43% of crime victims). The data were analyzed with multivariate analysis of variance for repeated measures. The effect that would test the hypothesized crime-illness link was the sample-by-time interaction, which would demonstrate that groups differed across time in their level of use.

In fact, a significant sample-by-time interaction was found for the dependent variable of physician visits. Whereas victims had been lower users than nonvictims prior to victimization, their level of use overtook that of nonvictims following victimization. In the year during which the crime occurred, all victims increased their physician usage. Specifically, visits increased 24% among noncontact crime victims, 15% among assault victims, and 18% among rape victims compared with the average yearly number of visits each group had made during the 2 previous years. During the comparable time period, nonvictims' medical visits decreased by 13%. Increases in physician visits were most marked in the year following the crime, when all crime groups made more visits than nonvictims. Visits made by noncontact crime victims increased 41% over the previous 2 years' baseline (from an average of 3.6 visits per year during the 2 years before the crime to 6.1 visits in the year following the crime). Similarly, rape victims increased physician visits 56% (from an average of 4.1 visits per year before the crime to 7.3 visits in the year following the crime). By comparison, nonvictims increased their use only 2% during year 4 over their baseline for the 2 previous years. Increases in crime victims' physician visits were still apparent in the last year of the study, which was 3 years following the crime: 31% among noncontact crime victims, 15% among assault victims, and 31% among rape victims, compared with a 1% increase among nonvictims over their 2-year baseline.

Although similar trends were seen for outpatient medical expenses, the sample-by-time interaction did not reach statistical significance. Visits may be more likely to show the impact of victimization because patients themselves control the initiation of appointments. Medical costs, however, vary according to the type of complaint and physician's behavior in ordering tests

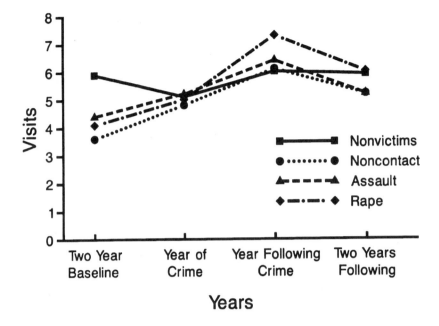

Figure 18.3. Outpatient Visits Across 5 Years Surrounding Crime Victimization

and making specialist referrals. Multivariate analysis of covariance also was performed on physician visits and outpatient costs to rule out the possibility that any health impact might have been attributable to potential effects of other major life stressors, income, or differences in ethnic makeup among the groups. However, none of these covariates made significant contributions to the prediction of the use criteria in these data.

Comment

The findings clearly demonstrate deleterious effects of crime as reflected by substantial increases in victimized women's use of medical services, an effect that prevailed for up to 3 years following the crime. However, the present study was unable to illuminate the processes by which these victimizations influenced health. At least 5 viable possibilities could be entertained. The first is stressor-linked changes in immune functioning, which are the most heuristic to account for infectious diseases that follow shortly after the trauma (Cohen, Tyrell, & Smith, 1991; Cohen & Williamson, 1991). Many domestic assaults and rapes are repetitive and could set up a continuing state of stress. A second possibility is alterations in health behaviors initiated in the aftermath of trauma to cope with distress (Cohen & Williamson, 1991; Kiecolt-Glaser & Glaser, 1987). To the extent that changes in health behaviors endure, they could influence disease susceptibility many years subsequent to termination of the violence. A third mechanism by which the health effects of a trauma could be prolonged is the post-traumatic stress disorder (PTSD) that victims may experience (Baum, 1990). Characteristic of PTSD is intrusive reexperiencing of the trauma, which may be accompanied by reactivation of the physiological responses that occurred during victimization. Reexperiencing both may prolong the state of active stress and may also be the source of physical sensations that are troubling to the patient. A forth process is intensified focus on bodily sensations and heightened concerns about bodily integrity, which some writers suggest may be created as a result of the fear of death or serious injury that occurs during most contact crimes (Wickramasekera, 1986).

Patients cannot discern whether the source of their distress stems from undetected physical injury from the crime, stress-induced disease, emotional reactions to trauma, physiological reexperiencing, or magnification and focus on normal physical sensations. All a patient can do is trigger a physician visit once her discomfort and concern exceed some threshold. Therefore no analysis of the processes by which victimization influences health is complete without taking into account the patient's interaction with the medical care system. If medical practitioners fail to elicit relevant psychosocial experiences, they miss opportunities to identify the etiology of the symptoms. If the physician forces some subset of the presenting complaints into a narrow biomedical diagnosis, the patient's misattributions about the significance of the physical sensations are reinforced, and she is put at risk for the iatrogenic effects of inappropriate medical interventions (Katon, Ries, & Kleinman, 1984).

Implications for Health Care Practitioners

The results suggest a role for the primary care medical system in assisting crime victims that transcends the traditional focus on emergency and forensic intervention. Crime victims in the present study uniformly used medical care during each of the 2 years following victimization. This pattern is a stark contrast to crime victims' very low levels of usage of specialty mental health or victim assistance services (Koss, Woodruff, & Koss, 1991). Unfortunately, the likelihood is low that physicians currently realize their potential to initiate service provision for traumatized crime victims because they don't screen for violence exposure even in psychiatric settings (Jacobson & Richardson, 1987). The failure to screen for victimization by violence communicates a lack of permission to discuss these issues in the medical setting. Not only does this omission preclude identification of the underlying etiology of the physical symptoms, patients experiencing ongoing violence are left at continuing risk of additional injury (American College of Obstetrics and Gynecologists, 1989; Flitcraft et al., 1992). As well, opportunities will be missed to facilitate simple confiding in a caring person, which is a simple task that has demonstrated therapeutic effects on immune response (Pennebaker, Kiecolt-Glaser, & Glaser, 1988). In response to confidences shared, practitioners must validate the women's experience. To ensure this outcome will require education of medical providers. Without training, physicians often react to revelations of rape just as lay people do—by questioning the credibility or culpability of the victim. The finding that the most significant changes in health care use were delayed until the second year following victimization suggests that a window of opportunity exists during which appropriate intervention might forestall or mitigate the severity of victimization-induced illness.

References

American College of Obstetrics and Gynecologists. (1989). *The battered woman* (ACOG Technical Bulletin No. 124). Washington, DC: American College of Obstetricians and Gynecologists.

Baum, A. (1990). Stress, intrusive imagery, and chronic distress. *Health Psychology, 9,* 653-675.

Brook, R. H., Ware, J. E., Davies-Avery, A., et al. (1979). *Conceptualization and measurement of health for adults in the Health Insurance Study.* Santa Monica, CA: RAND.

Bureau of Justice Statistics. (1992). *Criminal victimization in the United States, 1990.* Washington, DC: U.S. Department of Justice.

Cohen, S., Tyrell, D. A., & Smith, A. P. (1991). Psychological stress and susceptibility to the common cold. *New England Journal of Medicine, 325,* 606-612.

Cohen, S., & Williamson, G. M. (1991). Stress and infectious disease in humans. *Psychological Bulletin, 109,* 5-24.

Council on Scientific Affairs. (1992). Violence against women: Relevance for medical practitioners. *Journal of the American Medical Association, 267,* 3184-3189.

Flitcraft, A. H., Hadley, S. M., et al. (1992). American Medical Association diagnostic and treatment guidelines on domestic violence. *Archives of Family Medicine, 1,* 39-47.

Goldberg, W. G., & Tomlanovich, M. C. (1984). Domestic violence in the emergency department. *Journal of the American Medical Association, 251,* 3259-3264.

Hicks, D. J. (1988). The patient who's been raped. *Emergency Medicine, 20,* 106-122.

Hicks, D. J. (1990). Sexual battery: Management of the patient who has been raped. In J. J. Sierra (Ed.), *Gynecology and obstetrics* (Vol. 6, pp. 1-11). Philadelphia: Harper & Row.

Hochbaum, S. R. (1987). The evaluation and treatment of the sexually assaulted patient. *Obstetrical and Gynecological Emergency, 5,* 601-621.

Jacobson, A., & Richardson, B. (1987). Assault of 100 psychiatric patients: Evidence of the need for routine inquiry. *American Journal of Psychiatry, 144,* 908-913.

Katon, W., Ries, R. K., & Kleinman, A. (1984). The prevalence of somatization in primary care. *Comprehensive Psychiatry, 25,* 208-215.

Kiecolt-Glaser, J. K., & Glaser, R. (1987). Psychosocial moderators of immune function. *Annals of Behavioral Medicine, 9,* 16-20.

Koss, M. P. (1993). Detecting the scope of rape: A review of prevalence research methods. *Journal of Interpersonal Violence, 8,* 198-222.

Koss, M. P., & Heslet, L. (1992). Somatic consequences of violence against women. *Archives of Family Medicine, 1,* 53-59.

Koss, M. P., Koss, P. G., & Woodruff, W. J. (1991). Deleterious effects of criminal victimization on women's health and medical utilization. *Archives of Internal Medicine, 151,* 342-347.

Koss, M. P., Woodruff, W. J., & Koss, P. G. (1991). Criminal victimization among primary care medical patients: Prevalence, incidence, and physician usage. *Behavioral Science and the Law, 9,* 85-96.

Leymann, H. (1985). Somatic and psychological symptoms after the experience of life threatening events: A profile analysis. *Victimology, 10,* 512-538.

Martin, C. A., Warfield, M. C., & Braen, R. (1983). Physician's management of the psychological aspects of rape. *Journal of the American Medical Association, 249,* 501-503.

Pennebaker, J. W., Kiecolt-Glaser, J. K., & Glaser, R. (1988). Disclosure of traumas and immune function: Health implications for psychotherapy. *Journal of Consulting and Clinical Psychology, 56,* 239-245.

Sorenson, S. B. (1988). Health service utilization following sexual assault. *American Journal of Community Psychology, 16,* 625-643.

Steinwachs, D. M., Weiner, J. P., Shapiro, S., Batalden, P., Coltin, K., & Wasserman, F. (1986). A comparison of the requirements for primary care physicians in HMOs with projections made by GMENAC. *New England Journal of Medicine, 314,* 217-222.

Strickland, B. R. (1989). Sex-related differences in health and illness. *Psychology of Women Quarterly, 12,* 381-390.

U.S. Department of Health and Human Services. (1985). *Women's health: Report of the Public Health Service Task Force on Women's Health* (HHS publication [PHS] 85-50206). Washington, DC: Government Printing Office.

U.S. Department of Health and Human Services, U.S. Department of Justice. (1986). *Surgeon General's Workshop on Violence and Public Health.* Washington, DC: U.S. Department of Health and Human Services, Public Health Service.

U.S. Department of Justice. (1984). *Attorney General's Task Force on Family Violence: Final report.* Washington, DC: Author.

Verbrugge, L. M. (1985). Gender and health: An update on hypotheses and evidence. *Journal of Health and Social Behavior, 26,* 156-182.

Waigandt, C. A., & Miller, D. A. (1986). Maladaptive responses during the reorganization phase of rape trauma syndrome. *Research on Victimization of Women and Children, 9,* 20-21.

Waldron, I. (1983). Sex differences in illness incidence, prognosis, and mortality. *Social Science and Medicine, 17,* 321-333.

Wickramasekera, I. (1986). A model of people at high risk to develop chronic stress-related somatic symptoms: Some predictions. *Professional Psychology: Research and Practice, 17,* 437-447.

Wolfgang, M., Figlio, R., Tracey, P., & Singer, S. (1985). *Wolfgang Crime Severity Index.* Washington, DC: U.S. Department of Justice, Bureau of Justice Statistics.

19

Domestic Violence: Challenges to Medical Practice

Carole Warshaw

Over the past two decades, gender-based trauma has emerged as one of the most serious public health problems facing women in this country. For most women, the greatest risk of physical, emotional, and sexual violation will be from a man they have known and trusted, often an intimate partner. Although organized medicine has recently begun to address this issue, it has largely been the ongoing work of a grassroots battered women's movement that has generated the increased awareness we are now beginning to see (Flitcraft, 1991).

While it is possible for some women to escape after the first episode of violence, for most the abuse is ongoing, escalating in both frequency and severity (AMA, 1992), and carries significant social, psychological, and medical consequences. In the United States, where up to 25% of women will experience physical violence, sexual assault, or both at the hands of a current or former partner (Gelles & Straus, 1988; Shulman, 1979; Teske & Parker, 1983) and where over 50% of women who are murdered are killed by male intimates (Browne, 1992), it is not surprising to see such a high prevalence of abuse histories among women seeking medical care.

SOURCE: This chapter originally appeared in modified form in *Journal of Women's Health,* Vol. 2, No. 1, 1993, pp. 73-80; used by permission of Mary Ann Liebert, Inc., 1651 Third Ave., New York, NY 10128.

AUTHOR'S NOTE: I wish to acknowledge the support and/or editorial assistance of Elaine Carmen, Alice Dan, Barbara Seaman, Terri Randall, Michelle Citron, Barbara Engel, Pat Rieker, Mardge Cohen, Maryse Richards, Amy Rassen, Kathy Goggin, Ora Schub, Sara Hemphill, Barry Barnett, and Terrence Conway as well as the Chicago Abused Women Coalition, particularly Vickii Coffey and Beatrice Burgos, who have greatly enriched my own experience and understanding.

Intimate violence is also an important issue in gay and lesbian relationships (Island & Letellier, 1991; Kanuha, 1990; Lobel, 1986), but because most available data at this time only address male violence against women, I will refer to batterers as *he* and victim/survivors as *she*.

Health Care Implications

The connection between domestic violence and women's health becomes most clear, however, when we pull together the clinical data, thus underscoring the need for routine screening in all clinical settings. Studies indicate that battered women constitute 22%-35% of women seeking care for any reason in emergency departments (Appleton, 1980; Goldberg & Tomlanovich, 1984; McLeer & Anwar, 1989; Stark, Flitcraft, & Frazier, 1979; Stark et al., 1981), 14%-28% of women seen in ambulatory medical clinics (Gin, Rucker, Frayne, Cygan, & Hubbell, 1991; Warshaw et al., 1993), and 23% of women seeking routine prenatal care (Helton, Anderson, & McFarlane, 1987). In psychiatric settings, the prevalence appears to be even higher, accounting for 25% of women who attempt suicide or who use a psychiatric emergency service (Stark et al., 1981), 50% of women psychiatric outpatients (Hilberman & Munson, 1977-1978), and 64% of women psychiatric inpatients (Jacobsen & Richardson, 1987). In one study, 58% of women over 30 who had been raped were raped in the context of a battering relationship (Stark et al., 1981), and in 45%-59% of child abuse cases, the mother is also being beaten (McKibben, De Vos, & Newberger, 1989; Stark & Flitcraft, 1988). These data highlight the need to develop integrated child protection-battered women's programs that are neither punitive nor endangering to the mother, who may also be at risk for abuse. Among battered women who are first identified in a medical setting, 75% will go on to suffer repeated abuse (Stark et al., 1981).

Nonrecognition of Abuse
in Clinical Settings

Despite the fact that this information has been available since the late 1970s, health care providers have routinely avoided asking about domestic violence (Carmen, Rieker, & Mills, 1984; Helton et al., 1987; Hilberman, 1980; Hilberman & Munson, 1977-1978; Jacobsen & Richardson, 1987; McLeer & Anwar, 1989; Raskin & Warshaw, 1990; Stark, Flitcraft, & Frazier, 1979). Even in hospitals with established domestic violence protocols, this issue is often ignored, except when battering is most obvious and its recognition becomes inescapable (McLeer, 1989; Warshaw, 1989).

What happens when a woman who is being battered does reach out for help? Stark et al., in their landmark (1979) study, give one of the most elegant descriptions of the progression of symptomatology that develops in battered women through encounters with an unresponsive health care system. Through a careful analysis of emergency room records over time, they began to see a repetitive and disturbing pattern. Initially, a woman seeking medical attention for an isolated injury would be treated only symptomatically. When the underlying problem was not addressed, she would continue to seek help for recurrent injuries and the many medical consequences of ongoing abuse. Eventually, however, she herself would be defined as the problem and would be given such pejorative labels as "crock" or "hysteric," or more recently the pejorative psychiatric diagnostic labels of "somatization disorder," "self-defeating personality disorder," or, if she happened to express too much anger, "borderline personality disorder."[1] Her credibility would be further diminished if she developed any of the posttraumatic sequelae of abuse such as anxiety, depression, psychosis, or substance abuse. For some women, this repeated nonrecognition led to death by serious injury, homicide, or suicide. Having posttraumatic stress-related symptoms (Houskamp & Foy, 1991; Kemp, Rawlings, & Green, 1991; Walker, 1991) that are not recognized as such do not increase a woman's likelihood of being taken seriously. On the other hand, conceptualizing her symptoms as being caused by overwhelming trauma does begin to incorporate context into diagnosis, making her responses more understandable and ours potentially more empathic.

What is so significant about the pattern Stark et al. describe is that the long-term sequelae of even the sublethal violence and intimidation (Conway, Hu, Kim, Bullon, & Warshaw, 1993; Koss, in press; Wilson & Daly, 1992) associated with ongoing abuse may in part be a function of thwarted help seeking and negative responses on the part of the health care system and the hopelessness and despair that ensue from a woman's feeling she is at fault and without viable alternatives to remaining in an abusive relationship. This progression of events could be regarded as a form of iatrogenic retraumatization.

While there are women who remember being afraid or unwilling to discuss what was happening to them with an unresponsive or judgmental clinician, there are others who remember the concern of the one nurse or physician who said, "I can't let you go home like this. I don't think it's safe," or "Of course you feel that way. You're not the one who's crazy," which changed their lives and opened the door to ending the abuse.

Many women, in fact, make repeated attempts to get help only to be told that the violence must be their own fault and that "they" should just try harder to make "their" marriages work. Poor women and women of color often face others' assumptions that violence is normal and to be expected, while women who are more privileged face the problems of invisibility from helping professionals who cannot tolerate seeing abuse too close to home. One woman (who is still in danger and must maintain her anonymity) describes how for years she would go to emergency rooms with injuries inflicted by her husband, a prominent lawyer. When she told the nurses or physicians what had happened, they would either ask what she'd done to provoke him or say that her husband seemed so concerned and remorseful that she should just let it go. She realized that telling the truth about what had happened made people so uncomfortable that she received far worse treatment if she was honest than if she just lied and said she had had an accident. When she told their pediatrician that her daughter's injuries were inflicted by her husband, her husband was subsequently able to convince the pediatrician that the "assault" had been an "accident." When she tried to file police reports, her complaints were written up as accidental injuries rather than as battery. When she sought help from her family, they turned their backs. It was only recent public attention to this issue and the realization that her husband was not going to change that convinced her to try again.

Medicalization of Domestic Violence: New Questions, New Dangers

The question facing us today is no longer whether domestic violence is a problem of sufficient importance for health care providers to address but why this issue has not received adequate attention. What has made it so difficult for clinicians to ask about abuse and violence? And now that the scope of this issue is finally being recognized, what new dangers do we face?

Becoming aware of our own use of language begins to illuminate some of these difficulties. Just by making the shift from talking about the "impact of abuse and violence on our lives as women" to describing the "prevalence of abuse histories in women patients," we begin to move from a social framework that includes our own experiences to a medicalized one that serves to distance and protect. In this framework, socially condoned abuse and violence directed toward women are transformed into aspects of individual case histories that then become linked to the pathology and problems of "patients." As we think about reframing women's health, it is important to recognize how the institutional structures and conceptual frameworks in which we function serve to shape our thinking and practice.

It took years of struggle on the part of feminists to have domestic violence recognized as a sociopolitical issue rather than regarded as a private family matter or as evidence of individual psychopathology (Bograd, 1984; Brown, 1989, 1992; Gordon, 1988; Hamilton & Jensvold, 1992; Hilberman, 1989;

Kurz, 1987; Rieker & Carmen, 1984, 1986; Schechter, 1982; Stark et al., 1979; Yllö, 1988). As organized medicine begins to see "family" violence as a public health problem, we are again faced with the potential dangers that come with medicalizing social problems and pathologizing important aspects of our own lives. In our efforts to legitimize domestic violence as a condition to diagnose and treat, even the term *battered women* risks becoming a new diagnostic category that merges the culturally diverse and particular experiences of women into a generic battered woman and fails to recognize the individual difficulties women face. For example, women who are already marginalized, women with physical disabilities, and women who have chronic mental illness or substance abuse problems may be even more vulnerable to abuse yet face forms of discrimination that decrease their likelihood of being taken seriously or of finding programs willing and able to accommodate them. Cultural differences in gender socialization affect women's perceptions of abuse, their ability to access services, and their expectations of family support. In gay and lesbian relationships, domestic violence has been seriously underrecognized and intervention may be complicated by homophobic attitudes and lack of community resources (Hamilton, 1989; Kanuha, 1990; Lobel, 1986).

The issue of domestic violence is a particularly subversive one. Taking it seriously forces us to challenge the power dynamics inherent in the current structure of medicine. While organizations such as the AMA, ANA, JCAHO, and CDC may truly consider intimate violence to be a major health problem for women, one might question whether they will be able to fully acknowledge that abuse of power or domination and control in any form is unhealthy or to make the abolition of unequal power relationships a major priority. It is precisely these contradictions that we need to examine.

Why We Don't Identify Abuse: Constraints of the Medical Model

Structuring Our Interactions and Perceptions

Observing how women who seek help for abuse-related symptoms are treated in medical settings reveals the limits of the medical model for providing appropriate care. By examining the ways in which medicine is both taught and practiced, we can see how the objectification process intrinsic to its discourse transforms people—in this case women, with lives and agency of their own—into patients who only fit medical or psychiatric diagnostic categories. By showing how this model functions through techniques that institutionalize socially sanctioned hierarchies of domination and control, techniques that mimic the dynamics of abuse and battering, we begin to see why clinicians trained within that framework may find it difficult to provide the kinds of empowering responses that would be most supportive to women who have been abused.

The language and framework of medicine structure interactions in ways that make it almost impossible for battered women to voice their concerns. By looking at how the experience of battered women is actively dismantled through emergency room encounters, we can see how this process works at the level of the written text of medicine—the medical record. This record comes from a study of 52 emergency room charts over a 2-week period of women who had been deliberately injured by another person. Although these women gave strong indications about the presence of abuse in their lives, the signs were not appropriately read by the physicians who saw them. The information they gave, although recorded on the charts, was addressed directly in only one situation and in most cases was specifically avoided (Warshaw, 1989).

Nurse Triage Note: Hit by a fist to Rt. eye. Seeing white flashes in both eyes x 2 mos.

MD History: Pt 42 y/o BF c Hx head trauma but presents with complaint of flashing lights in peripheral vision. Pt. first noticed it after blunt trauma to R eye. It has since spread to the L eye. Pt. symptoms assoc. c tingling over the head. Not assoc c position. No risk factor for vascular disease except HTN.

MD Physical Exam: Mild swelling R eye, Eye—EOMI, PERRLA Fundus—Neg, Visual field intact, Vision 11/100 bilaterally. No bruits, No murmur, S1S2 RR nl, lungs—clear

Discharge DX: BLUNT TRAUMA FACE, HTN

DISPOSITION: Opthalmology clinic appt., return in 1 week for BP check

Not only does the physician fail to deepen or expand the level of information already described by the triage nurse, he actually further obscures what has happened to this woman. Thus, even when information was available on the chart, it was not integrated into the discharge diagnosis or reflected in the outcome. No intervention was made that would have been appropriate to someone who was being beaten by her partner.

Even if this record were complete from a medical point of view, there would still be glaring omissions. First of all, the woman herself is missing. In the triage note, she has already been removed from the picture and only her right eye remains. What happens when she sees the physician, who is supposed to deepen the level of understanding and further develop the history? She is transformed into a "patient," a "42 y/o BF," ensuring, in this case, that her life outside the medical context will be deemed irrelevant.

This process of devaluing the patient's perspective actually begins with the standard medical language of *patient "complains" of* and continues in the SOAP format in which "subjective" information, the devalued position in a "scientific" discourse, is that which the patient relates while what is truly "objective" is that which the clinician observes (Donnelly & Braumer, 1992).

Significantly, the perpetrator is also missing. The fist is no longer connected to the person who wielded it. In fact, the physician's note does not even mention "hit by a fist" but instead refers to "history of head trauma," something that now exists in her body and is no longer connected to something that happened in her life, much less something that a particular person, most likely the one she's returning home to, did to her. More important, this interaction does not leave room for the woman to discuss what may have been her most pressing reason for seeking care (Warshaw, 1989).

By focusing on the physical trauma, the physician makes a choice that obscures both the etiology and the meaning of the woman's symptoms. In contrast, the physician could choose to say, "Mrs. Johnson states that her husband punched her in the right eye with his fist 2 months ago, after which she began to experience flashing lights in her peripheral vision and tingling over her head. The physical abuse began 10 years ago, after their first child was born and has become more frequent and severe over time," or "Her husband locked her and their 6 children out of the house for a week, preventing her from taking her blood pressure medication." These statements, rather than obscuring the etiology of her symptoms, begin to tell us explicitly what is going on and what issues need to be addressed.

This narrowing of focus to what is happening only within the patient's body is further complicated by the presence of specialization. Each specialty adapts this framework to its own categories of significance. Given similar presentations of complex medical and social problems, information is reduced to the diagnoses deemed valid and treatable by each discipline.

OB/GYN: Hx: G2P2, 16 weeks by dates, kicked in abdomen
Dx: IUP, Blunt trauma to abdomen
Rx: Prenatal vitamins, f/u clinic appt.

MED: Hx: Listing of vague medical complaints including chest pain, problems with husband
Dx: Atypical chest pain
Rx: Clinic appointment, analgesics

PSYCH: Hx: Mention of abuse, sx of anxiety

Dx: Adjustment disorder with anxious mood

Rx: Referral to MHC, librium

It is not just the surgical record that reduces our experience in this way. Trouble at home with an alcoholic mate is translated into a medical diagnosis of atypical chest pain rather than pain secondary to this woman's husband punching her in the chest or pain secondary to panic attacks that began after he threatened to kill her if she ever tried to leave.

What happens in psychiatry where practitioners are presumably more attuned to these dimensions? In a study of over 200 emergency psychiatric records, we found similar charting patterns and inability to integrate context into diagnosis and treatment (Raskin & Warshaw, 1990). Even when information about an abusive event was explicitly recorded, clinician thinking was bound by *DSM-III-R* categories. In this case and in many others, a woman's difficulty "adjusting" properly to being beaten leads to a psychiatric diagnosis of adjustment disorder and the questionable prescribing of a benzodiazepine rather than the accessing of resources that could help her address the abuse (Stark et al., 1979; Warshaw, 1989).

Functions of the Medical Model

In a number of ways, the biomedical framework actively obscures and discounts the lived experience of the very people it attempts to serve. For example, it reduces information to standard diagnostic categories or problems that can be readily manipulated and controlled. It does not formulate a general assessment that links the patient's context with her symptoms and, by failing to do so, constructs a history that is no longer historical. When symptoms are seen as isolated events in the body rather than as a response to ongoing social conditions outside the context of medicine, the notion that this was a solitary episode that will not recur is reinforced. What is potentially lethal for any battered woman is not necessarily her current injuries or symptoms but her return home to a situation of escalating violence. Physicians, when offered complex sets of information, selectively attend to the "physical" (Mishler, 1981, 1984). In doing so, they extract information from the context in which it has meaning for the patient and reconfigure it into a medical event that has meaning for the physician. While it is the task of medical history taking to do precisely that, we can see how much is missed (Warshaw, 1989).

The objectification inherent in this methodology creates an encounter in which the concerns of the patient are not recognized or taken seriously and her needs are once again subordinated to those of a more powerful other.

Perhaps more important is how this kind of model helps us maintain distance and protects us from potentially disturbing information by fostering the belief that our own subjectivity is a danger to the "objectivity" of our practice. This is what Keller (1985) has referred to as the protective motivation behind the so-called neutral stance of the Western scientific paradigm, a position that has been challenged by a number of other theorists (Collins, 1990; Flax, 1990; Fraser & Nicholson, 1990; Harding, 1986, 1990; Harstock, 1990; MacKinnon, 1987).

Structuring the Personal
and Our Ability to Acknowledge Feelings

Any attempt to challenge this model requires not only a change in how we learn to think but also a change that supports our ability to tolerate our own feelings while functioning in a professional mode. Neither alone will address these issues. Although health care providers often acknowledge that they do not routinely ask about domestic violence, they frequently cite practical reasons for not doing so. In training programs, however, where residents have ongoing support for discussing their own feelings about painful clinical situations, they do acknowledge how overwhelmed and confused they sometimes feel when they actually let themselves listen to a woman talk about her experiences (Warshaw & Poirier, 1991). Under conditions that do not allow room for us to acknowledge our own feelings, we rationalize, telling ourselves, "There isn't enough time"; "It is not really part of our role"; "Asking is too intrusive"; "We do not know what to do or say"; or "It probably wouldn't make a difference anyway" (Sugg & Inui, 1992).

In fact, at the practical level, intervention is not that difficult. Once we have a basic understanding of the issues, are able to create a safe environment in which to talk, feel we can express genuine interest and concern, and learn to ask appropriate questions, domestic violence intervention mainly involves assessing immediate and ongoing safety, discussing options, developing liaisons with community groups, and offering resources. The true difficulties, though, are deeper and more complex. What we do not allow ourselves to know is often what we do not feel we can tolerate knowing. When we examine these reasons more closely, we see that they are part of two interrelated phenomena structured directly into the medical paradigm. These phenomena affect the ways we relate both to ourselves and to the people we see as patients and involve the need to maintain our own sense of power and control and to avoid the feelings of vulnerability and helplessness that often arise when we cannot.

Feeling Personally Overwhelmed

As clinicians, we may be shocked and overwhelmed when faced with the prevalence data and the possibility that somewhere between every second and every fifth woman we see may be abused. We may attempt to deal with these feelings by telling ourselves that, if the prevalence is that high, it really will be impossible to find time to address these issues. At a time when cutting health care costs has become a national priority and the danger of losing "nonessential" services imminent, it is important to recognize that the time spent on repeated visits for undiagnosed sequelae of violence is far greater than the time it would take for appropriate intervention. In fact, the long-term social, psychological, and physical as well as financial costs of nonrecognition are staggering. It is more likely, however, that we are attempting to cope with feeling personally overwhelmed by knowing that these are not just isolated events in disturbed families but are happening to large numbers of women we see and care for every day. When we look, however, at the number of women who have been victims of some form of gender-based trauma, we are forced to acknowledge that violence against women is actually a normative social experience for most of us rather than a problem for some women patients. If we happen to believe in a just world (Janoff-Bulman & Frieze, 1983), the extent of abuse and violence in this society may be impossible to apprehend. If our own experiences make this issue far too real, we may find it difficult to have feelings of anger, despair, or helplessness evoked while trying to function in a professional role.

The stated fear that asking about abuse will take too much time, will be perceived as intrusive, or will open a Pandora's box (Sugg & Inui, 1992) can also mask the fear of being professionally overwhelmed. Even if our own personal experiences have not generated these responses, our expectations as health care providers leave little tolerance for the feelings of helplessness and professional inadequacy that arise when we cannot do something to "fix" a battered woman's situation. This leaves us feeling uncomfortable and incompetent in an arena that is systematically devalued during much of our training (Williamson, Beitman, & Katon, 1981). In fact, being trained in an environment that leaves little room for doubt or uncertainty leads us to want to avoid areas in which we do not feel sufficiently skilled. One way of avoiding these more vulnerable feelings in ourselves is to become angry and frustrated with the woman for not responding to our need to make her better. At a practical level, however, feelings of discomfort and intrusiveness can be overcome in the same way that discomfort with sexual history taking has been addressed—with practice and by understanding that it is both legitimate and important to ask.

Addressing the issue of domestic violence may also force us to confront attitudes of which we were not even aware but through which we maintain our own sense of power or safety. Personal bias can take many forms based on our own experiences and our individual needs to disidentify with certain feelings and behaviors. It may be difficult for us to identify with someone who is being victimized when, throughout our training, we ourselves have struggled so hard to be in control. When functioning within a system that devalues feelings and creates a hierarchy in which some people get to be in control at the expense of others, it is difficult not to want to identify with the more powerful position. When we have a hard time empathizing with a woman's "choosing" to stay with her partner, we in effect blame[2] her for his violent behavior by implying that it is her responsibility to get him to stop. When we use these kinds of techniques to protect ourselves, we are in danger of re-creating an abusive dynamic between ourselves and our patients.

It is not easy to acknowledge that people we could know and like are capable of this kind of behavior and we may inadvertently be protective of people we perceive as being like ourselves. Battered women often find it very difficult to elicit appropriate responses from anyone in their own professions or in their partners'. Police have been notoriously reluctant to intervene when the abuser is a fellow officer; women married to lawyers typically have great difficulty in court battles, particularly when their husbands have political connections; and women whose partners are doctors may have to make many attempts before finding a physician who is willing to intervene and document the abuse. We may find it difficult to resist being taken in by the assailant when he seems likable, charming, concerned, and solicitous and believe him when he seems sorry, says it was an accident, or blames the woman for provoking his behavior.

How We Relate Versus What We Do

If we have never learned that the way we relate to a woman who has been abused is as important as what we do, it is easy to feel that it is not worth bothering or that our attempts to help her will not do any good. Whether or not a woman chooses to access services or leave her partner when we first see her, our intervention is still important. It takes most women a long time and multiple attempts before they feel safe enough to leave, able to manage on their own, or ready to give up hope that a person they have loved and a relationship they are invested in will change. Just knowing that someone is concerned, that she is not alone, that intimidation and violence are never justified, and that resources are available can make a tremendous difference over time. When an abused woman who is treated in a health care setting experiences respect, caring, and interest in her thoughts, perceptions, concerns, and well-being and finds that she can make her own choices without fear of retaliation, she may begin to change how she experiences herself and what she feels she can expect from others.

When we are forced to deny our own personal feelings and experience, it becomes more difficult to recognize the feelings and assumptions that shape our perceptions and interactions. What we cannot acknowledge or accept in ourselves becomes difficult to tolerate or relate to in others and what we learn to do to ourselves, we by necessity do to our patients. Acknowledging our own feelings provides access to one of our most valuable clinical tools: the ability to know and understand through our own capacity for empathy.

Patients often provide clues to their real concerns, but as they are often exquisitely attuned to the power dynamics of a medical encounter, they may retreat if their attempts at communication are not well received. A woman who is being abused may already feel shame and humiliation at how she has been treated, and revelation of her situation may be difficult to initiate unless she is asked directly in a genuinely concerned and open way. This doctor-patient power differential is compounded by differences in race, gender, and class.

A health care provider's inability to tolerate hearing women talk about abuse because of the feelings evoked in him or her makes it almost impossible for patients to discuss these issues. An attitude that is judgmental or blaming may cause a woman to withdraw and perhaps avoid seeking help another time. A provider's anger or frustration may either anger or intimidate the woman, causing further hurt and despair. A physician's lack of conviction that violence is never a legitimate way for her partner to express anger, or the implication that she must have done something to provoke the abuse, reconfirms what the abuser has said all along—its her fault, her responsibility, and she deserves to be treated that way.

Most of us in fact will have strong feelings when listening to women describe their experiences of abuse and will respond in many different ways. It is not the having of feelings that is problematic but the failure to recognize the impact of feelings that remain unacknowledged. Thus dismantling these structures involves not just expanding our conceptual paradigm but also creating environments that both allow and encourage us to take time for self-reflection and discussion with people we trust, and that leave room for us to understand our own feelings so that an unconscious need to deny them does not interfere with our own perceptions and ability to provide care.

Recontextualizing Abuse:
Changing the Framework of Medical Practice

Some of the most intriguing work in this area has developed precisely where the issues of abuse and victimization challenge these models. A number of authors have addressed the need to recontextualize and make sense of abusive experiences rather than merely label or pathologize (Rieker & Carmen, 1986; Warshaw, 1989; Warshaw & Poirier, 1991). Others have described the revictimization that takes place under the guise of therapeutic encounters, the increased burden of victimization in women facing other forms of oppression, and the role of victimization in the doubled prevalence of depression in women versus men (Bograd, 1984; Brown, 1989; Hamilton, 1989; Hamilton & Jensvold, 1992; Kurz, 1987; Rieker & Carmen, 1984; Stark et al., 1979). In their attempts to expand the post-traumatic stress disorder framework to incorporate the experiences of women who have been chronically victimized since childhood (complex PTSD; Fraser & Nicholson, 1990), during a battering relationship as adults (intercurrent traumatic stress; Anne Flitcraft, personal communication), or as part of the ongoing microtraumatization of social disenfranchisement (abuse and oppression artifact disorder; Hamilton & Jensvold, 1992), feminist clinicians are trying to bring the social context into psychiatric conceptualizations.

For women in battering relationships, however, this diagnosis is still problematic (Campbell, 1990; Figley, 1992; Woods & Campbell, 1993). First of all, (having) any psychiatric diagnosis, including PTSD, can be used to prevent a woman from maintaining custody of her children (Susan Schechter, personal communication). Second, most abused women are still in danger at the time they seek help and, if they decide to leave, the danger may increase significantly. For them the stress is not "post," the trauma is ongoing, and symptoms may be an adaptive response to danger. Even if the abuse stops, an overwhelming response to "minor" stimuli is still considered part of the disorder. This framework fails to consider that, once a person has been traumatized, it becomes difficult for that person not to be aware of what the more subtle forms of objectification and victimization can mean about abuse of power and disregard. Such heightened sensitivity may make it harder to function in a world filled with daily violations and is viewed as pathological, rather than as a reflection of acute social awareness; it is this awareness, however, that allows us to recognize the kinds of behavior and attitudes that are potentially dangerous and unacceptable before they reach the levels of actual violence seen everyday in emergency rooms.[3]

Changing Ourselves:
Acknowledging Our Own Experiences

How do we begin to bridge these gaps between our own experiences and those of others? Listening to women who have been battered talk about their lives creating oppertunities outside of the clinical setting for listening to women who have been battered talk about their lives, can allow us to temporarily free ourselves from our clinician mode and attend to our own responses. The capacity to listen to a woman who has been battered and learn from what she has to say requires that we understand our own experience. It may be difficult to acknowledge that we too could be seduced, trapped, or terrorized into remaining in a situation that we know is harmful to ourselves. Although medical training is not the same as being in a battering relationship, there are a number of parallels.

How Is Medical Training
Like an Abusive Relationship?

Medicine is an arena in which we want to succeed, especially once we have invested a lot of our time and energy, and we know that we would feel like failures if we left. When our efforts are not responded to, it becomes easy to blame ourselves for not working hard enough, not knowing enough, or not being sufficiently dedicated, particularly when those feelings are continually reinforced. As we become more isolated from friends and family and have less access to other valued parts of ourselves, our self-esteem starts to diminish. As our attention begins to revolve around daily survival, it gets harder even to think about mobilizing the energy it would take to leave or change our lives. Medical training is physically punishing, emotionally draining, and socially isolating. It is often abusive and humiliating and we may feel anxious, exhausted, overwhelmed, depressed, and traumatized. Our lives become insidiously controlled by it, despite our original intentions. As we slowly begin to reorient our identities in terms of its values, we find ourselves internalizing its constructs and judging ourselves by its terms. People who care about us may become frustrated and wonder how we could have allowed this to happen.

These parallels between medical training and battering relationships are, however, double edged. They are precisely what can, if acknowledged, help to bridge our experiences, while, if avoided and denied, re-create the problems described above.

Ultimately, however, the objectification inherent in the theory and structure of medicine, continually reinforced by external factors and internal needs, is played out in the doctor-patient dynamic in ways that subtly diminish the patient and are often abusive and disempowering. This practice makes it not only possible but acceptable to relate to another person as a nonperson. Understanding our own experience allows us to recognize the needs generated from the conceptual paradigms in which we have been trained, the institutional hierarchies in which we practice, and the current economic priorities of the health care system.

The issue of domestic violence raises important questions about the limitations and dangers of the framework in which we practice and demands that we create room for the complexity and mutuality required to provide genuine care as well as technical expertise. As organized medicine begins to take up the pressing issues of women's health and violence against women, we must have a voice in how this is done and use this opportunity to challenge not only which clinical issues are considered priorities but also the very framework in which research and practice take place.

Notes

1. Flitcraft makes an important distinction between "diagnosis," which leads to treatment and access to resources, versus "labeling," which leads largely to dismissal (Houskamp & Foy, 1991). All too often in medical settings, however, psychiatric "diagnoses" function as "labels."

2. Again, pathologizing can provide a less overt form of distancing and ultimately blaming ("I would never let this happen to me, so what is 'wrong with her' that makes her more vulnerable or susceptible to being abused?").

3. This is not to say that the long-term impact of chronic violation and betrayal by someone we have trusted is not devastating but that our solutions must be collective and preventive as well as individual and treatment oriented.

References

AMA. (1992). *Diagnostic and treatment guidelines on domestic violence.* Chicago: American Medical Association.

Appleton, W. (1980). The battered women syndrome. *Annals of Emergency Medicine, 9,* 84-91.

Atwood, G., & Stolorow, R. (1984). *Structures of subjectivity: Explorations in psychoanalytic phenomenology.* Hillsdale, NJ: Analytic.

Bograd, M. (1984). Family systems approaches to wife battering: A feminist critique. *American Journal of Orthopsychiatry, 54,* 558-568.

Brown, L. S. (1989, August). *The contribution of victimization as a risk factor for the development of depressive symptomatology in women.* Paper presented at the 97th Annual Convention of the American Psychological Association, New Orleans, LA.

Brown, L. S. (1992). A feminist critique of personality disorders. In L. S. Brown & M. Ballou (Eds.), *Personality and psychopathology: Feminist reappraisals.* New York: Guilford.

Browne, A. (1992). Violence against women: Relevance for medical practitioners (Council on Scientific Affairs Report). *Journal of the American Medical Association, 267*(23), 3184-3189.

Campbell, J. C. (1990, December). Battered woman syndrome: A critical review. *Violence Update.* Newbury Park, CA: Sage.

Carmen, E., Rieker, P., & Mills, T. (1984). Victims of violence and psychiatric illness. *American Journal of Psychiatry, 141,* 378-383.

Collins, P. H. (1990). *Black feminist thought: Knowledge, consciousness, and the politics of empowerment.* Boston: Unwin Hyman.

Conway, T., Hu, T. C., Kim, P., Bullon, A. E., & Warshaw, C. (1993). *Health impact of violence on the victim.* Unpublished abstract.

Donnelly, B., & Braumer, D. (1992). Why SOAP is bad for the medical record. *Archives of Internal Medicine, 152*(3), 481-484.

Figley, C. R. (1992, May). Posttraumatic stress disorder Part II: Relationship with various traumatic events. *Violence Update.* Newbury Park, CA: Sage.

Flax, J. (1990). Postmodernism and gender relations in feminist theory. In L. J. Nicholson (Ed.), *Feminism/postmodernism.* London: Routledge.

Flitcraft, A. (1991). [AMA scientific statement]. Chicago: American Medical Association.

Fraser, N., & Nicholson, L. (1990). Social criticism without philosophy: An encounter between feminism and postmodernism. In L. J. Nicholson (Ed.), *Feminism/postmodernism.* London: Routledge.

Gelles, R. J., & Straus, M. A. (1988). *Intimate violence.* New York: Simon & Schuster.

Gin, N. E., Rucker, L., Frayne, S., Cygan, R., & Hubbell, A. (1991). Prevalence of domestic violence among patients in three ambulatory care internal medicine clinics. *Journal of General Internal Medicine, 6*(4), 317-322.

Goldberg, W. G., & Tomlanovich, M. C. (1984). Domestic violence victims in the emergency department: New findings. *Journal of the American Medical Association, 251,* 3259-3264.

Gordon, L. (1988). *Heroes of their own lives: The politics and history of family violence: Boston 1880-1960.* New York: Viking.

Hamilton, J. A. (1989). Emotional consequences of victimization and discrimination in special populations of women. *Psychiatric Clinics of North America, 12,* 35-51.

Hamilton, J. A., & Jensvold, M. (1992). Personality, psychopathology and depressions in women. In L. S. Brown & M. Ballou (Eds.), *Personality and psychopathology: Feminist reappraisals.* New York: Guilford.

Harding, S. (1986). *The science question in feminism.* Ithaca, NY: Cornell University Press.

Harding, S. (1990). Feminism, science and the anti-enlightenment critiques. In L. J. Nicholson (Ed.), *Feminism/postmodernism.* London: Routledge.

Harstock, N. (1990). Foucault on power: A theory for women. In L. J. Nicholson (Ed.), *Feminism/postmodernism.* London: Routledge.

Helton, A. S., Anderson, E., & McFarlane, J. (1987). Battered and pregnant: A prevalence study with intervention measures. *American Journal of Public Health, 77,* 1337-1379.

Herman, J. (1992). *Trauma and recovery: The aftermath of violence—from domestic abuse to political terror.* New York: Basic Books.

Hilberman, E. (1980). Overview: The "wife-beater's wife" reconsidered. *American Journal of Psychiatry, 137*(11), 1336-1347.

Hilberman, E., & Munson, K. (1977-1978). Sixty battered women. *Victimology, 2,* 460-470.

Houskamp, B. M., & Foy, D. (1991). The assessment of posttraumatic stress disorder in battered women. *Journal of Interpersonal Violence, 6*(3), 367-375.

Island, D., & Letellier, P. (1991). *Men who beat the men who love them: Battered gay men and domestic violence.* New York: Harrington Park.

Jacobsen, A., & Richardson, B. (1987). Assault experiences of 100 psychiatric inpatients: Evidence of the need for routine inquiry. *American Journal of Psychiatry, 144,* 908-913.

Janoff-Bulman, R., & Frieze, I. H. (1983). A theoretical perspective for understanding reactions to victimization. *Journal of Social Issues, 39*(2), 1-17.

Kanuha, V. (1990). Compounding the triple jeopardy: Battering in lesbian of color relationships. In L. S. Brown & M. P. Root (Eds.), *Diversity and complexity in feminist therapy.* New York: Harrington Park.

Keller, E. F. (1985). *Reflections on gender and science.* New Haven, CT: Yale University Press.

Kemp, A., Rawlings, E. I., & Green, B. L. (1991). Post-traumatic stress disorder (PTSD) in battered women: A shelter sample. *Journal of Traumatic Stress, 4*(1), 137-148.

Koss, M. P. (in press). The impact of crime victimization on women's medicalization. *Journal of Women's Health.*

Kurz, D. (1987). Emergency department responses to battered women: Resistance to medicalization. *Social Problems, 3*(1), 69-81.

Lobel, K. (Ed.). (1986). *Naming the violence: Speaking out about lesbian battering.* Seattle: Seal.

MacKinnon, C. (1987). *Feminism unmodified: Discourses on life and law.* Cambridge, MA: Harvard University Press.

McKibben, L., De Vos, E., & Newberger, E. (1989). Victimization of mothers of abused children: A controlled study. *Pediatrics, 84*(3), 531-535.

McLeer, S. V. (1989). Education is not enough: A systems failure in protecting battered women. *Annals of Emergency Medicine, 18,* 651-653.

McLeer, S. V., & Anwar, R. (1989). A study of battered women presenting in an emergency department. *American Journal of Public Health, 79,* 65-66.

Mishler, E. (1981). Viewpoint: Critical perspectives on the biomedical model. In E. Mishler (Ed.), *Social contexts of health, illness and patient care.* Cambridge, MA: Harvard University Press.

Mishler, E. (1984). *The discourse of medicine: Dialectics of medical interviews.* Norwood, NJ: Ablex.

Raskin, V. D., & Warshaw, C. (1990, May). *Emergency room complaints of victimization: Evidence of inattention.* Poster session presented at the American Psychiatric Association meeting.

Rieker, P. P., & Carmen, E. (1984). Violence and psychiatric disorder. In P. P. Rieker & E. Carmen (Eds.), *The gender gap in psychotherapy: Social realities and psychological processes.* New York: Plenum.

Rieker, P., & Carmen, E. (1986). The victim-to-patient process: The disconfirmation and transformation of abuse. *American Journal of Orthopsychiatry, 56*(3), 360-370.

Schechter, S. (1982). *Women and male violence: The visions and struggles of the battered women's movement.* Boston: South End.

Shulman, M. (1979). *A survey of spousal violence against women in Kentucky.* Washington, DC: U.S. Department of Justice, Law Enforcement Assistance Administration.

Stark, E., & Flitcraft, A. (1988). Women and children at risk: A feminist perspective on child abuse. *International Journal of Health Services, 18,* 97-118.

Stark, E., Flitcraft, A., & Frazier, W. (1979). Medicine and patriarchal violence: The social construction of a "private" event. *International Journal of Health Services 9,* 461-492.

Stark, E., Flitcraft, A., Zuckerman, D., Gray, A., Robison, J., & Frazier, W. (1981). *Wife abuse in the medical setting: An introduction for health personnel* (Monograph 7). Washington, DC: Office of Domestic Violence.

Sugg, N. K., & Inui, T. (1991). Primary care physician's response to domestic violence opening Pandora's box. *Journal of the American Medical Association, 267*(23), 3157-3160.

Teske, R. H., & Parker, M. L. (1983). *Spouse abuse in Texas: A study of women's attitudes and experiences.* Huntsville, TX: Sam Houston State University, Criminal Justice Center.

Walker, L. E. (1991). Post-traumatic stress disorder in women: Diagnosis and treatment of battered woman syndrome. *Psychotherapy, 28,* 21-29.

Warshaw, C. (1989). Limitations of the medical model in the care of battered women. *Gender and Society, 3*(4), 506-517.

Warshaw, C., Conway, T., Hu, T. C., Coffey, V., Bullon, A. E., & Kim, P. (1993). *Prevalence of victimization amongst women patients in an ambulatory walk-in clinic.* Unpublished abstract.

Warshaw, C., & Poirier, S. (1991). Case and commentary: Hidden stories of women. *Second Opinion, 17*(2), 48-61.

Williamson, P., Beitman, B., & Katon, W. (1981). Beliefs that foster physician avoidance of psychosocial aspects of health care. *Journal of Family Practice, 13,* 999-1003.

Wilson, M., & Daly, M. (1992). Till death us do part. In J. Radford & D. E. H. Russell (Eds.), *Femicide: The politics of woman killing.* New York: Twayne.

Woods, S. J., & Campbell, J. C. (1993). Post-traumatic stress in battered women: Does the diagnosis fit? *Issues in Mental Health Nursing, 14,* 173-193.

Yl|ö, K. (1988). Political and methodological debates in wife abuse research. In K. Yllö & M. Bograd (Eds.), *Feminist perspectives on wife abuse.* Newbury Park, CA: Sage.

20

Gender Entrapment:
An Exploratory Study

Beth E. Richie

Given the increasing rate of imprisonment of women in the United States, especially lower income women of color, further exploration of women's participation in criminal activities is essential to broaden feminist scholarship to include the experiences of all women in this country, no matter what their social position or life experiences. The purpose of this chapter is to describe the results of an exploratory study that seeks to provide an alternative explanation of battered women's involvement in illegal activities. The proposed social paradigm, called "gender entrapment," links culturally constructed, gender-identity development to violence against women in their intimate relationships and, ultimately, to their participation in crime. Specifically, the research describes the interaction between gender inequality, violence, biased criminal justice practices, and cultural conditioning as well as how this process may cause certain women to be more vulnerable to violence and participation in criminal activities.

A number of academic and social trends informed the research for this chapter. This study was based partly on the new scholarship that emphasizes the interaction between race/ethnicity, gender, and class as a more useful approach to understanding societal and cultural experiences. In particular, it draws from feminist epistemological approaches to research on African American women and the black family, which suggest that, to produce an accurate knowledge base about an understudied, marginalized group, an "interested" standpoint must be assumed (Collins, 1990). Finally, this research is in response to the belief that the grassroots feminist movement has had limited success in creating the necessary social changes to end violence against women partly because it has failed to address the needs of those whose lives are most marginalized (Dobash & Dobash, 1992)—in this case, lower income, battered women of color who have been incarcerated.

Ultimately, it is hoped that this study will contribute to the movement to end violence against women in American society. Further, it is hoped that the theoretical model of gender entrapment will influence criminal justice reform efforts so that fewer women will be battered and subsequently incarcerated.

The Theoretical Paradigm:
Gender Entrapment

The term *gender entrapment* is borrowed from the legal notion of entrapment, which implies a circumstance whereby an individual is lured into a compromising act. From the study described in this chapter, the gender-entrapment theoretical paradigm is conceptualized as a dynamic process of cumulative experiences, which begins with the organization of the individual's gender-identity development in her family of origin, leading to her experiences of violence in her intimate relationships, and culminating in forced involvement in illegal activities. I argue that gender entrapment results in some battered women being penalized for activities they engage in and emotions they express even when those behaviors are a logical extension of their gender identities, their culturally expected gender roles, and the violence they experience in their intimate relationships.

The theory of gender entrapment developed in this study assumes that social relationships and institutional practices are organized in such a way as to regulate the behavior of social actors according to their gender. It also assumes that there is a dynamic interaction between the public and private spheres of human life, and that historical and ongoing cultural practices influence and are influenced by internal psychological processes. Emotional expression, identity development, and the meaning social actors give to family life play an important role in gender entrapment by influencing the ways in which women establish and maintain intimate, social, and institutional relationships.

The gender entrapment theoretical model that I developed from this study incorporates four levels of analysis. First, on the *social* level, the model explains how social structures, institutional practices, and dominant ideology influence human behavior. Second, on the *individual* or interpersonal level, the theoretical model of gender entrapment considers how human behavior is influenced by the dynamics and meaning of intimate relationships. Third, the model suggests that the dynamics of gender entrapment operate at the *community* level, where historically specific norms influence the emotional life and subsequent behavior of social actors. Fourth, the gender entrapment theoretical model incorporates the influence of the *intrapsychic* level to explain the ways internal psychological processes affect the meanings social actors give to experiences and the circumstances of their lives. Based on these four levels of understanding, the gender entrapment theory described in this chapter constitutes a complex social process incorporating not only the combined effect of gender identity, violence, cultural determinants of behavior, and crime but the *intersection* of these variables: the ways that the aforementioned factors influence each other in dynamic and dramatic ways.

The study attempted to fill the empirical gaps in the research on domestic violence and women's criminality by looking beyond the superficial, unidirectional explanations that prevail in the social science literature to a deeper level of analysis where the intersections of gender identity, emotional attachments, race/ethnicity, and violence create a subtle yet profoundly effective system of organizing women's behavior into patterns that leave them vulnerable to private and public subordination, to violence in their intimate relationships, and in turn to incarceration for the illegal activities in which they subsequently engage. As such, the gender entrapment theory helps to explain how some women who participate in illegal activity do so in response to domestic violence, the threat of violence, and other forms of coercion by their male partners. The study showed how these battered women were invisible to mainstream social service programs, legal advocacy groups, and feminist antiviolence projects because the nature of their abuse resulted in their being labeled "criminals" rather than "victims" of a crime.

The Research Design

This exploration of the theoretical paradigm that links gender-identity development, violence, race/ethnicity, and crime used the life-history interview method and the grounded theory method of data analysis. The specific research questions that this study of gender entrapment sought to answer are as follows:

1. How were the subjects' gender identities socially constructed in response to the combined effect of their emotional developments in their households of origin and their interpretations of the cultural norms and values?

2. How was gender identity and the consequent emotional work of the sample population influenced by (a) dominant ideology, (b) broader social circumstances, and (c) ongoing institutional practices in a society that is hierarchically organized by gender and race/ethnicity?

3. What "emotional work" did the subjects do in response to being abused or threatened by their male partners?

4. How did this "emotional work" represent efforts to manage the discrepancy between cultural reality and cultural ideals?

5. What circumstances influenced the subjects' paths from being abused to their participation in illegal activities?

6. What social, institutional, and emotional factors contributed to the subjects' being arrested and detained in the Rose M. Singer Center on Rikers Island?

7. How did the subjects believe the criminal justice system, social services, and other institutional responses mediated or exacerbated their negative experiences as battered women?

8. How do the factors explored in questions 1-7 constitute a unique social experience for this particular population, heretofore referred to as *gender entrapment*?

9. How did the *gender entrapment* process of African American women who were battered compare with that of two other populations at Rikers Island: (a) African American women who were not battered and (b) white women who were battered?

The Setting

The study was conducted at the Rose M. Singer Center, the women's jail at Rikers Island Correctional Facility in New York City. As the largest detention center in the United States, Rikers Island detains more than 125,000 inmates each year, with an average daily census of more than 16,000. Most of the inmates in the custody of New York City jails are detainees awaiting adjudication, having been arrested and charged but not yet tried, convicted, and/or sentenced. The population of women detained on Rikers Island has risen precipitously in the past few years. In 1987 women made up 7% of the inmate population; currently, they constitute 12%, with an average daily census of 2,000. The women detained on Rikers Island typically come from New York City's most destitute neighborhoods, where violence, poverty, and lack of health and human services have come to symbolize the institutional and governmental neglect of inner cities in this country. The fact that a disproportionate number of women inmates at Rikers Island are economically disenfranchised, undereducated, and unemployed women of color is related to the general rise in crime, more stringent criminal justice policies, and biased practices in the criminal justice system (Currie, 1985). Some criminologists suggest that the purpose of jails in contemporary society is to "manage the underclass in American society" (Irwin, 1985). The women detained at Rikers Island have experiences in jail that reflect that purpose.

The Sample

The particular focus of this study was the population of African American battered women incarcerated on Rikers Island Correctional Facility. This group was chosen because I hypothesized that they were uniquely vulnerable to the social process of gender entrapment for a number of reasons, including (a) culturally determined gender roles, (b) prevailing social conditions in African American communities, (c) hierarchical institutional arrangements in contemporary society based on race/ethnicity, and (d) biased practices within the criminal justice system. The selection of the sample population for this study was therefore purposeful and deliberate. The original interviewed sample consisted of 26 African American women who self-identified as battered women or having had a history of violence in their intimate relationship(s).

The experiences of the original group of African American battered women were compared with two other groups of women detained at Rikers Island: five African American women who were not battered and six white battered women. (See Table 20.1 for the demographic summary.) The comparative analysis of the life-history interviews of these three subgroups of women helped to refine the gender entrapment theory by isolating the effects of race/ethnicity and violence in an intimate relationship to highlight the ways that these particular variables influenced some women's experiences. While the sample obviously did not reflect the universe of experiences, by expanding the original sample to include racial/ethnic variation and experiential variations, a more complex and textured analysis of gender entrapment was possible.

The Methods of Data Collection and Analysis

The principal method of data collection used in the study was the life-history interview, following a schedule of open-ended questions. The life-history method was selected for this study because it is particularly useful in gathering information about stigmatized, uncomfortable, or difficult circumstances in subjects' lives (Marshall & Rossman, 1989), and it offered a more intense opportunity to learn about subjects' backgrounds, opinions, feelings, and the meanings they give to the mundane events and the exceptional experiences in their lives (Mishler, 1986; Watson & Franke, 1985). A review of sociological studies of similar populations that have successfully used the life-history method of data collection further established the advantage of this type of qualitative methodology (Ladner, 1972; Miller, 1986; Rollins, 1985).

TABLE 20.1 Demographic Summary

	African American		White
	Battered	*Nonbattered*	*Battered*
N	26	5	6
Household of Origin:			
Socioeconomic status			
poor/public assistance	18	4	3
working poor/working class	8	1	3
Composition of household			
adult woman and man	10	2	4
woman only	11	1	1
more than one woman	4	2	0
institutional setting	1	0	1
Number of siblings			
0	4	0	0
1-3	15	4	4
4-6	4	0	2
> 7	3	1	1
Subjects' level of education			
7-11 grade	10	4	3
graduated high school	3	1	2
earned GED	9	0	0
1-3 years of college	4	0	1
Experience of Violence:			
Early childhood abuse			
physical only	4	0	0
sexual only	12	1	0
both	0	1	5
no abuse	10	3	1
Observed mother abused	14	1	4
Battered as adults			
physical abuse	26	NA	6
sexual abuse also	20	NA	5
Use of services			
police/victims services	3	NA	5
health care providers	7	NA	5
battered women's program	1	NA	4
extended family/friends	5	NA	6
other services			
(drug programs, counseling,			
religious organizations)	1	NA	5
Illegal activity:			
Number of past incarcerations			
0	15	0	4
1	3	2	0
2-4	6	0	2
> 5	2	3	0

TABLE 20.1 Continued

	African American		White
	Battered	Nonbattered	Battered
Paths to illegal activity			
Path 1: child murder	4	0	0
Path 2: assaulted other men	4	0	0
Path 3: illegal sexual acts	6	0	3
Path 4: crime during assault	3	0	2
Path 5: economic crime	5	1	0
Path 6: illegal drug activity	4	4	1

The grounded theory methodology was used to analyze the data from the life-history interviews. Commonly employed when the goal of a study is to generate a theory that accounts for a pattern of behavior that is relevant and problematic for those involved, the grounded theory method of analysis was useful for uncovering the key elements of the theoretical paradigm of gender entrapment—the complex interactions of events and ongoing social processes associated with gender-identity development (Schwartz & Jacobs, 1979), emotional work in the public and private spheres (Hochschild, 1983), intimate violence (McGuire, 1987), and the circumstances that led to arrest (Miller, 1986). This method of analysis allowed for a discussion of the findings within a broader sociological context (Taylor & Bogdan, 1984) to illuminate the complex social process of gender entrapment.

Results

The findings revealed that the subjects' paths to illegal activities were determined by a multiplicity of factors, including their early childhood experiences as girls in their households, the construction of a cultural/racial identity, and critical events in the public sphere. A pattern emerged from the data that showed how these factors varied by race/ethnicity and experience of abuse, thereby distinguishing the backgrounds of the three subgroups and their vulnerabilities to gender entrapment.

The African American Battered Women:
Gender Entrapment

For the African American battered women, a central factor in their gender entrapment was the series of shifts in their identities in response to conditions in the private sphere and experiences in the public domain. The African

American battered women grew up as relatively privileged children in their households of origin. Despite social and economic limitations and compared with other children in their households, the women in this subgroup received more attention and a greater proportion of material resources and emotional interest from the adults around them. They developed an optimistic sense of their future and felt the expectation of social success generated by their privileged status.

While their early childhood was characterized by a sense of being competent and desirable African American girls, when they entered the public sphere, they felt the limitations of their gender, race/ethnicity, and class status. They felt unable to actualize their dreams for social success when educational and occupational opportunities were unavailable or withheld, and they felt the stigma of discrimination based on hierarchical institutional arrangements. The gender-entrapment process began here, where the African American battered women's identities developed in their households of origin were contradicted by their experiences and treatment in the public sphere. The contradiction had a particularly gendered and racial aspect, which was an important finding from this study.

While the African American battered women's public identity became more fragile, they continued to feel that a "successful" family life, as defined by dominant ideology, was within their reach. The more they became socially disenfranchised, the more they longed for respect and a sense of accomplishment that they had come to believe was possible. The African American battered women held firmly to their interest in establishing traditional nuclear families and hegemonic intimate relationships with men; however, the African American men with whom they were involved were also marginalized and thus unable to assume the traditional patriarchal roles as "head of their households."

Subsequently, the African American battered women described feeling compelled to provide opportunities for the African American men to feel powerful in the domestic sphere by relinquishing some of their status and authority. The discrepancy between the women's reality and their socially constructed ideals required them to work hard to manage the contradictions they felt and left them vulnerable to gender entrapment.

The nature of the trauma associated with the onset of abuse in their intimate relationships caused another shift in the African American battered women's identities. Violence from their intimate partners effectively destroyed their sense of themselves as "successful" women and eroded their hopes for an ideologically "normal" private life. They felt betrayed, abandoned, disoriented, and yet ironically loyal to the African American men who were abusing them. Few reached out directly for assistance, attempting instead to manage the violent episodes and conceal the signs of abuse. Their avoidance of criminal justice intervention, in particular, was noteworthy and consistent with the general sense of the hostile relationship between communities of color and the police in cities like New York.

Typically, the violence escalated over time, reaching extreme levels. The subjects were threatened with constant emotional, physical, and sexual abuse; they were seriously injured, permanently disfigured, and fearful that their batterers would eventually kill them. The shifts in their identities once again—as powerless, fearful women at serious risk of losing their lives—cemented their vulnerability to gender entrapment, leading them to participate in illegal activities for which they were eventually arrested and detained at Rikers Island Correctional Facility.

The data revealed that there were six categories of crimes or "paths" that led the African American battered women to Rikers Island Correctional Facility. Four subjects in this sample were being detained for failing to protect their children, whom their husbands killed while the women were virtually held hostage in their homes; six were arrested for prostitution or other illegal work in the sex industry, into which they were forced by their abusive husbands; three of the African American battered women were charged with property damage or arson, which occurred during a violent encounter with their batterer; four were arrested for symbolic or projected retaliation for past abuse, illustrated by the case of a woman who killed a stranger standing on her fire escape whom she thought was her abusive husband; five African American battered women were arrested for economic crimes such as shoplifting, forging checks, or robbery, which were sources of family income; and four were arrested for selling the illegal drugs they became addicted to in response to the violence.

In each of the unique life histories, the dynamics of gender entrapment led the battered women to commit crimes. Deeply invested in and committed to their relationships, the women were surprised by and denied the seriousness of the abuse. They felt compelled to accept the violence because they had a sense of themselves as relatively privileged over the men who were abusing them. The abuse reached very dangerous levels, yet the African American battered women did not reach out for help given their mistrust of the criminal justice system. When their batterer lured, threatened, or forced them into illegal activities, they felt that they had no other options but to comply. Ironically, for some women, being in jail was safer than being in the "free world."

The African American Battered
and Nonbattered Women: The Impact of Violence

A comparison of the gender identity development in both samples of African American battered and nonbattered women showed that both groups

VIOLENCE, ABUSE, AND WOMEN'S HEALTH

were influenced in significant ways by the organization of their households of origin. However, the nonbattered women interviewed for this study were less affected by the dominant ideology; their families were more isolated from social institutions in the dominant social structure; and they had looser networks of social support in their communities. The African American women who were not battered were less likely to be influenced by hegemonic values than either of the other two groups.

Additionally, the African American women who were not battered expressed less sensitivity to the social and economic position of African American men and they identified more strongly as members of an oppressed group rather than the relatively privileged women in this sample did. They understood that some African American men used their experiences of racial discrimination as an excuse to subordinate African American women, which led the women in this subgroup to establish a more oppositional stance toward the men in their lives. The African American nonbattered women grew up expecting to be treated badly by men and were therefore less likely to do the emotional work necessary to tolerate or excuse physical abuse.

The one area in which the African American nonbattered women *did* express solidarity with African American men was in their distrust of the criminal justice system. However, because the women were not victimized by the men, they did not need to depend on its agents for protection. Ironically, the African American nonbattered women identified themselves as "victims of the system" more than "criminals" or "offenders," whereas the African American battered women had a more complex analysis of their multiple identities, which shifted over time.

The paths that African American nonbattered women took to criminal activities included arrests for drug-related offenses, robbery, or burglary. As such, they were more similar to the profile of the "typical" woman detained in correctional institutions in the United States.

The African American and the
White Battered Women: The Impact of Race

Further refinement of the gender entrapment model developed in this study was gained from a comparison between the African American battered women and the white battered women in this sample. For the white battered women, gender identity was also constructed in their families of origin. Their household arrangements most closely mirrored the ideological norm in structure as generally patriarchal and rigidly organized by gender and generation, and in most cases they were oppressive environments. As such, the white battered women's attempts to attain the ideologically normative family structure were characterized by less failure and therefore created less internal tension and less ambivalence about their roles, responsibilities, and privileges as women.

Another significant difference between the white battered women and the African American battered women was the absence of a culturally constructed sensitivity to men's needs. From a very early age, the white women interviewed for this study felt inferior to the men in their lives. Unlike the African American battered women, they did not feel that they had the means to, strength to, or interest in protecting their men. When they were battered, they felt less ambivalent and confused; they understood their risks immediately; and they were more likely to reach out for help. Without overstating the availability of services for the white battered women, documentation and public recognition of the abuse were symbolic and practical in decreasing their sense of isolation and shame. In terms of the relationship to the legal system, the white battered women developed mistrust of the criminal justice system *after* being arrested, in contrast to either group of African American women, who felt mistrustful even *before* their involvement in it as criminals and/or victims.

The paths the white women took to criminal activities were also distinct from the African American battered women. They were not held hostage or terrorized in the same way that the African American battered women were; nor did they attack their batterers or other men who reminded them of their batterers. They were less likely to be arrested for arson, other property damage, or assault because they had some external protection and support.

Discussion

While the research design for this study did not require the use of a random sample or control group, through the use of the two "comparison groups" and a "model group," as directed by the principles of theoretical sampling (Strauss & Gelles, 1990), the specific mechanisms of gender entrapment with regard to race/ethnicity and violence were uncovered. Although the comparison groups were relatively small, the theory of gender entrapment, as an alternative explanation of some women's involvement in illegal activity, was strengthened by a closer analysis of the impact of race/ethnicity and violence.

The theoretical model that the study illuminated explains how some were lured, threatened, or forced into illegal activity. The African American battered women felt the impact of their gender-identity development, their family expectations and cultural loyalty, and their experiences in the public sphere in particular ways. The social, community, individual, and intrapsychic dimensions of their lives—and the emotional work they did to manage the complex and sometimes contradictory forces—constituted their gender entrapment.

Three policy issues were raised by this exploratory study of the social process I call gender entrapment.

The Stigma of Deviant Identities

First, the findings from the study point to the ways that gender, race/ethnicity, and violence interact with social stigma and deviance to negatively affect some social actors. In this sample, the women who experienced gender entrapment had six stigmatized identities—as *women* in a patriarchal society, as *African American* women who experienced ethnic stigma and discriminatory treatment (Lewis, 1990; Morton, 1991), as *poor* women, and then as *battered women*, which symbolized their failure to accomplish the socially constructed expectations and desires for safety and comfort in their domestic sphere. When the African American battered women became *criminals* (Schur, 1984), they violated still another normative standard based on the assumption of obedience and morality, which led to their experiences of the stigma of *incarceration* (Crew, 1991). The policy implications support development of strategies to counter the emotional, cultural, social, economic, and political forces that led to "deviance" that would subsequently reverse the long-term effects of stigma based on gender, race/ethnicity, and the experiences of violence and crime.

The Legal Implications
of the Question of Agency

The theoretical model of gender entrapment, which is based on the understanding that some women are lured, threatened, or forced into compromising acts, raises the legal questions of intentionality and duress. From a philosophical perspective, the question is this: "What are the limits of free will and individual choice?" While their involvement in crime could be considered an exercise of their agency, it may be possible to interpret the African American battered women's illegal activities in *legal* terms that would limit their culpability. This policy issue suggests the need for further analysis of gender entrapment from the perspective of feminist legal scholarship to explore the utility of the theory in the defense of some battered women who commit crimes.

The Relationship Between
a Gendered and Racial Analysis

The third issue that the gender entrapment theoretical model raises is related to the current sociological and political question about the "plight of black men" in contemporary society (Wilson, 1987). The facts that surround the question include the rising incarceration and homicide rates, troubling unemployment statistics, and highly publicized cases of police brutality toward young African American men (National Research Council, 1989). These concerns reflect a larger social, political, and economic crisis that is disproportionately affecting the African American community, resulting in a sense of collective devastation and individual despair. The underlying causes of this crisis situation require critical attention, policy reform, and the infusion of resources.

The framework for the analysis and construction of the response, however, will be seriously flawed without attention to the intersection of institutionalized racism, discrimination, *and gender* inequality. Without a gender analysis of this crisis, African American women's experience will be rendered invisible and/or insignificant, and the potential solutions will reproduce relationships of gender domination within the African American community. Instead, my hope is that the gender entrapment theoretical model will expand the terms of the debate and deepen the analysis to include a critical feminist perspective.

Conclusion

This chapter described the findings of an exploratory study designed to develop the theoretical model of gender entrapment, an alternative explanation of some women's involvement in illegal activity. It described the extreme consequences in which gender inequality, violence, biased criminal justice practices, and cultural conditioning intersect. It could be argued that had the dynamics between the circumstances in the public and the private spheres of their lives been different, some of the African American battered women in this study might have been extraordinarily successful. Instead of positioning them for success, their idealism, emotional skills, their families' investment in their future, and the African American battered women's loyalty converged with their stigmatized identities and marginalized status in the public sphere to leave them vulnerable to violence and crime. My hope is that the theoretical model of gender entrapment will influence criminal justice reform so that fewer women will be battered and incarcerated and so that such a contribution to the body of feminist scholarship can create change on behalf of those women whose experiences are most invisible or misunderstood by the dominant social science paradigms.

References

Collins, P. H. (1990). *Black feminist thought: Knowledge, consciousness and the politics of empowerment.* Boston: Unwin Hyman.

Crew, K. B. (1991). Sex differences in criminal sentencing: Chivalry or patriarchy. *Justice Quarterly, 8*(1), 59-82.

Currie, E. (1985). *Confronting crime: An American challenge.* New York: Pantheon.

Dobash, R. E., & Dobash, R. P. (1992). *Women, violence and social change.* New York: Routledge.

Hampton, R. (Ed.). (1987). *Violence in the black family: Correlates and consequences.* Lexington, MA: Lexington.

Hochschild, A. (1983). *The managed heart: Commercialization of feeling.* Berkeley: University of California.

Irwin, J. (1985). *The jail: Managing the underclass in American society.* Berkeley: University of California.

Ladner, J. (1972). *Tomorrow's tomorrow: The black woman.* New York: Doubleday.

Lewis, D. (1990). A response to inequality: Black women, racism and sexism. In M. Malson et al. (Eds.), *Black women in America: Social science perspectives.* Chicago: University of Chicago.

Marshall, C., & Rossman, G. (1989). *Designing qualitative research.* Newbury Park, CA: Sage.

McGuire, P. (1987). *Doing participatory research: A feminist approach.* Amherst: University of Massachusetts, Center for International Education.

Miller, E. (1986). *Street women.* Philadelphia: Temple University Press.

Mishler, E. G. (1986). *Research interviewing: Context and narrative.* Cambridge, MA: Harvard University Press.

Morton, P. (1991). *Disfigured images: The historical assault on Afro-America women.* New York: Greenwood.

National Commission on Crime and Delinquency. (1989, December). *Focus,* p. 1.

National Research Council. (1989). *A common destiny: Blacks and American society.* Washington, DC: National Academy Press.

Rollins, J. (1985). *Between women: Domestics and their employers.* Philadelphia: Temple University Press.

Schur, E. (1984). *Labeling women deviant: Gender, stigma and social control.* New York: Random House.

Schwartz, H., & Jacobs, J. (1979). *Qualitative sociology: A method to the madness.* New York: Free Press.

Strauss, M. A., & Gelles, R. J. (1990). *Physical violence in American families: Risk factors and adaptations to violence in 8,145 families.* New Brunswick, NJ: Transaction.

Taylor, S., & Bogdan, R. (1984). *Introduction to qualitative research.* New York: Wiley.

Watson, L., & Franke, M. B. W. (1985). *Interpreting life histories.* New Brunswick, NJ: Rutgers University Press.

Wilson, W. J. (1987). *The truly disadvantaged: The inner city, the underclass and public policy.* Chicago: University of Chicago.

21

Gender-Based Abuse: The Global Epidemic

Lori L. Heise

Prologue

Wife beating is an accepted custom . . . we are wasting our time debating the issue.

Comments made by a parliamentarian during floor debates on wife battering in Papua New Guinea ("Wife Beating," 1987)

A wife married is like a pony bought; I'll ride her and whip her as I like.

Chinese proverb (Croll, 1980)

Women should wear *purdah* [head to toe covering] to ensure that innocent men do not get unnecessarily excited by women's bodies and are not unconsciously forced into becoming rapists. If women do not want to fall prey to such men, they should take the necessary precautions instead of forever blaming the men.

Comment made by a parliamentarian of the ruling Barisan National Party during floor debates on rape reform in Malaysia (Heise, 1991)

The boys never meant any harm to the girls. They just wanted to rape.

Statement by the deputy principal of St. Kizito's boarding school in Kenya after 71 girls were raped and 19 others died when the boys attacked the girls for refusing to join them in a strike against the school's headmaster (Perlez, 1991)

Breast bruised, brains battered,
Skin scarred, soul shattered,

Can't scream—neighbors stare,
Cry for help—no one's there.

Stanza from a poem by Nenna Nehru,
a battered Indian woman (APDC, 1989)

The child was sexually aggressive.

Observation made by a Canadian judge in British Columbia,
who suspended a 33-year-old man for sexually assaulting
a 3-year-old girl (House of Commons, 1991)

Are you a virgin? If you are not a virgin, why do you complain? This is normal.

Response by the assistant to public prosecutor in Peru when nursing
student, Betty Fernandez, reported being sexually molested by police
officers while in custody (Kirk, 1993)

Gender-based violence—including rape, domestic violence, mutilation, murder, and sexual abuse—is a profound health problem for women across the globe. Although a significant cause of female morbidity and mortality, gender violence is almost never seen as a public health issue. Recent World Bank estimates of the global burden of disease indicate that in Established Market Economies gender-based victimization is responsible for *one out of every five healthy days of life lost to women of reproductive age.* On a per capita basis, the health burden imposed by rape and domestic violence is roughly equivalent in both the industrial and the developing world, but because the overall burden is so much greater in the developing world, the percentage attributable to gender-based victimization is smaller (World Bank, 1993). Nonetheless, on a global basis, the health burden from gender-based victimization among reproductive-age women is comparable to that posed by other conditions already high on the world agenda (see Table 21.1).

Female-focused violence also represents a hidden obstacle to economic and social development. By sapping women's energy, undermining their confidence, and compromising their health, gender violence deprives society of women's full participation. As the United Nations Fund for Women (UNIFEM) recently observed: "Women cannot lend their labor or creative ideas fully if they are burdened with the physical and psychological scars of abuse" (Carrillo, 1992, p. 11).

In recent years, the world community has taken some tentative, yet important, steps toward urging greater attention to the issue of gender-based abuse. Various U.N. bodies, including the Commission on the Status of Women, the

TABLE 21.1 Estimated Health Burden of Various Conditions for Women
Aged 15 to 44, Globally

Conditions	DALYs (in millions)
Maternal conditions	29.0
a sepsis	10.0
b obstructed labor	7.8
STDs excluding HIV	15.8
a PID	12.8
Tuberculosis	10.9
HIV	10.6
Cardiovascular disease	10.5
Rape and domestic violence	9.5
All cancers	9.0
a breast	1.4
b cervical	1.0
Motor vehicle accidents	4.2
War	2.7
Malaria	2.3

NOTE: DALY (disability adjusted life year) = a measure of healthy years of life lost due to health-related morbidity or premature death. Every year lost to death is counted as 1 DALY and every year spent sick or incapacitated is counted as a fraction of a DALY, based on the severity of the disability. (For further explanation, see World Bank, 1993.)

Economic and Social Council, the Committee on Crime Prevention and Control, and the General Assembly, have all passed resolutions recognizing violence against women as an issue of grave concern. Negotiations are also under way through the Organization of American States to draft a Pan American Treaty Against Violence Against Women.

This international attention, however, comes on the heels of over two decades of organizing by women's groups around the world to combat gender-based abuse. In country after country, women have started crisis centers, passed laws, and worked to change the cultural beliefs and attitudes that undergird men's violence. A recent directory published by the Santiago-based ISIS International lists 379 separate organizations working against gender violence in Latin America alone (ISIS, 1990).

The Magnitude of the Problem

Domestic violence. The most pervasive form of gender violence is abuse of women by intimate male partners. More than 30 well-designed surveys are now available from a wide range of countries showing that between one fifth to over half of women interviewed have been beaten by a male partner (see Table 21.2). The majority of these women are beaten at least three times a year with many experiencing persistent psychological and sexual abuse as well.

According to a recent review in the *Journal of the American Medical Association*, "women in the United States are more likely to be assaulted and injured, raped or killed by a current or ex-male partner than all other assailants combined" (Council on Scientific Affairs, 1992, p. 3185). The same could be said of women elsewhere in the world. In Papua New Guinea (PNG), 18% of *all* urban wives surveyed had received hospital treatment for injuries inflicted by their husbands (Toft, 1987). In Alexandria, Egypt, domestic violence is the leading cause of injury to women, accounting for 28% of all visits to area trauma units (Graitcer, personal communication). And in countries as diverse as Brazil, Israel, Canada, and PNG, over half of all women murdered are killed by a current or former partner (Heise, 1994).

Rape and sexual abuse. Regrettably, statistics suggest that sexual coercion is also a common reality in the lives of women and girls. An islandwide survey of women in Barbados revealed that one in three women had been sexually abused as a child or adolescent (Handwerker, 1993a). In Seoul, South Korea, 17% of women report being a victim of attempted or completed rape (Shim, 1992). And in the United States, 78 adult women—and at least as many girls and adolescents—are raped each hour, according to a national survey (Kilpatrick, Edmunds, & Seymour, 1992).

Rape survivors exhibit a variety of trauma-induced symptoms including sleep and eating disturbances, depression, feelings of humiliation, anger and self-blame, fear of sex, and inability to concentrate (Koss, 1990). Survivors also run the risk of becoming pregnant or contracting STDs, including HIV. A rape crisis center in Bangkok, Thailand, reports that 10% of their clients contract STDs as a result of rape and 15% to 18% become pregnant, a figure consistent with data from Mexico and Korea (Archavanitkui & Pramualratana, 1990; COVAC, 1990; Shim, 1992). In countries where abortion is illegal or unavailable, victims often resort to illegal abortion, greatly increasing their chance of future infertility or even death.

Why Focus Specifically on Violence Against Women?

Although men *are* victims of street violence, brawls, homicide, and crime, violence directed at women is a distinctly different phenomenon. Men tend to be attacked and killed by strangers or casual acquaintances, whereas women are most at risk at home from men whom they trust (Kellermann & Mercy, 1992). Violence against women is grounded in power imbalances

(*text continued on page 243*)

TABLE 21.2 Prevalence of Wife Abuse, Selected Countries

Country	Sample Size	Sample Type	Findings	Comments
Barbados (Handwerker, 1993a)	264 women and 243 men aged 20-45	Islandwide national probability sample	30% of women battered as adults	Women and men report 50% of their mothers beaten
Antigua (Handwerker, 1993b)	97 women aged 20-45	Random subset of national probability sample	30% of women battered as adults	Women report 50% of mothers beaten.
Uganda (Wakabi & Mwesigye, 1991)	80 women; 16 women from each of Kampala's five divisions	House-to-house written survey; 7 women refused to answer	46% of women responding ($n = 73$) reported being physically abused by a partner	An additional 7 women reported beatings by family members and another 5 assaults or rapes by outsiders
Kenya (Raikes, 1990)	733 women from Kissi District	Districtwide cluster sample	42% "beaten regularly"	Taken from contraceptive prevalence survey
Tanzania (Sheikh-Hashim & Gabba, 1990)	300 women from Dar-es-Salaam	Convenience sample from three districts—Ilala, Temeke, and Kinondoni (interviews)	60% had been "physically abused" by a partner	
Zambia (Phiri, 1992)	171 women aged 20 to 40	Convenience sample of women from shanty compounds, medium- and high-density suburbs of Lusaka and Kafue Rural	40% "beaten" by a partner; another 40% "mentally abused"	17% said they thought that physical or mental abuse was a normal part of marriage
Papua New Guinea (Toft, 1987)	Rural: 736 men; 715 women; Urban low income: 368 men; 298 women; Urban elite: 178 men; 99 women	Rural survey in 19 villages in all regions and provinces; Urban survey with over sample of elites	67% rural women "beaten" 56% urban low-income women 62% urban elite women	Almost perfect agreement between percentage of women who claim to have been beaten and percentage of men who admit to abuse

237

TABLE 21.2 Continued

Country	Sample Size	Sample Type	Findings	Comments
Sri Lanka (Sonali, 1990)	200 mixed ethnic, low-income women from Colombo	Convenience sample from low-income neighborhood	60% have been beaten	51% of those beaten said husbands used weapons
Korea (Kim & Cho, 1992)	707 women and 609 men who had lived with a partner for at least 2 years	Three-stage, stratified random sample of entire country; face-to-face interviews	37.5% of wives report "being battered" by their spouse in *last year*	12.4% report serious physical abuse within last year (N to R on the Conflict Tactics Scale)
Korea (Shim, 1988)	708 women in Suwon and Seoul	Convenience sample; based on distributed questionnaires	42.2% have been "beaten by husband after marriage"	14% report being "beaten by their husband" within the last year
India (V. Rao, University of Michigan, personal communication, 1993)	170 women of childbearing age in 3 villages in rural southern Karnataka	100% sample of potter community in each village based on previous census	22% of women report being "physically assaulted" by their husbands; 12% report being beaten within the last month, on average 2.65 times	Author notes that informal interviews and ethnographic data suggest that prevalence rates are "vastly underreported."
India (Mahajan, 1990)	109 men and 109 women from village in Jullundur District, Punjab	50% sample of all scheduled caste households & 50% of nonscheduled caste houses	75% of scheduled caste men admit to beating their wives; 22% of higher caste men admit to beatings	75% of scheduled (lower) caste wives report being beaten "frequently"
Malaysia (WAO, 1992)	713 women and 508 males over 15 years old	National random sample of peninsular Malaysia	39% of women have been "physically beaten" by a partner in 1989	Note: This is an annual figure; 15% of adults consider wife beating acceptable (22% of Malays).

Study	Sample	Sample method	Findings	Notes
Japan (Domestic Violence Research Group, 1993)	796 women from all over Japan (17% return on 4,675 questionnaires)	Convenience sample based on survey distributed nationally through women's groups, adult education classes, media, and so on	58.7% report physical abuse by a partner; 65.7 report emotional abuse; 59.4 report sexual abuse	44% of sample experienced all three types of abuse simultaneously. Note: This is not a representative sample.
Colombia (PROFAMILIA, 1992)	3,272 urban women 2,118 rural women	National random sample	20% physically abused; 33% psychologically abused; 10% raped by husband	Part of Colombia's Demographic and Health Survey (DHS)
Costa Rica (Chacon et al., 1990)	1,388 women	Convenience sample of women attending child welfare clinic (for reasons not related to violence)	50% report being physically abused	
Guatemala (Coy, 1990, cited in Castillo et al., 1992)	1,000 women	Random sample of women in Sacatepequez	49% abused, 74% by an intimate male partner	Includes physical, emotional, and sexual abuse in adulthood; sponsored by UNICEF/PAHO
Mexico (Ramirez & Vazquez, 1993)	1,163 rural women; 427 urban women in the state of Jalisco	Random household survey of women on DIF (social welfare) register	56.7% of urban women and 44.2% of rural women had experienced some form of "interpersonal violence"	In more than 60% of cases, the principal aggressor was the husband.
Mexico (Shrader Cox & Valdez Santiago, 1992)	342 women aged 15 years or older, low to middle income	Random sample of households in Mexico City periurban neighborhood	33% had lived in a "violent relationship"; 6% had experienced marital rape	Of abused women, 66% had been physically abused, 76% psychologically abused, and 21% sexually abused.
Ecuador (CEPLAES, 1992)	200 low-income women	Convenience sample of Quito barrio	60% had been "beaten" by a partner	37% of those beaten were assaulted once a month or more

(continued)

TABLE 21.2 Continued

Country	Sample Size	Sample Type	Findings	Comments
Chile (Larrain, 1993)	1,000 women in Santiago ages 22 to 55 years involved in relationship of 2 years or more	Stratified random sample with a maximum sampling error of 3%	60% have been abused by a male intimate; 26.2% have been physically abused (severe violence on the CTS, i.e., more severe than pushes, slaps, or having object thrown at you)	70% of those abused are abused more than once a year
Belgium (Bruynooghe et al., 1989, as cited in Garcia, 1991)	956 women between the ages of 30 and 40	Random sample from 62 municipalities throughout the country	3% had experienced "very serious violence"; 13% "moderately serious violence"; and 25% "less serious" violence	Survey queried women on 15 types of physical violence ranging from blows with the hand to life-threatening forms such as strangulation and gun wounds.
Norway (Schei & Bakketeig, 1989)	150 women aged 20 to 49 years in Trondheim	Random sample selected from census data	25% had been physically or sexually abused by a male partner	Definition includes only forms of violence more severe than pushing, slapping, or shoving (severe violence on the CTS).
The Netherlands (Romkens, 1989)	1,016 women aged 20 to 60 years	Face-to-face interviews	20.8% experienced physical violence in a heterosexual relationship	Half (11%) experienced severe, repeated violence.
New Zealand (Anderson et al., in press)	3,000 women in Otago sent questionnaire; 497 women interviewed (half sexually abused and half control group)	Random sample of women selected from electoral rolls; all figures weighted back from interview sample to main postal sample	22.4% had been physically abused since age 16, 76% by a male intimate (i.e., 17% of total)	

240

New Zealand (Mullen et al., 1988)	2,000 women sent questionnaire; stratified random sample of 349 women selected for interview	Random sample selected from electoral roles of five contiguous parliamentary constituencies	20.1% report being "hit and physically abused" by a male partner; 58% of these women (> 10% of sample) were battered more than 3 times	11.3% report abuse within last year
United States (Straus & Gelles, 1986)	2,143 married or cohabiting couples	National probability sample using random digit dialing	28% report at least one episode of physical violence	
United States (Grant, Preda, & Martin, 1989)	6,000 women statewide from Texas; 1,539 usable questionnaires returned	Statewide random sample based on women holding valid driver's licenses	39% have been abused by male partner after age 18; 31% have been physically abused	> 12% have been sexually abused by male partner after age 18
United States (Teske & Parker, 1983)	3,000 rural women in Texas	Random sample from communities with 50,000 people or less	40.2% have been abused after age 18; 31% have been physically abused	22% abused within the last 12 months
Canada (Smith, 1987)	604 presently or formerly married or cohabiting women aged 18 to 50 in metropolitan Toronto	Random digit dialing phone survey	36.4% report being physically abused ever in a relationship; 11.3% report severe physical abuse (items 16-19 on CTS)	14.4% report physical abuse within the last year
Canada (Haskell & Randall, 1993)	Face-to-face interviews with 402 women between the ages of 18 and 64 years in Toronto	Random sample of all residential addresses (including apartments) in Toronto	27% report being physically assaulted ever by an intimate partner	In 36% of the cases, women reported fearing that they would be killed by the man who assaulted them
Canada (Lupri, 1989)	426 married or cohabiting women	Random sample using face-to-face interviews and mailed questionnaire	17.8% of women report physical violence by a partner within the last year	Note: This is a 1-year rate

(continued)

TABLE 21.2 Continued

Country	Sample Size	Sample Type	Findings	Comments
Canada (Statistics Canada, 1993)	Nationally representative sample of 12,300 women 18 and older	Indepth interview by phone using random digit dialing	25% of women (29% of ever married women) report being physically assaulted by a current or former male partner since age 16	65% of victims were assaulted more than once; 32% more than 11 times; 45% of wife assault incidents resulted in injury
Canada (Kennedy & Dutton, 1989)	1,045 men and women in Alberta, Canada	454 face-to-face interviews with residents of households randomly selected from census enumerations; 244 telephone interviews with Calgary residents and 347 from rest of province, selected by random digit dialing	11.2% of respondents report physical abuse within last year according to the CTS	Note: This is a 1-year rate

between men and women and is caused and perpetuated by factors different than violence against men. As such, the violence must be analyzed and addressed differently. While women are occasionally violent against intimates, research has shown that female violence is usually in self-defense and that it is women who suffer the bulk of injury (Dobash et al., 1992).

Impact on Health Care Use

In addition to injury, physical and sexual abuse provide the primary context for many other health problems. Victims of sexual abuse, rape, and domestic violence are at increased risk of suicide, depression, drug and alcohol abuse, STDs, hypertension, chronic pelvic pain, irritable bowel syndrome, asthma, gynecological problems, and a variety of psychiatric disorders (Heise, 1994; Koss & Heslet, 1992). Most victims of violence first seek medical care for the secondary sequelae of abuse rather than for the initial abuse-related trauma.

Not surprisingly, victims of violence require a significant portion of scarce health resources. Studies reveal that 22% to 35% of women presenting with any complaint to U.S. emergency rooms are there because of symptoms related to partner abuse (Council on Scientific Affairs, 1992). Another study at a major U.S. HMO found that a history of rape or assault was a stronger predictor of physician visits and outpatient costs among women than were age or other health risks, such as smoking. Women who had been raped or assaulted had medical costs two and half times higher in the index year than nonvictimized women, even after controlling for other health, stress, and demographic factors (Koss, Koss, & Woodruff, 1991). A similar study by Feletti (1991) found that, among women enrolled in an HMO plan, 22% of those who had a history of childhood molestation or rape had visited a physician 10 or more times a year compared with 6% of nonvictimized women. Such expenditures could be drastically reduced through preventive actions.

Implications for International Development

Violence presents a powerful obstacle to achieving other goals high on the development agenda. Violence during pregnancy, for example, threatens the goal of "safe motherhood" for all women. Among 80 battered women seeking judicial intervention in San Jose, Costa Rica, 49% report being beaten during pregnancy (Ugalde, 1988). Battered women run twice the risk of miscarriage and four times the risk of having a low birth weight infant (Bullock & McFarlane, 1989; Stark et al., 1981). In some regions, violence also accounts for a sizable portion of maternal mortality. In Matlab Thana, Bangladesh, intentional injury—motivated by dowry disputes or stigma over rape and unwed pregnancy—accounted for 6% of all maternal deaths between 1976 and 1986 (Faveau & Blanchet, 1989).

New evidence from the United States suggests that sexual abuse may serve as a direct break on socioeconomic development by affecting a woman's educational and income levels. A recent study shows that women who have been sexually abused during childhood achieve an annual income 3% to 20% lower than women who have not been abused depending on the type of abuse experienced and the number of perpetrators (after controlling for all known income factors) (Hyman, 1993). Violence has also been shown to interfere with women's participation in development projects. A study commissioned by UNIFEM/Mexico found that a primary reason women dropped out of projects was threats and violence by husbands who disapproved of their wives' empowerment (cited in Carrillo, 1992).

Likewise, fear of male violence can interfere with efforts to curb population growth and to control the spread of AIDS. According to research generated by USAID's Women and HIV project, women are frequently afraid to raise the issue of condom use for fear of abandonment, accusations of infidelity, or physical reprisal (G. Rao Gupta, Institute for Research on Women, Washington, DC, personal communication, April 1993). In some cultures, men assert that use of any birth control implies promiscuity or a woman's desire to be unfaithful. In Kenya, women regularly forge their partner's signature on spousal consent forms for contraception rather than ask their partner's permission (Banwell, 1990). When family planning clinics in Ethiopia removed their requirement for spousal consent, clinic use rose 26% in just a few months (Cook & Maine, 1987).

Response of the Health Sector

As the only public institution likely to interact with all women at some point in their lives, the health system is particularly well placed to identify and refer victims of violence. This access is important because experience has shown that, even in countries with a strong movement against violence, many women never choose to call the police or a crisis hot line, the two most widely developed sources for referral. Advocates in the state of Connecticut, for example, estimate that only 10% of battered women living there ever come in contact with the state's extensive network of legal advocates, shelters, and crisis centers, because the system relies primarily on the justice system and word of mouth to notify victims of available services (Heise & Chapman,

1992). In politically repressive countries, the likelihood of the police serving as an adequate source of referral is even more unrealistic.

Women unable or unwilling to seek help from the police or other governmental authorities may nonetheless admit abuse when questioned gently, in private, by a supportive health care provider. Providers have found that, contrary to their expectations, women have proven quite willing to admit abuse when asked directly in a nonjudgmental way. When Planned Parenthood of Houston and Southeast Texas added four abuse assessment questions to their standard intake form, for example, 8.2% of women self-identified as physically abused. When asked the same questions in person by a provider, 29% of women reported abuse (Bullock et al., 1989).

Despite the potentially critical role of health care professionals, evidence indicates that few providers identify and respond appropriately to victims of abuse (Kurz, 1987). Health facilities can greatly enhance their staff's sensitivity to gender-based violence by introducing training and standardized protocols on how to respond to abuse. At the emergency department of the Medical College of Pennsylvania, the percentage of female trauma patients found to be battered increased more than fivefold, from 5.6% to 30%, after training and protocols were introduced (McCleer & Anwar, 1989). Providers can emphasize that no one deserves to be beaten or raped, and help women think through future options for protecting themselves (e.g., seeking safety at a friend's house). There are also a growing number of services in both the industrial and the developing world to which providers can refer women for legal or psychological support. Even where no external support exists, having a sympathetic individual acknowledge and denounce the violence in a woman's life offers considerable relief from isolation and self-blame.

Despite their utility, protocols and training are still uncommon in the United States. Only 20% of emergency departments in Massachusetts—one of the better organized states—had a written protocol for domestic violence in 1991 (Isaac & Sanchez, 1992). That same year, however, two important initiatives were launched that should encourage greater health care involvement in the issue of violence. First, the American Medical Association (AMA) initiated a major campaign to educate the public and physicians about family violence and devoted an entire issue of their prestigious *Journal of the American Medical Association* to the theme. The U.S. Joint Commission on Hospital Accreditation also passed new standards including emergency room protocols and training on family violence among the criteria used to evaluate hospitals for accreditation (Heise & Chapman, 1992). This policy change should encourage more active screening and referral of victims of abuse. A new project sponsored by the Family Violence Prevention Fund in San Francisco and the Pennsylvania Coalition Against Domestic Violence hopes to help institutionalize the new hospital accreditation standards by developing model protocols, training programs, and dissemination strategies that can be applied throughout the country.

What Can Be Done?

Cross-cultural research indicates that, although violence against women is an integral part of the vast majority of cultures, there *are* isolated examples of societies where gender-based abuse does not exist (Levinson, 1989; Sanday, 1981). Such societies stand as proof that social relations can be organized in such a way as to minimize or eliminate violence against women. Low-violence cultures share the following key features:

- strong sanctions against interpersonal violence
- community support for victims
- flexible gender roles for men and women
- equality of decision making and resources in the family
- a cultural ethos that condemns violence as a means to resolve conflict
- female power and autonomy outside of the home

Even where supportive social factors do not exist, experience has shown that strategic intervention on the part of the community, women's organizations, and the state can save lives, reduce injury, and lessen the long-term impact of victimization on women and their children.

Any response to violence must meet the immediate needs of victims while working to combat the attitudes, beliefs, and social structures that encourage gender-based abuse. Important first steps include (a) reforming laws that discriminate against women; (b) expanding legal, medical, psychological, and advocacy services for victims; (c) enacting and enforcing laws against battering, rape, and sexual abuse; (d) training professionals in how to identify and respond to abuse; (e) expanding the availability of shelters and safe home networks; (f) incorporating gender awareness training, parenting skills, and nonviolent conflict resolution into family life curricula; (g) eliminating gratuitous violence from the media; and (h) ensuring alternatives for women by expanding access to low-income housing, credit, child care, and divorce.

There is also urgent need for more and better data on the social and economic costs of violence, its impact on women's health and well-being, and the effectiveness of various interventions designed to curb abuse. Ongoing research efforts, such as focus groups and surveys being conducted on sexuality for the purposes of developing AIDS prevention programs, should use these opportunities to explore the role that violence and coercion plays in women's sexual and reproductive decision making.

Program Implications

It is time that governments and the international community recognize that women have a right to live free from physical and psychological abuse. The most important step forward is to support the nascent antiviolence initiatives already under way at both the governmental and the nongovernmental levels. Much of the leadership to date has come from autonomous women's organizations who have fought tirelessly to open crisis centers, change laws, and challenge the cultural beliefs that perpetuate violence against women. These groups could easily be strengthened with only a minimal investment of resources.

A growing number of governments also have important new initiatives in need of support. Both the Brazilian and Colombian constitutions now have articles establishing the state's responsibility to combat family violence. Other governments—including Papua New Guinea, Chile, Canada, and Ecuador—have sponsored research, opened shelters, or sponsored national media campaigns. The women's health community can play an important role in holding governments accountable to these commitments. At the recent World Conference for Human Rights held in Vienna, Austria, a coalition of 950 women's organizations demanded and got, for the first time, official recognition of violence against women as an abuse of women's human rights. As the women's statement to the Government Assembly observed, "Putting violence high on the world agenda is not appeasing the interests of a 'special interest' group, it is restoring the birthright of half of humanity."

References

Anderson, J., et al. (in press). Violence against women in New Zealand: The Otago Women's Health Survey. *Journal of the American Academy of Child and Adolescent Psychiatry.*

APDC (Asian and Pacific Development Center) (1989). *Asian & Pacific Women's Resource and Action Series: Health.* Kuala Lumpur: Author.

Archavanitkui, K., & Pramualratana, A. (1990, October 29-31). *Factors affecting women's health in Thailand.* Paper presented at the Workshop on Women's Health in Southeast Asia, the Population Council, Jakarta, Indonesia.

Banwell, S. S. (1990). *Law, status of women and family planning in Sub-Saharan Africa: A suggestion for action.* Nairobi, Kenya: Pathfinder Fund.

Bruynooghe, R., et al. (1989). *Study of physical violence against Belgian women.* Limburgs, Belgium: Limburgs Universitair Centrum, Department des Sciences Humaines et Sociales.

Bullock, L. F., & McFarlane, J. (1989). The birth/weight battering connection. *American Journal of Nursing, 89*(9), 1153-1155.

Bullock, L., et al. (1989). The prevalence and characteristics of battered women in a primary care setting. *Nurse Practitioner, 14*, 47-54.

Carrillo, R. (1992). *Battered dreams: Violence against women as an obstacle to development.* New York: U.N. Fund for Women.

Castillo, D., et al. (1992, March 11-13). *Violencia hacia la mujer en Guatemala.* Paper prepared for the First Central American Seminar on Violence Against Women as a Public Health Problem, Managua, Nicaragua.

CEPLAES (Centro de Planificacion y Estudios Sociales). (1992). *Proyecto educativo sobre violencia de genero en la relacion domestica de pareja.* Quito, Ecuador: Author.

Chacon, K., et al. (1990). *Caracteristicas de la mujer agredida atendida en el Patronato Nacional de la Infancia (PANI).* San Jose, Costa Rica: Author.

Cook, R., & Maine, D. (1987). Spousal veto over family planning services. *American Journal of Public Health, 77*(3), 339-344.

Council on Scientific Affairs, American Medical Association. (1992). Violence against women: Relevance for medical practitioners. *Journal of the American Medical Association, 267*(23), 3184-3189.

COVAC. (1990). *Evaluacion de Proyecto para Educacion, Capacitacion, y Atencion a Mujeres y Menores de Edad en Materia de Violencia Sexual, Enero a Diciembre 1990.* Mexico City: Asociacion Mexicana Contra la Violencia a las Mujeres.

Croll, E. (1980). *Feminism and socialism in China.* New York: Schocken.

Dobash, R., et al. (1992). The myth of sexual symmetry in marital violence. *Social Problems, 39*(1), 71-91.

Domestic Violence Research Group. (1993, June 12-25). *A study on violence precipitated by husbands (boyfriends) in Japan: Preliminary findings.* Paper presented at the NGO parallel activities at the U.N. Conference on Human Rights, Vienna, Austria.

Fauveau, V., & Blanchet, T. (1989). Deaths from injuries and induced abortion among rural Bangladeshi women. *Social Science and Medicine, 29*(9), 1121-1128.

Garcia, A. (1991). *Sexual violence against Belgian women: Contribution to strategy for countering the various forms of such violence in the Council of Europe member states.* Strasbourg: European Committee for Equality Between Women and Men.

Grant, R., Preda, M., & Martin, J. D. (1989). *Domestic violence in Texas: A study of statewide and rural spouse abuse.* Wichita Falls, TX: Midwestern State University, Bureau of Business and Government Research.

Handwerker, P. (1993a). Gender power differences between parents and high risk sexual behavior by their children: AIDS/STD risk factors extend to a prior generation. *Journal of Women's Health, 2*(3), 301.

Handwerker, P. (1993b). *Power, gender violence, and high risk sexual behavior: AIDS/STD risk factors need to be defined more broadly.* Unpublished manuscript, Humboldt State University, Arcata, CA.

Haskell, L., & Randall, M. (1993). *The Women's Safety Project: Summary of key statistical findings.* Ottawa: Canadian Panel on Violence Against Women.

Heise, L. (1991, December 13). When women are prey. *Washington Post*, Outlook sec., pp. C1-C3.

Heise, L., & Chapman, J. R. (1992). Reflections on a movement: The U.S. battle against woman abuse. In M. Schuler (Ed.), *Freedom from violence: Women's strategies from around the world* (pp. 257-294). Washington, DC: OEF International. (Available through UNIFEM, New York)

Heise, L., with Pitanguy, J., & Germaine, A. (1994). *Violence against women: The hidden health burden.* Washington, DC: World Bank.

House of Commons. (1991). *The war against women* (Report of the Standing Committee on Health and Welfare, Social Affairs, Seniors and the Status of Women). Ottawa, Canada: Author.

Hyman, B. (1993). *Economic consequences of child sexual abuse in women.* Unpublished doctoral dissertation, Heller School of Policy, Brandeis, University, Waltham, MA.

ISIS International. (1990). *Violencia en contra de la mujer en America Latina y El Caribe: Directorio de programas.* Santiago, Chile: Author.

Isaac, N., & Sanchez, R. (1992, November). *Emergency department response to battered women in Massachusetts.* Paper presented at the APHA Conference, Washington, DC.

Kellermann, A. L., & Mercy, J. A. (1992). Men, women, and murder: Gender-specific differences in rates of fatal violence and victimization. *The Journal of Trauma, 33*(4), 1-5.

Kennedy, L. W., & Dutton, D. G. (1989). The incidence of wife assault in Alberta. *Canadian Journal of Behavioral Science, 21,* 40-54.

Kilpatrick, D. G., Edmunds, C. N., & Seymour, A. K. (1992). *Rape in America: A report to the nation.* Arlington, VA: National Victim Center.

Kim, K., & Cho, Y. (1992). Epidemiological survey of spousal abuse in Korea. In E. C. Viano (Ed.), *Intimate violence: Interdisciplinary perspectives* (pp. 277-283). Washington, DC: Hemisphere.

Kirk, R. (1993). *Untold terror: Violence against women in Peru's armed conflict.* New York: Human Rights Watch.

Koss, M. (1990). The women's mental health research agenda: Violence against women. *American Psychologist, 45*(3), 374-380.

Koss, M., & Heslet, L. (1992). Somatic consequences of violence against women. *Archives of Family Medicine, 1,* 53-59.

Koss, M., Koss, P., & Woodruff, J. (1991). Deleterious effects of criminal victimization on women's health and medical utilization. *Archives of Internal Medicine, 151,* 342-347.

Kurz, D. (1987). Emergency department response to battered women: Resistance to medicalization. *Social Problems, 34*(1), 69-81.

Larrain, S. (1993). *Estudio de frecuencia de la violencia intrafamiliar y la condicion de la mujer en Chile.* Santiago, Chile: Pan American Health Organization.

Levinson, D. (1989). *Violence in cross-cultural perspective.* Newbury Park, CA: Sage.

Lupri, E. (1989). Male violence in the home. *Canadian Social Trends, 14,* 19-21.

Mahajan, A. (1990). Instigators of wife battering. In S. Sood (Ed.), *Violence against women* (pp. 1-10). Jaipur, India: Arihant.

McCleer, S. V., & Anwar, R. (1989). A study of women presenting in an emergency department. *American Journal of Public Health, 79,* 65-67.

Mullen, P. E., Romans-Clarkson, S. E., Walton, V. A., & Herbison, P. G. (1988). Impact of sexual and physical abuse on women's mental health. *Lancet, 1,* 841.

Perlez, J. (1991, July 29). Kenyans do some soul-searching after the rape of 71 schoolgirls. *The New York Times,* p. A1.

Phiri, E. (1992). *Violence against women in Zambia.* Luska: YWCA.

PROFAMILIA. (1990). *Encuestra de prevalencia, demografia y salud* (DHS). Bogotá, Colombia: Author.

Raikes, A. (1990). *Pregnancy, birthing and family planning in Kenya: Changing patterns of behavior: A health utilization study in Kissi District.* Copenhagen: Centre for Development Research.

Ramirez Rodriguez, J. C., & Uribe Vasquez, G. (1993). Mujer y violencia: Un hecho cotidiano. *Salud Publica de Mexico, 35*(2), 148-160 (Cuernavaca: Instituto Nacional de Salud Publica).

Romkens, R. (1989). *Violence in heterosexual relationships: A national research into the scale, nature, consequences and backgrounds.* Amsterdam: University of Amsterdam, Foundation for Scientific Research on Sexuality and Violence.

Sanday, P. R. (1981). The socio-cultural context of rape: A cross cultural study. *Journal of Social Issues, 37*(4), 5-27.

Schei, B., & Bakketeig, L. S. (1989). Gynecological impact of sexual and physical abuse by spouse: A study of a random sample of Norwegian women. *British Journal of Obstetrics and Gynecology, 96,* 1379-1383.

Sheikh-Hashim, L., & Gabba, A. (1990). *Violence against women in Dar es Salaam: A case study of three districts.* Dar es Salaam: Tanzania Media Women's Association.

Shim, J. K. (1988). Family violence and aggression. In K. I. Kim (Ed.), *Family violence: The fact and management.* Seoul: Tamgudang.

Shim, Y. (1992, June 21-27). *Sexual violence against women in Korea: A victimization survey of Seoul women.* Paper presented at the conference on International Perspectives: Crime, Justice and Public Order, St. Petersburg, Russia.

Shrader Cox, E., & Valdez Santiago, R. (1992). *Violencia hacia la mujer Mexicana como problema de salud publica: La incidencia de la violencia domestica en una microregion de Ciudad Nexahualcoyotl.* Mexico City: CECOVID.

Smith, M. (1987). The incidence and prevalence of woman abuse in Toronto. *Violence and Victims, 2,* 33-37.

Sonali, D. (1990). *An investigation into the incidence and causes of domestic violence in Sri Lanka.* Colombo, Sri Lanka: Women in Need (WIN).

Stark, E., Flitcraft, A., Zuckerman, B., Grey, A., Robinson, J., & Frazier, W. (1981). *Wife abuse in the medical setting: An introduction for health personnel* (Monograph 7). Washington, DC: Office of Domestic Violence.

Straus, M. A., & Gelles, R. J. (1986). Societal change and change in family violence from 1975 to 1985 as revealed by two national surveys. *Journal of Marriage and the Family, 48,* 465-479.

Teske, R., Jr., & Parker, M. (1983). *Spouse abuse in Texas: A study of women's attitudes and experiences.* Austin: Texas Department of Human Resources.

Toft, S. (Ed.). (1987). *Domestic violence in Papua New Guinea* (Occasional Paper No. 19). Port Morseby, Papua New Guinea: Law Reform Commission.

Ugalde, J. G. (1988). Sindrome de la mujer agredida. *Mujer, 5,* p. 41. (San Jose, Costa Rica: Cefemina).

Wakabi, Y., & Mwesigye, H. (1991). *Violence against women in Uganda: A research report.* Kampala: Association of Ugandan Women Lawyers (FIDA).

Wife beating. (1987, June 15). *World Development Forum.*

Women's AID Organization. (1992). *Draft report of the National Study on Domestic Violence.* Kuala Lampur, Malaysia: Author.

World Bank. (1993). *The world development report 1993: Investing in health.* Washington, DC: World Bank.

PART V

Research in Women's Health

22

Gender Bias in Clinical Research:
The Difference It Makes

Sue V. Rosser

In scientific research, whether in the behavioral, biomedical, or physical sciences, researchers rarely admit that data have been gathered and interpreted from a particular perspective. Because research in biology, chemistry, and physics centers on the physical and natural world, it is presumed "objective"; therefore the term *perspective* does not apply to it. The reliability and repeatability of data gathered and hypotheses tested using the scientific method convince researchers that they are obtaining unbiased information about the physical, natural world.

In the past two decades, feminist historians and philosophers of science (Fee, 1981, 1982; Haraway, 1978, 1989; Harding, 1986; Longino, 1990) and feminist scientists (Birke, 1986; Bleier, 1984, 1986; Fausto-Sterling, 1985; Keller, 1983, 1985; Rosser, 1988) have pointed out a source of bias and absence of value neutrality in science, particularly biology. By the exclusion of females as experimental subjects, a focus on problems of primary interest to males, faulty experimental designs, and interpretations of data based in language or ideas constricted by patriarchal values, experimental results in several areas of biology are biased or flawed. These flaws and biases were permitted to become part of the mainstream of scientific thought and were perpetuated in the scientific literature for decades because most scientists were men, who did not detect or acknowledge bias. Values held by male scientists were seen as synonymous with the "objective" view of the world (Keller, 1982, 1985).

A first step of feminist scientists was recognition of the possibility of androcentric bias that resulted from having virtually all theoretical and decision-making positions in science held by men (Keller, 1982). It was not until a critical mass of women existed in the profession (Rosser, 1986) that the bias of androcentrism began to emerge. As long as only a few women were scientists, they had to demonstrate or conform to the male view of the world to be successful and have their research meet the criteria for "objectivity."

Gender Bias in Traditional
Approaches to Clinical Research

Once androcentric bias was discovered, feminist scientists set out to explore the extent to which it had distorted science. They recognized potential distortion on a variety of levels of research and theory: the choice and definition of problems to be studied, exclusion of females as experimental subjects, bias in methodology used to collect and interpret data, and bias in theories and conclusions drawn from the data. They also began to realize that, because the practice of modern medicine depends heavily on clinical research, any flaws and ethical problems in this research are likely to result in poorer health care and inequity in the medical treatment of disadvantaged groups.

Androcentric bias in defining priorities for medical research. Recent evidence suggests that gender bias may have flawed some medical research. The choice of problems for study in medical research is substantially determined by a national agenda that defines what is worthy of study. As Marxist (Zimmerman et al., 1980), African American (McLeod, 1987), and feminist critics (Hubbard, 1983) of scientific research have pointed out, the scientific research that is undertaken reflects the societal bias toward the powerful, who are overwhelmingly white, middle- to upper-class men in the United States. Obviously, the members of Congress who appropriate the funds for the National Institutes of Health (NIH) and other federal government agencies are overwhelmingly white, middle- to upper-class men; they are more likely to vote for funds for research they view as beneficial to health needs as defined from their perspective. It may be argued that actual priorities for medical research and allocations of funds are not set by members of Congress but by the leaders in medical research who are employees of the NIH or other federal government agencies or who are brought in as consultants. Unfortunately, the same descriptors—white, middle- to upper-class men—must be used to characterize the individuals in the theoretical and decision-making positions within the medical hierarchy and scientific establishment.

Lack of funding for clinical research on women. Research on conditions specific to females receives low priority, funding, and prestige, although females make up half of the population and receive more than half of the health care. With the expense of sophisticated equipment, maintenance of laboratory animals and facilities, and salaries for qualified technicians and researchers, virtually no medical research is undertaken today without federal government or foundation support. In fiscal 1989 the NIH funded approximately $7.1 billion of research (*Science and Government Report*, 1990). Private foundations and state governments funded a smaller portion of the research (*National Science Foundation Science and Engineering Indicators*, 1987, App. table 4-10). However, in 1988 the NIH allocated only 13.5% of its total budget to research on illnesses of major consequence for women (Narrigan, 1991).

Responding to this neglect of women's health issues by the scientific community, in 1991 Congress created the Office of Research on Women's Health to address specific issues in women's health. Also in 1991, the NIH launched the Women's Health Initiative, attempting to raise the priority of women's health and provide baseline data on previously understudied causes of death in women (Pinn & LaRosa, 1992). The Women's Health Initiative to date has focused on research regarding cardiovascular diseases, cancers, and osteoporosis. Additional examples that might be targeted for future research include dysmenorrhea, incontinence in older women, and nutrition in postmenopausal women. Effects of exercise level and duration upon alleviation of menstrual discomfort, as well as the length and amount of exposure to video display terminals that have resulted in the "cluster pregnancies" of women giving birth to deformed babies in certain industries, also have received low priority.

In contrast, significant amounts of time and money are expended upon clinical research on women's bodies in connection with aspects of reproduction. In this century, up until the 1970s, considerable attention was devoted to the development of contraceptive devices for women rather than for men (Cowan, 1980; Dreifus, 1978). Furthermore, substantial clinical research has resulted in increasing medicalization and control of pregnancy, labor, and childbirth. Feminists have criticized (Ehrenreich & English, 1978; Holmes, 1981) the conversion of a normal, natural process controlled by women into a clinical, often surgical, procedure controlled by men. More recently, new reproductive technologies such as amniocentesis, in vitro fertilization, and artificial insemination have become heavily emphasized, as means are sought to overcome infertility. Feminists have warned of the extent to which these technologies place pressure upon women to produce the "perfect" child while placing control in the hands of the male medical establishment (Arditti, Duelli Klein, & Shelley, 1984; Corea & Ince, 1987; Corea et al., 1987; Klein, 1989).

Additionally, contraceptive research exclusively on women is problematic. Specifically, this type of biased research has produced birth control methods that permit men to have sexual pleasure without the risk of impregnating women and without the risk of deleterious pharmacological side effects now experienced by women.

These examples suggest that considerable resources and attention are devoted to women's health issues when those issues are directly related to men's interest in controlling production of children.

Failure to recognize the effects of gender. The immense preponderance of male leaders setting the priorities for medical research results in definite effects on the choice and definition of problems for research: Hypotheses are not formulated to focus on gender as a crucial part of the question being asked. Because many diseases have different frequencies (heart disease, lupus erythematosus), symptoms (gonorrhea), or complications (most sexually transmitted diseases) in the two sexes, scientists should routinely consider and test for differences or lack of differences based on gender in any hypothesis being tested. For example, the study of how a drug is metabolized should routinely include both males and females.

Five dramatic, widely publicized recent examples demonstrate that sex differences are *not* routinely considered as part of the question asked. In a longitudinal study of the effects of cholesterol-lowering drugs, gender differences were not tested: The drug was tested on 3,806 men and no women (Hamilton, 1985). The Multiple Risk Factor Intervention Trial Group (1990) examined mortality from coronary heart disease in 12,866 men only. The Health Professionals Follow-Up Study (Grobbee et al., 1990) explored the association between coffee consumption and heart disease in 45,589 men. The Physician's Health Study (Steering Committee of the Physician's Health Study Group, 1989) found that low-dose aspirin therapy reduced the risk of myocardial infarction in 22,071 men. A study published in September 1992 in the *Journal of the American Medical Association* surveyed the literature from 1960 to 1991 on clinical trials of medications used to treat acute myocardial infarction. Women were included in only 20% of those studies; elderly people (over 75 years of age) were included in only 40% of such studies (Gurwitz, Nananda, & Avorn, 1992).

The scientific community has often failed to include females in animal studies in basic research as well as in clinical research unless the research centered on reproductive control. The reasons for the exclusion (to prevent interference from estrus or menstrual cycles, to avoid the fear of induction of fetal deformities in pregnant subjects, and to take advantage of the higher incidence of some diseases in males) may be financially practical, but such exclusion results in drugs that have not been adequately tested in female subjects before being marketed and in lack of information about the etiology of some diseases in women.

Using the male as the experimental subject not only ignores the fact that females may respond differently to the variable tested, it may, ironically, lead to less accurate models even in the male. Models that more accurately simulate functioning complex biological systems may be derived from using female, not male, rats as experimental subjects. Scientists such as Joan Hoffman (1982) have questioned the tradition of using male rats or primates as subjects. As Hoffman points out, the rhythmic cycle of hormone secretion as portrayed in the cycling of female rat reproductive hormones appears to be a more accurate model for the secretion of most hormones. With the exception of insulin and the female reproductive hormones, most of the 20-odd human hormones were assumed by endocrinologists to remain at constant levels in both males and females. Thus the male of the species, whether rodent or primate, was chosen as the experimental subject because of his noncyclicity. However, new techniques of measuring blood hormone levels have demonstrated episodic rather than steady patterns of secretion of virtually all hormones in both males and females.

Some diseases that affect both sexes are defined as male diseases. Heart disease is the best example of a disease that has been so designated because heart disease occurs more frequently in men at younger ages than women. Therefore most of the funding for heart disease has been appropriated for research on predisposing factors for the disease (such as cholesterol level, lack of exercise, stress, smoking, and weight) using white, middle-aged, middle-class men.

This "male disease" designation has resulted in very little research being directed toward high-risk groups of women. Heart disease is a leading cause of death in older women (Healy, 1991; Kirschstein, 1985), who live an average of 8 years longer than men (Boston Women's Health Book Collective, 1984). It also is frequent in poor black women who have had several children (Manley, Lin-Fu, Miranda, Noonan, & Parker, 1985). Virtually no research has explored predisposing factors for these groups, who fall outside the disease definition established from an androcentric perspective.

Recent data indicate that the designation of AIDS as a disease of male homosexuals and intravenous (IV) drug users has led researchers and health care practitioners to fail to understand the etiology and diagnosis of HIV/ AIDS in women (Norwood, 1988). Currently, women constitute the group in which HIV/ AIDS is increasing most rapidly, and women with HIV/AIDS have symptoms that differ from those of men. However, it was not until October 1992 that the Centers for Disease Control (CDC) announced a case definition that includes gynecological conditions and other symptoms related to HIV/AIDS in women; this case definition was enacted in January 1993

(Nora Bell, Board of the National Leadership Coalition on AIDS, personal communication). This androcentric bias has had serious consequences: Most health care workers are unable to diagnose HIV/ AIDS in women until the disease has advanced significantly. The average death after diagnosis of AIDS in a man is 30 months; for a woman, it is 15 weeks.

These types of bias raise ethical issues. Because of the paucity of research on women, health care practitioners today must treat the majority of the population, which is female, based on information gathered from clinical research in which drugs may not have been tested on females, in which the etiology of the disease in women has not been studied, and in which women's experiences have been ignored.

Interaction between gender, ethnicity, and class in research. When women are used in experimental studies, often they are not accorded the respect due to any human being. In his attempts to investigate the side effects of nervousness and depression attributable to oral contraceptives, Goldzieher (Goldzieher, Moses, Averkin, Scheel, & Taber, 1971a, 1971b) gave placebos to 76 women who sought treatment at a San Antonio clinic to prevent further pregnancies. None of the women was told that she was participating in research or receiving placebos (Cowan, 1980; Veatch, 1971). The women in Goldzieher's study were primarily poor, multiparous, Mexican Americans. Research that raises similar issues about the ethics of informed consent was carried out on poor Puerto Rican women during the initial phases of testing the effectiveness of the pill as a contraceptive (Zimmerman et al., 1980). Recent data have revealed that at certain clinics routine testing of pregnant women for HIV positivity was carried out without their informed consent (Chavkin, Driver, & Forman, 1989; Marte & Anastos, 1990). Subsequently, pressure was placed on those women who were HIV positive to abort their fetuses (Selwyn et al., 1989).

Admittedly, it is difficult to determine whether the treatment of these women stems more from attitudes about gender or ethnicity and class. From the Tuskegee Syphilis Experiment, in which the effects of untreated syphilis were studied in 399 men over a period of 40 years (Jones, 1981), it is clear that lower income, African American men may not receive appropriate treatment or information about experiments in which they are participating. Feminist scholars (Dill, 1983; Ruzek, 1988) have begun to explore the extent to which gender, ethnicity, and class become complex, interlocking political variables that may affect access to and quality of health care.

Reciprocal relationship between research and female subjects. Most current clinical research sets up a distance between the observer and the human subject. Several feminist philosophers (Haraway, 1978; Harding, 1986; Hein,

1981; Keller, 1985) have characterized this distancing as an androcentric approach. Distance between the observer and experimental subject may be more comfortable for men, who are more comfortable with autonomy and distance (Keller, 1985), than for women, who tend to value relationship and interdependency (Gilligan, 1982).

Suggestions for relevant research questions based on the personal experiences of women also have been neglected. In the health care arena, women have often reported (and accepted among themselves) experiences that could not be documented by scientific experiments or were not accepted as valid by the researchers of the day. For example, for decades dysmenorrhea was attributed by most health care researchers and practitioners to psychological or social factors despite the reports from an overwhelming number of women that these were monthly experiences in their lives. Only after prostaglandins were "discovered" was there widespread acceptance among the male medical establishment that this experience reported by women had a biological component (Kirschstein, 1985). Thus researchers should make an effort to include qualitative experiences and insights of women in the design and implementation of research on women. Using only traditional scientific methods may result in failure to obtain sufficient information about the problems being studied. Ironically, this is particularly true of the research on pregnancy, childbirth, menstruation, and menopause because these experiences, which are exclusive to women, have been studied almost entirely by methodologies created by men.

Androcentrism in theories and conclusions in research. An androcentric perspective may lead to the formulation of theories and conclusions drawn to support the status quo of inequality for women and other oppressed groups. Building upon their awareness of these biases, female scientists have criticized the studies of brain-hormone interaction (Bleier, 1984) because they were based on the theory of biological determinism, which was used to justify women's socially inferior position. Bleier has repeatedly warned against extrapolating from one species to another with regard to biochemical as well as behavioral traits.

The traditional rationale to support "objective" methods is that they prevent bias. Emphasis upon traditional quantitative approaches that maintain the distance between observer and experimental subject ostensibly removes the bias of the researcher. Ironically, to the extent that these "objective" approaches are in fact synonymous with a masculine perspective of the world, they may introduce bias. Specifically, androcentric bias may permeate the theories and conclusions drawn from the research in several ways.

Theories may be presented in androcentric language. Much feminist scholarship has focused on problems of sexism in language and the extent to which patriarchal language has excluded and limited women (Kramarae & Treichler, 1986; Lakoff, 1975; Thorne, 1979). Because language shapes our concepts and provides the framework through which we express our ideas, sexist language is a reflection of underlying sexism. An awareness of sexism as expressed through patriarchal language enables feminist researchers to describe their observations in less gender-biased terms. Such an awareness must be extended to all researchers, both men and women. Further, an awareness of language should aid experimenters in avoiding the use of terms that often permeate behavioral descriptions in clinical research, including *tomboyism* (Money & Erhardt, 1972), *aggression,* and *hysteria,* as they tend to reflect assumptions about gender-appropriate behavior (Hamilton, 1985). The limited research on HIV/AIDS in women focuses on women as prostitutes or mothers. Describing the woman as a vector for transmission to men through prostitution or to the fetus has produced little information on the progress of HIV/AIDS in women themselves (Rosser, 1991). Once the bias in the terminology is exposed, the next step is to ask whether that terminology leads to a constraint or bias in the theory itself.

Theories and conclusions drawn from all research endeavors should be examined to determine to what extent they represent and reinforce sexism, racism, and classism harmful to women. As Swigonski (1993) suggests, researchers should carefully consider how particular research questions or theories contribute to the oppression of the participants, how the conclusions of their research will be used, and how they can ensure that the research findings are beneficial to the participants and women in general.

Inequities in health care practices for women. Not a surprise, androcentric bias in research has resulted in differences in management of disease and access to health care procedures based on gender. In a 1991 study in Massachusetts and Maryland, Ayanian and Epstein (1991) demonstrated that women were significantly less likely than men to undergo coronary angioplasty, angiography, or surgery when admitted to the hospital with the diagnosis of myocardial infarction, unstable angina, chronic ischemic heart disease, or chest pain. This significant difference remained even when variables such as ethnicity, age, economic status, and other chronic diseases such as diabetes and heart failure were controlled.

A similar study (Steingart et al., 1991) revealed that women have angina before myocardial infarction as frequently and with more debilitating effects than men, yet women are referred for cardiac catheterization only half as often. The 1992 *Journal of the American Medical Association* study concluded that the exclusion of women from 80% of the trials and the elderly from 60% of the trials for medication for myocardial infarction limits the ability to generalize study findings to the patient population that experiences the most morbidity and mortality from acute myocardial infarction (Gurwitz et al., 1992). Gender bias in cardiac research has therefore been translated into bias in management of disease, leading to inequitable treatment for life-threatening conditions in women.

Overcoming Gender Bias in Clinical Research

Recognizing gender bias is the first step toward understanding the difference it makes. Perhaps male researchers are less likely to see flaws in and question biologically deterministic theories that provide scientific justification for men's superior status in society because they gain social power and status from such theories. Researchers from outside the mainstream (feminists, for example) are much more likely to be critical of such theories that prevent their empowerment. To eliminate bias, the community of scientists undertaking clinical research must include individuals from as many diverse backgrounds as possible (Rosser, 1988). Only then is it less likely that the perspective of one group will bias research design, approaches, subjects, and interpretations.

Similarly, researchers need to consider the influence that they have on the design, implementation, and conclusions of their studies, based on a variety of personal characteristics including their own ethnicity/culture, class, age, education, functional ability, and gender (Swigonski, 1993). In other words, researchers should acknowledge that most scientific endeavors, even one's own, are value laden. Biases, as well as their possible effects on the research, should be identified throughout the research process (Swigonski, 1993).

Cross-disciplinary or multidisciplinary research methods are needed to ensure a comprehensive understanding of women's experiences from a variety of perspectives. For example, if the topic of research is occupational exposures that present a risk to the pregnant woman working in a plant where toxic chemicals are manufactured, it would be best to use a combination of methods traditionally used in social science research with those frequently used in biology and chemistry. Checking the chromosomes of any miscarried fetuses, chemical analysis of placentas after birth, as well as Apgar Scores and blood samples of the newborns to determine trace amounts of the toxic chemicals would be appropriate biological and chemical methods to gather data. Methods used in social science research such as in-depth interviews with women to determine how they are feeling and any irregularities they detect during each month of the pregnancy would be appropriate as well. Evaluations using weekly written questionnaires regarding the pregnancy progress also would enhance the research process. Jean Hamilton (1985) has called for interactive models that draw on both the social and the natural sciences to explain complex problems:

> Particularly for understanding human, gender-related health, we need more interactive and contextual models that address the actual complexity of the phenomenon that is the subject of explanation. One example is the need for more phenomenological definitions of symptoms, along with increased recognition that psychology, behavioral studies, and sociology are among the "basic sciences" for health research. Research on heart disease is one example of a field where it is recognized that both psychological stress and behaviors such as eating [sic] and cigarette smoking influence the onset and natural course of a disease process. (p. VI-62)

Perhaps if more women held positions that enabled them to make decisions regarding the design and funding of clinical research, there would be more interdisciplinary research on menstruation, pregnancy, childbirth, lactation, and menopause. The interdisciplinary approaches developed to solve these problems might then be applied to other complex problems to benefit all health care consumers, both male and female. Given that the overall agenda for research and policies concerning access to health care is set in the political arena, politicians also must reflect the diversity and needs of the American population. Then we can work together to overcome gender bias in health research and the difference it makes.

References

Arditti, R., Duelli Klein, R., & Shelley, M. (1984). *Test-tube women: What future for motherhood?* London: Pandora.

Ayanian, J. Z., & Epstein, A. M. (1991). Differences in the use of procedures between women and men hospitalized for coronary heart disease. *New England Journal of Medicine, 325,* 221-225.

Birke, L. (1986). *Women, feminism, and biology.* New York: Methuen.

Bleier, R. (1984). *Science and gender: A critique of biology and its theories on women.* New York: Pergamon.

Bleier, R. (1986). Sex differences research: Science or belief? In R. Bleier (Ed.), *Feminist approaches to science.* New York: Pergamon.

Boston Women's Health Book Collective. (1984). *The new our bodies, ourselves.* New York: Simon & Schuster.

Chavkin, W., Driver, C., & Forman, P. (1989). The crisis in New York City's perinatal services. *New York State Journal of Medicine,* 685-663.

Corea, G., Hanmer, J., Hoskins, B., Raymond, J., Duelli Klein, R., Holmes, H. B., Keshwar, M., Rowland, R., & Steinbacker, R. (Eds.). (1987). *Man-made women: How new reproductive technologies affect women.* Bloomington: Indiana University Press.

Corea, G., & Ince, S. (1987). Report of a survey of IVG clinics in the USC. In P. Spallone & D. L. Steinberg (Eds.), *Made to order: The myth of reproductive and genetic progress.* Oxford: Pergamon.

Cowan, B. (1980). Ethical problems in government-funded contraceptive research. In H. Holmes, B. Hoskins, & M. Gross (Eds.), *Birth control and controlling birth: Women-centered perspectives* (pp. 37-46). Clifton, NJ: Humana.

Dill, B. T. (1983). Race, class and gender: Prospects for an all-inclusive sisterhood. *Feminist Studies, 9,* 1.

Dreifus, C. (1978). *Seizing our bodies.* New York: Vintage.

Ehrenreich, B., & English, D. (1978). *For her own good.* New York: Anchor.

Fausto-Sterling, A. (1985). *Myths of gender.* New York: Basic Books.

Fee, E. (1981). Is feminism a threat to scientific objectivity? *International Journal of Women's Studies, 4,* 213-233.

Fee, E. (1982). A feminist critique of scientific objectivity. *Science for the People, 14*(4), 8.

Gilligan, C. (1982). *In a different voice: Psychological theory and women's development.* Cambridge, MA: Harvard University Press.

Goldzieher, J. W., Moses, L., Averkin, E., Scheel, C., & Taber, B. (1971a). A placebo-controlled double-blind crossover investigation of the side effects attributed to oral contraceptives. *Fertility and Sterility, 22*(9), 609-623.

Goldzieher, J. W., Moses, L., Averkin, E., Scheel, C., & Taber, B. (1971b). Nervousness and depression attributed to oral contraceptives: A double-blind, placebo-controlled study. *American Journal of Obstetrics and Gynecology, 22,* 1013-1020.

Grobbee, D. E., Rimm, E. B., Giovannucci, E., Colditz, G., Stampfer, M., & Willett, W. (1990). Coffee, caffeine, and cardiovascular disease in men. *New England Journal of Medicine, 321,* 1026-1032.

Gurwitz, J. H., Nananda, F. C., & Avorn, J. (1992). The exclusion of the elderly and women from clinical trials in acute myocardial infarction. *Journal of the American Medical Association, 268*(2), 1417-1422.

Hamilton, J. (1985). Avoiding methodological biases in gender-related research. In *Women's health report of the Public Health Service Task Force on Women's Health Issues.* Washington, DC: U.S. Department of Health and Human Services Public Health Service.

Haraway, D. (1978). Animal sociology and a natural economy of the body politic, Part I: A political physiology of dominance; and animal sociology and a natural economy of the body politic, Part II: The past is the contested zone: Human nature and theories of production and reproduction in primate behavior studies. *Signs: Journal of Women in Culture and Society, 4*(1), 21-60.

Haraway, D. (1989). Monkeys, aliens, and women: Love, science, and politics at the intersection of feminist theory and colonial discourse. *Women's Studies International Forum, 12*(3), 295-312.

Harding, S. (1986). *The science question in feminism.* Ithaca, NY: Cornell University Press.

Healy, B. (1991). Women's health, public welfare. *Journal of the American Medical Association, 264*(4), 566-568.

Hein, H. (1981). Women and science: Fitting men to think about nature. *International Journal of Women's Studies, 4,* 369-377.

Hoffman, J. C. (1982). Biorhythms in human reproduction: The not-so-steady states. *Signs: Journal of Women in Culture and Society, 7*(4), 829-844.

Holmes, H. B. (1981). Reproductive technologies: The birth of a women-centered analysis. In H. B. Holmes et al. (Eds.), *The custom-made child?* Clifton, NJ: Humana.

Hubbard, R. (1983). Social effects of some contemporary myths about women. In M. Lowe & R. Hubbard (Eds.), *Woman's nature: Rationalizations of inequality.* New York: Pergamon.

Jones, J. H. (1981). *Bad blood: The Tuskegee Syphilis Experiment.* New York: Free Press.

Keller, E. (1982). Feminism and science. *Signs: Journal of Women in Culture and Society, 7*(3), 589-602.

Keller, E. F. (1983). *A feeling for the organism: The life and work of Barbara McClintock.* New York: Freeman.

Keller, E. F. (1985). *Reflections on gender and science.* New Haven, CT: Yale University Press.

Kirschstein, R. L. (1985). *Women's health: Report of the Public Health Service Task Force on Women's Health Issues* (Vol. 2). Washington, DC: U.S. Department of Health and Human Services Public Health Service.

Klein, R. D. (1989). *Infertility.* London: Pandora.

Kramarae, C., & Treichler, P. (1986). *A feminist dictionary.* London: Pandora.

Lakoff, R. (1975). *Language and woman's place.* New York: Harper & Row.

Longino, H. (1990). *Science as social knowledge: Values and objectivity in scientific inquiry.* Princeton, NJ: Princeton University Press.

Manley, A., Lin-Fu, J., Miranda, M., Noonan, A., & Parker, T. (1985). Special health concerns of ethnic minority women in women's health. In *Report of the Public Health Service Task Force on Women's Health Issues.* Washington, DC: U.S. Department of Health and Human Services Public Health Service.

Marte, C., & Anastos, K. (1990). Women: The missing persons in the AIDS epidemic. Part II. *Health/PAC Bulletin, 20*(1), 11-23.

McLeod, S. (1987). *Scientific colonialism: A cross-cultural comparison.* Washington, DC: Smithsonian Institution Press.

Money, J., & Erhardt, A. (1972). *Man and woman, boy and girl.* Baltimore: Johns Hopkins University Press.

Multiple Risk Factor Intervention Trial Research Group. (1990). Mortality rates after 10.5 years for participants in the Multiple Risk Factor Intervention Trial: Findings related to a prior hypotheses of the trial. *Journal of the American Medical Association, 263,* 1795-1801.

Narrigan, D. (1991, March-April-May). Research to improve women's health: An agenda for equity. *The Network News: National Women's Health Network,* pp. 3, 9.

National Science Foundation Science and Engineering Indicators (NSB-1). (1987). Washington, DC: NSF.

Norwood, C. (1988, July). Alarming rise in deaths. *Ms.,* pp. 65-67.

Pinn, V., & LaRosa, J. (1992). *Overview: Office of Research on Women's Health.* Bethesda, MD: National Institutes of Health.

Rosser, S. V. (1986). *Teaching science and health from a feminist perspective: A practical guide.* Elmsford, NY: Pergamon.

Rosser, S. V. (1988). Women in science and health care: A gender at risk. In S. V. Rosser (Ed.), *Feminism within the science of health care professions: Overcoming resistance.* Elmsford, NY: Pergamon.

Rosser, S. V. (1991). AIDS and women. *AIDS Education and Prevention, 3*(3), 230-240.

Ruzek, S. (1988, February 27). *Women's health: Sisterhood is powerful, but so are race and class.* Keynote address delivered at Southeast Women's Studies Association Annual Conference, University of North Carolina—Chapel Hill.

Science and Government Report, 18(4), 1. (1990, March 1). Washington, DC.

Selwyn, P. A., et al. (1989). Prospective study of human immunodeficiency virus infection and pregnancy outcomes in intravenous drug users. *Journal of the American Medical Association, 261,* 1289-1294.

Steering Committee of the Physician's Health Study Group. (1989). Final report on the aspirin component of the ongoing physician's health study. *New England Journal of Medicine, 321,* 129-135.

Steingart, R. M., Packes, M., Hamm, P., et al. (1991). Sex differences in the management of coronary artery disease. *New England Journal of Medicine, 325*, 226-230.

Swigonski, M. E. (1993). Feminist standpoint theory and the questions of social work research. *Affilia: Journal of Women and Social Work, 8*(2), 171-183.

Thorne, B. (1979, September 13-15). *Claiming verbal space: Women, speech and language in college classrooms.* Paper presented at the Research Conference on Educational Environments and the Undergraduate Women, Wellesley College, Wellesley, MA.

Veatch, R. M. (1971). Experimental pregnancy. *Hastings Center Report, 1*, 2-3.

Zimmerman, B., et al. (1980). People's science. In R. Arditti, P. Brennan, & S. Cavrak (Eds.), *Science and liberation* (pp. 299-319). Boston: South End.

23

Real and Perceived Legal Barriers to the Inclusion of Women in Clinical Trials

Michelle Oberman

In 1990 the General Accounting Office issued a report that finally acknowledged and successfully documented the neglect of women's health that activists and health care providers who specialize in women's health had been complaining about for decades (Nadel, 1990). This neglect takes a variety of forms: failure to fund research on health issues unique to women, failure to study diagnosis and treatment of women suffering from diseases that afflict both genders, and failure to adequately ensure safety of medical products and treatments that women routinely use.

Responding to public outcry against the now-documented, seemingly systematic neglect of women's health issues by the scientific community, Congress created the Office of Research on Women's Health and began to allocate funding to address specific women's health problems (National Institutes of Health Revitalization Amendments, 1991). Yet little effort has been made to understand the underlying causes of the neglect of women's health issues. The explanations most commonly cited for women's exclusion from the scientific agenda suggest that the problem lies with the male-dominated research community. As the columnist Ellen Goodman put it, "They fund what they fear" (Goodman, 1990, p. 74). Upon closer scrutiny, however, the problem is not simply garden-variety gender bias but a more complex reincarnation of the age-old phenomena of male normativity, complemented by the somewhat more modern obsession with potential legal liability. This chapter illustrates how these two factors have joined to perpetuate a system that not only neglects to develop safe and effective medical treatments for women but neglects to do so in the name of protecting women from harm.

In the area of medical research, women are often measured against a male norm, by which they are found either similar or dissimilar, problematic or deserving of special protection. Perhaps the clearest illustration of this may be seen in the regulation of clinical trials related to new drug development. This chapter focuses therefore on the Food and Drug Administration's regulation of fertile women's inclusion in drug trials so as to illustrate a much broader problem. This example demonstrates the manner in which women came to be marginalized by the scientific community, the surface and underlying justifications for such exclusion, and the response of the community and the federal government to the growing demands for change.

A Brief History of Regulation of Clinical Trials and the Federal Mandate to Exclude Women

One of the ironies of women's underrepresentation in clinical trials is that the federal regulations limiting women's participation as subjects in drug trials were promulgated not in the nineteenth or early twentieth centuries but as recently as 1977 (U.S. Department of Health, Education, and Welfare [HEW], 1977). Historically, women were popular subjects of medical research for precisely the same reasons that render them problematic subjects today. Specifically, women's reproductive capacity has always intrigued scientists and has thus been the subject of countless studies and treatments. In centuries past, this research took the form of subjecting women to various "cures," such as hysterectomy, clitoridectomy, forced pregnancy, and electroshock treatments. During this century, the dominant focus has shifted to controlling reproduction through contraception and various medications designed to manage the pregnancy process by controlling nausea, minimizing miscarriage, and halting premature labor (Ikemoto, 1992).

In the 1960s and 1970s, the combination of scientific curiosity about women's reproductive capacity and the burgeoning pharmaceutical industry led to a series of catastrophic medical escapades. Perhaps the most celebrated crisis involved thalidomide, a drug used to prevent early miscarriages. In 1962, while thalidomide was still pending drug approval in the United States, it was revealed that thalidomide had caused over 1,000 birth-related defects in Europe (Janssen, 1980; Temin, 1980). Then, in 1973, it was further revealed that the U.S. Public Health Service had itself engaged in a 40-year study in which syphilitic black men were deprived of medical treatment without their consent. These two experiences, taken together with disclosures of exploitative medical experimentation on vulnerable groups (Beecher, 1966; U.S.

Public Health Service, 1973), led to a demand for tighter regulation of clinical research in the United States. The Nuremberg trials had sensitized many to the danger of medical experimentation becoming bound up with exploitation of vulnerable persons; the thalidomide and Tuskegee disasters seemed therefore to touch an especially sensitive nerve of the American people.

In the early 1970s, Senate hearings on "biomedical research with human subjects" resulted in the creation of the National Commission for the Protection of Human Subjects of Biomedical and Behavioral Research (*Public Law 93-348*, 1974). The commission's first charge was to investigate research practices affecting pregnant women and fetuses, which reflected the then widely held perception of the fetus as the "most vulnerable" research subject (McCarthy, 1993). The consensus regarding the fetus was the result of an odd coalition of activists: antiabortion conservatives, who, 6 to 12 months after *Roe v. Wade* (1973), were just emerging as a group with a national identity and agenda (Luker, 1984), and liberals, who were eager to establish a powerful regulatory system that would prevent pharmaceutical catastrophes from recurring.

The commission was given 4 months in which to complete its report, which ultimately advocated, without any detailed explanations, that pregnant and fertile women be excluded from research. In 1977 the FDA, following the commission's guidance, promulgated a policy banning fertile women from toxicity studies and from initial safety and efficacy studies. The regulations permitted, but did not mandate, women's inclusion in final studies of safety, efficacy, and dosage (*General Considerations for the Clinical Evaluation of Drugs*, U.S. HEW, 1977).

The Pharmaceutical Industry's Response: Fear-Based Exclusionary Policies Take Hold

While the FDA policy only mandated the exclusion of women from early phases of drug testing, the research community generally responded by excluding women from testing altogether (McCarthy, 1993). Given the general perception that research was risky and onerous, there was no real public outcry against this practice until, 15 years later, research demonstrating metabolical gender differences led women's health advocates to urge that the policy be changed (Rosser, this volume).

The pharmaceutical industry's embracing of the policy excluding women from testing was somewhat puzzling, because most of these drugs, once approved, ultimately would be prescribed for and used by women. At first glance, one might have expected that the industry would have rallied against the regulations, which precluded drug manufacturers from determining new drug safety in women, who account for 52% of the population and often constitute the majority of the general population consuming a new drug. The fact is, though, that the pharmaceutical industry welcomed the FDA regulations because, for the reasons I will now address, they corresponded well with the industry's independent desire to limit women's exposure to experimental drugs.

The Products Liability Revolution and the Emergence of Women as Liability Time Bombs

In the years leading up to the 1976 FDA guidelines, the pharmaceutical industry experienced a series of legal liability crises that led those engaged in drug research and development to conclude that women represented liability time bombs to those engaged in biomedical research. Thalidomide was the first and most dramatic example. Then, in 1971, evidence emerged regarding diethylstilbestrol, or DES, a popular antimiscarriage drug that had been approved by the FDA in 1941. Unlike thalidomide, whose harmful effects were made apparent in the form of severe birth defects, daughters born of mothers who ingested DES during pregnancy did not typically manifest the carcinogenic and other effects of the drug until decades into their lives (Herbst, Ulfelder, & Poskanzer, 1971; Siegler, 1987). During the years following the news about DES, hundreds of lawsuits were filed on behalf of the daughters of the women who ingested DES while pregnant (*Bichler v. Eli Lilly*, 1981; *Sindell v. Abbott Lab.*, 1980).

Another example of the liability climate that prevailed in the period surrounding the promulgation of the FDA guidelines is the initial birth control pill, Enovid. By the late 1960s, after the pill had been FDA approved and was being used or had been used by one in four married American women under age 45 (Vaughan, 1970), the FDA confirmed British reports that linked Enovid use to deep vein thrombosis or pulmonary embolism (Silverman & Philip, 1974). Other reports linked pill use to increased cervical and endometrial cancer rates, diabetes, liver troubles, hair loss, and depression (Silverman & Philip, 1974). Although the amount of pill-related litigation never approached that of other pharmaceutical disasters of the era, the industry felt threatened by the obstacles that were placed in the way of a drug that they perceived as nothing short of a revolutionary technological breakthrough. Rather suddenly, manufacturers realized that developing drugs for fertile women, especially healthy fertile women, was a highly risky enterprise. Peter Huber's study of the products liability "revolution" notes that "research expenditures by U.S. companies working on contraceptives peaked in 1973 and plummeted 90% in the next decade" (Huber, 1988).

Just as the controversy over the pill was heating up, a plastic intrauterine device called the Dalkon Shield came on the market. By 1974 half of the nation's 4 million IUD users were using the Dalkon Shield (Schwartz, 1974). Yet, by late 1973, there were signs of trouble with the device. A. H. Robins Co. received numerous reports from physicians and from the Centers for Disease Control regarding deaths attributed to the Dalkon Shield as well as an unusually high incidence of septic midtrimester spontaneous abortions in women who had conceived while the Shield was in place and who attempted to carry the pregnancy to term (Christian, 1974; Schwartz, 1974). By 1990 A. H. Robins was in bankruptcy proceedings. In all, some 320,000 claims were filed against it, and the company was ordered to set aside $2.475 billion to cover damages to victims of the Dalkon Shield (Hilts, 1990). The growing perception that fertile women represented a potential threat to drug companies had only grown stronger as companies watched A. H. Robins's slow demise.

The Pharmaceutical Industry's
Cost-Benefit Analysis

The specter of massive, delayed liability that the thalidomide, DES, Enovid, and Dalkon Shield cases revealed make it easy to understand why the pharmaceutical industry might shy away from developing and marketing drugs specifically for pregnant or even fertile women. It is far less obvious, however, why the industry would exclude this same population from clinical trials designed to ascertain the safety and efficacy of new drugs prior to marketing. After all, it is statistically inevitable that huge numbers of fertile and pregnant women will ingest most drugs that are marketed for the general population. Why then would the industry respond to the potential danger that these drugs pose to women by excluding women from testing altogether? Wouldn't it make more sense to investigate drug risks in women during the research and development phases, thus avoiding postmarketing disasters? How is that the drug manufacturers benefit by putting their heads in the sand and pretending that the dangers to women and fetuses do not exist?

The answer to this riddle emerges from a complex analysis of factors that meet in that gray zone at the intersection of science, law, and pragmatism. In determining whether to include fertile women in a clinical study, the sponsor undertakes a cost-benefit analysis. Put simply, the study's sponsor will compare the potential costs associated with including fertile women, on the one hand, with the potential benefits that can be gained by including fertile women, on the other hand. The result of this comparison is not hard to predict.

Sponsors—whether manufacturers or researchers—perceive that they have very little to gain and much to lose by including fertile women in their study populations.

Let me first address what a study sponsor has to gain by including fertile women in a clinical trial. With the exception of certain rare drugs that are designed and marketed primarily for use in pregnancy, a drug manufacturer knows that, no matter how safe a drug appears to be in clinical studies, legal liability risks for *in utero* injuries make it foolhardy to actively market the drug to pregnant women. Indeed, the manufacturer knows that, no matter how safe a drug appears to be in clinical studies, it will make sense for it to market the drug with an explicit warning about its unknown effects on pregnancy and fetuses. (Approximately one third of the drugs currently listed in the *Physician's Desk Reference* carry such a warning.) This strategy allows the manufacturer to enjoy the best of both worlds. On the one hand, even without direct marketing to fertile and pregnant women, and even with the explicit warning, the manufacturer knows that the drug eventually *will* be used by fertile women, some of whom will be pregnant. On the other hand, though, by not having actively marketed the drug to fertile or pregnant women and by including a warning label, the manufacturer will be able to limit its liability for injuries associated with the drug's ingestion.

It is apparent, then, that there is not much to gain by doing clinical trial studies on fertile women. Even if the studies show no teratogenicity, the manufacturer will still be wary of marketing the drug without the usual warnings. Moreover, if the studies show some level of teratogenicity, the manufacturer will be put in the position of having created the scientific data showing teratogenicity upon which a potential plaintiff may seek to rely in a suit based on *in utero* injuries.

There is, of course, one scenario in which the sponsor will benefit considerably by the inclusion of fertile women. If a clinical study were to show an extremely high level of teratogenicity, then the manufacturer might decide that the drug should not be marketed at all or that, in the case of a prescription drug, an aggressive campaign should be mounted to warn physicians not to prescribe the drug to fertile women at risk of pregnancy. This potential benefit would appear to be more conjectural than real, however. If the level of teratogenicity is so high as to justify abandoning a drug or undertaking this kind of warning campaign, then this will generally become known through animal studies that precede the human studies. Moreover, the number of human subjects that are used in clinical studies is not so high that the inclusion of fertile women would be likely to yield fruitful data on rare teratogenic side effects. Thus we are left with the situation that there are not many benefits to prompt a clinical trial sponsor to test a drug's efficacy on fertile women.

While the benefits of including fertile women are minimal, the costs of doing so can be quite high under our current legal system. I am not talking here about the research costs associated with including fertile women in a clinical study. To be sure, a sponsor will recognize that including fertile women adds variables to the study that make it more difficult and, arguably, more costly to conduct the study. The hormonal variations associated with fertile women, combined with complicating factors associated with contraception, contraception counseling, and pregnancy, are all factors that add to a study's complexity and cost. Ideally, one would hope that researchers would consider these gender differences as important factors to be studied; realistically, though, they are often treated as methodological hurdles to be avoided.

The much greater perceived cost of including fertile women in clinical studies relates to the sponsors' fear that a woman will conceive while in the study, will choose to carry the pregnancy to term, and will give birth to a child with disabilities. Similarly, sponsors fear that any child born with any disability will seek to sue the sponsor of a clinical trial in which the child's mother participated, whether or not there is any real evidence that the disability relates to the drug that was administered. Both of these scenarios create strong disincentives to include fertile women in studies. Because of the sympathy factor generated by a disabled child, a jury may choose to find against a drug manufacturer without direct evidence of causation. And even if a child's suit for *in utero* injuries ultimately fails, the litigation costs can be enormous.

Sponsors' fear of legal liability is legitimate and is a problem that must be addressed if trial sponsors are expected to willingly include fertile women in their studies. The fear is not so much a lawsuit by the female subject: She, like a male subject, knowingly consents to participate in a study and waives the right to sue for injuries she suffers. A child injured *in utero* is different, however. Unlike the adult subject in a clinical trial who knowingly consents to risk and thereby waives the right to sue for injuries, a child who is harmed while *in utero* through a clinical study may well have a cause of action against those who caused the injury. The traditional legal rule is that, while a mother's informed consent will limit her own ability to sue for her injuries, her consent will not preclude claims by her child who is injured *in utero*.

Moreover, the child who is injured by a drug as part of a clinical trial may have a much stronger claim of liability than children in the general public whose mothers took the drug notwithstanding the warning labels about its unknown effects on pregnancy. Having *actively* administered the drug to the mother, the manufacturer cannot hide behind its warning labels and accuse the mother or a prescribing physician as having been the negligent party in taking or prescribing the medication.

There are, then, significant costs associated with including fertile women in a clinical study. And once these costs are compared with the minimal benefits that will accrue to the sponsor by including fertile women, it is not difficult to understand why women—particularly fertile women—have been so underrepresented. If the underrepresentation problem is to be solved, this current incentive structure must be reversed. One way of reversing it is to decrease the disincentives to including fertile women in studies. A second way is to increase the incentives associated with including women—particularly fertile women—in the studies.

The 1993 FDA Guidelines
and the Prospects for Change

The present system is no longer tenable. The various rationales for women's exclusion from clinical trials can be easily disposed of as being scientifically unsound and ethically problematic. Those who claim that women are essentially identical to men and need not be studied are silenced by the growing number of studies that demonstrate significant gender disparity in terms of clinical diagnoses, treatments, and outcomes (Rosser, this volume). Those who assert that women's physiological differences constitute distractions are forced to admit that this is only true to the extent that men's bodies are accepted as the norm—an odd presumption given that women constitute the majority of the population. And, finally, the claim that women should be protected from the hazards of clinical trials belies the obvious truth that such a policy in effect subjects all women to unofficial, uncontrolled medical experimentation whenever they seek medical treatment.

While exposing and demystifying the assumptions that have led to women's exclusion from clinical trials are of critical importance to promoting women's health, that will only constitute half the battle. What remains to be determined is exactly what changes in regulatory policy must be made to ensure that federally approved drugs truly are appropriate and safe for the entire population. After numerous hearings and conferences, the FDA has issued new guidelines, designed to replace the 1977 guidelines, which it acknowledges have come to seem "rigid and paternalistic, leaving virtually no room for the exercise of judgment by responsible female research subjects, physician investigators, and [Institutional Review Boards]" (*Guideline for the Study and Evaluation of Gender Differences in the Clinical Evaluation of Drugs*, U.S. Department of Health and Human Services, 1993).

The new guidelines are cause for optimism because they articulate the general expectation that drugs are to be studied in a sample representative of the full range of patients likely to receive the drug once marketed. More particularly, the FDA has enumerated three gender-specific factors to be considered during drug development:

1. the influence of menstrual status on the drug's pharmacokinetics, including both comparisons of premenopausal and post-menopausal patients and examination of within-cycle changes;
2. the influence of concomitant supplementary estrogen treatment or systemic contraceptives (oral contraceptives, long-acting progesterone) on the drug's pharmacokinetics; and
3. the influence of the drug on the pharmacokinetics of oral contraceptives. (U.S. Department of Health and Human Services, 1993)

Although guidelines represent a positive development, they are no panacea to the problem of women's underrepresentation in clinical trials. While the guidelines lift the ban on fertile women's participation in early phases of clinical trials, the agency stops short of mandating women's inclusion in the initial phases of particular trials (U.S. Department of Health and Human Services, 1993). Overall, the new policy studiously avoids setting quotas for the number of women to be included and, in fact, permits the investigators to determine how many women are needed to "allow detection of clinically significant gender-related differences in drug response" (U.S. Department of Health and Human Services, 1993).

Additionally, the new guidelines explicitly advocate the use of contraception and pregnancy tests in designing research protocols (U.S. Department of Health and Human Services, 1993). As a result, they perpetuate the exclusion of pregnant women from clinical trials, despite the lack of a scientific inquiry into the risks and benefits of this policy. Furthermore, their assumption that women in trials should be using effective contraception raises the very real possibility that only women who are perceived by investigators to be responsible contraceptors will be permitted to participate in trials. This may take the form of setting up a de facto criteria that all women in studies must use one of a small number of contraceptive options. It may also play into underlying problems of race and class bias, in that white, middle-class investigators may tend to view women of different race and class status as poor contraceptors.

While it remains to be seen how industry will react to these new guidelines, one problem with them can be anticipated already. They fail to take into consideration the source of the pharmaceutical industry's incentives to exclude women from drug trials. In 1986 the president of a major pharmaceutical company asked, "Who in his right mind would work on a product today that would be used by pregnant women?" (Huber, 1988). From the industry's perspective, nothing has changed since then. The industry will not be persuaded by the FDA assertion that, "in 1993, protecting the fetus from unanticipated exposure to potentially harmful drugs remains critically important, but the ban on women's participation in early clinical trials no longer seems reasonable" (Merkatz, 1993). If it is to succeed in promoting women's health, any attempt to build a new policy must give serious consideration to the motivating factors behind women's underrepresentation. While it is to be applauded for taking action on this urgent problem, the FDA's proposed regulations ultimately fail to address these factors, and thus, although they may prompt marginal numerical gains in terms of women's representation in clinical trials, they provide no definitive check on the underlying incentive to exclude fertile women.

References

Beecher, H. K. (1966). Ethics and clinical research. *New England Journal of Medicine, 274,* 1354-1360.

Bichler v. Eli Lilly and Co., 79 A.D. 317 (1981).

Christian, C. D. (1974). Maternal deaths associated with an IUD. *American Journal of Obstetrics and Gynecology, 119*(4), 441.

Goodman, E. (1990, June 23). [Personal column]. *New York Newsday,* p. 74.

Herbst, A. L., Ulfelder, H., & Poskanzer, D. C. (1971). Adenocarcinoma of the vagina: Association of maternal stilbestrol therapy with tumor appearance in young women. *New England Journal of Medicine, 284,* 878-881.

Hilts, P. J. (1990, December 16). Birth control backlash. *The New York Times, 6,* 41.

Huber, P. (1988). *Liability: The legal revolution and its consequences.* New York: Basic Books.

Ikemoto, L. C. (1992). The code of perfect pregnancy: At the intersection of the ideology of motherhood, the practice of defaulting to science, and the interventionist mindset of law. *Ohio State Law Journal, 53,* 5.

Janssen, W. F. (1980). The U.S. food and drug law: How it came; how it works. *Food Drug Cosmetic Law Journal, 35*(3), 132.

Levine, R. J. (1988). *Ethics and regulation of clinical research.* New Haven, CT: Yale University Press.

Luker, K. (1984). *Abortion and the politics of motherhood.* Berkeley: University of California Press.

McCarthy, C. R. (1993, June 28). Address given at the conference on the inclusion of women and minorities in clinical research. Washington, DC: Georgetown University Leavey Center.

Merkatz, R. (1993, June 28). Address given at the conference on the inclusion of women and minorities in clinical research. Washington, DC: Georgetown University Leavey Center.

Nadel, M. V. (1990). Summary of GAO testimony by Mark V. Nadel on problems in implementing the National Institutes of Health policy on women in study populations (GAO/T-HRD 90-38). Washington, DC: Government Accounting Office.

National Institutes of Health Revitalization Amendments of 1991, H.R. 2507, 10 Cong. 1st Sess. Sec. 141 (July 25, 1991), in 137 Cong. Rec. H. 5848.

Public Law No. 93-348 (codified as amended in scattered sections of 42 U.S.C.).

Roe v. Wade, 410 U.S. 113 (1973).

Schwartz, M. (1974). The Dalkon shield: Tale of a tail. *Family Planning Perspectives, 6*(4), 198-201.

Siegler, M. (Ed.). (1987). *Medical innovation and bad outcomes: Legal, social, and ethical responses.* Ann Arbor, MI: Health Administration Press.

Silverman, M., & Lee, P. R. (1974). *Pills, profits, and politics.* Berkeley: University of California Press.

Sindell v. Abbott Lab., 607 P. 924 (1980).

Temin, P. (1980). *Taking your medicine: Drug regulation in the United States.* Cambridge, MA: Harvard University Press.

U.S. Department of Health and Human Services. (1993). *Guideline for the study and evaluation of gender differences in the clinical evaluation of drugs* (58 FR 39406). Washington, DC: Author.

U.S. Department of Health, Education, and Welfare. (1977). *General considerations for the clinical evaluation of drugs* (Publication No. [FDA] 77-3040). Washington, DC: Author.

U.S. Public Health Service. (1973). *Tuskegee syphilis study ad hoc advisory panel: Final report.* Washington, DC: Author.

Vaughan, P. (1970). *The pill on trial.* London: Weidenfeld and Nicolson.

24

Health Policy and Breast Cancer Screening: The Politics of Research and Intervention

Renee Royak-Schaler

Breast cancer is a disease that has a profound psychological impact on one in nine American women and their families (American Cancer Society [ACS], 1991). It is the number 1 cause of death in women 40 to 55 years old and follows cardiovascular disease as the number 2 cause for women over 50 (U.S. Department of Health and Human Services, 1990). Of women who get breast cancer, 25% are premenopausal; the past decade has seen a 5% increase in mortality rates for women under 50 years old (ACS, 1988).

Acknowledging the enormous toll that breast cancer takes on American women and seeking to have an impact on this, the Congressional Caucus for Women's Issues of the U.S. Congress posed the Breast Cancer Challenge to the National Cancer Institute (NCI) and the medical research community in June 1991. This challenge specified five goals to be reached by the end of this century: (a) to understand the cause of and find a cure for breast cancer, (b) to reduce significantly the incidence of breast cancer, (c) to reduce the mortality rate of breast cancer by 50%, (d) to ensure that all women over the age of 40 get regular mammograms, and (e) to ensure that all mammograms are of the highest quality (Congressional Caucus for Women's Issues, 1991).

This challenge speaks for policymakers, researchers, and clinicians alike, in their efforts to influence breast cancer's impact and empower women in the face of it. This chapter will review the interface of health policy and research as related to breast cancer screening practices among American women. Areas of critical need will be identified for demonstration projects during the 1990s that will empower women and health professionals with information, skills, and services to reduce breast cancer mortality. Finally, health policies that will facilitate these goals will be suggested.

Breast Cancer Screening in the 1990s:
Its Roots and Future Directions

Despite major advances in the early detection of breast cancer, women are not compliant with recommended screening guidelines for either breast physical examination or mammography. Data from the National Health Interview Survey of 1987 indicate that more than 80% of women 40 years and older have had a breast physical exam at some time in their lives, although only one third report having had one in the past year, and 63% report being examined in the past 3 years. Women with higher education and higher income are more likely to have had a recent breast physical exam (Dawson & Thompson, 1989).

A similar situation is evident for mammography compliance. The NCI reports that, while 50% of eligible women in this country have had at least one mammogram, a considerably smaller percentage follow American Cancer Society guidelines (National Cancer Institute [NCI] Breast Cancer Screening Consortium, 1990). Higher education and income are positively associated with ever having had a mammogram and having had one recently. Younger women, 40 to 64 years old, are more likely to have had a mammogram than older women, 65 years old and up (Dawson & Thompson, 1989; NCI Breast Cancer Screening Consortium, 1990).

The first set of specific guidelines related to the early detection of breast cancer were developed in 1977 in a Consensus Development Meeting on Breast Cancer Screening held by the NCI (NCI, 1978). They reflected concern about the lack of demonstrable benefit of mammography in women under 50 from the Health Insurance Plan of Greater New York (HIP) study and possible radiation exposure risk for women participating in the ongoing Breast Cancer Detection Demonstration Project (BCDDP). The BCDDP was undertaken to demonstrate the feasibility of detecting very early breast cancer through mammography, clinical breast exam, and breast self-exam (Baker, 1982). The guidelines specified that all women older than 50 were to continue having annual mammograms; all women from 40 to 49 could have mammography if they, or their mothers or sisters, had breast cancer; and women from 35 to 39 years old could have mammography only with a personal history of breast cancer.

The 1980 guidelines of the American Cancer Society continued to reflect concern about mammography for younger women:

1. Women older than 20 years of age should perform breast self-examinations (BSE) monthly.

2. Women from 20 to 40 years of age should have a breast physical examination every 3 years.

3. Women older than 40 years of age should have a breast physical examination every year.

4. Women from 35 to 40 years of age should have a baseline mammogram.

5. Women younger than 50 years of age should consult their physicians about the need for mammography in their individual cases.

6. Women older than 50 years of age should have a mammogram every year.

7. Women with personal or family histories of breast cancer should consult their physicians about the value of more frequent examinations or about the need to begin mammography before 50 years of age.

The concern about mammography for younger women was alleviated with 1983 results from the BCDDP indicating that one third of breast cancers occurred in women 35 to 49 years old, that most did not involve lymph nodes, and most were detected by mammography rather than physical exam (Baker, 1982). When considered in conjunction with improvements in the quality and accuracy of mammography and significant decreases in amounts of radiation delivered to patients, there appeared to be favorable benefits for women 40 and older. The ACS therefore modified the 1980 guidelines for asymptomatic women 40 to 49 years old, recommending they have annual physical breast exams and mammograms every 1 to 2 years. Because of costs involved and the fact that only 25% of breast cancer occurred in women 40 to 49 years old, biannual screening was advised (Dodd, 1992).

During the latter half of the 1980s, use of mammography as a screening procedure increased rapidly. In 1988 the American College of Radiology convened a meeting of the major cancer organizations in this country to develop uniform guidelines. All participants agreed on the necessity for physical examination and the need for annual screening in women 50 and older. They did not agree on the usefulness of BSE, the need for a baseline mammogram between 35 and 39 years old, and the use of periodic screening with mammography in 40- to 49-year-olds. The guidelines adopted are as follows:

1. Clinical examination of the breast and mammography are the basic detection methods. The examinations are complementary and both are necessary to achieve maximum detection rates.

2. It is recommended that the screening process begin examinations with screening mammography performed at 1-year to 2-year intervals.

3. Beginning at 50 years of age, both clinical examination and mammography should be performed on an annual basis.

4. The recommendations apply only to women without signs or symptoms of breast cancer; the frequency and type of examination will vary for the individual with symptoms and should be determined by the responsible physician (Dodd, 1992).

Noncompliance with these guidelines by women 65 and older and their providers prompted the convening of the Forum for Breast Cancer Screening in Older Women in July 1990 (Costanza, 1992; Harris et al., 1991; NCI Breast Cancer Screening Consortium, 1990). Guidelines developed by this forum emphasized the importance of regular screening in women 65 and older and encouraged primary care physicians and medical organizations to implement national programs to increase screening in this age group. The forum recommended the following guidelines:

a. annual clinical breast examination and mammography every 2 years for women 65-74,
b. annual clinical breast examination and mammography every 2 years for women 75 and over whose general health and life expectancy are good, and
c. monthly BSE in women 65 and over to identify lesions and encourage seeking professional care (Costanza, 1992).

National Breast Cancer Screening Policies

Development of guidelines for the early detection of breast cancer has led to increased use of mammography, changes in payment practices, and legislative and regulatory activity. On the national level, a number of countries have adopted screening programs. In 1987 the United Kingdom recommended a policy of single-view mammography performed every 3 years in women 50 to 64 years old. In 1988 Canada recommended mammography be performed every 2 years in women between 50 and 69 years old. While similar policies have been instituted in Sweden, Finland, The Netherlands, and Australia, the United States is not actively considering a national program (Harris, Lippman, Veronesi, & Willett, 1992). What has been our policy as a nation in confronting the breast cancer epidemic?

Psychosocial research has significantly affected breast cancer screening policies in the United States. Recognition of barriers to screening—women's social and demographic characteristics, perceptions of screening efficacy, and provider's perceptions of patients—has influenced national policy. This is evident in congressional mandates to increase funding for breast cancer research by 40% annually—$90 million in 1991, $133 million in 1992, and $175 million in 1993. These mandates were partly stimulated by the Women's Health Equity Act of 1990. The Congressional Caucus for Women's Issues coalesced in the face of the threat of removal of Medicare coverage for mammography screening in 1989, prevented this action by Congress, and proposed an omnibus package of legislation designed to address research, services, and prevention deficiencies in women's health care. The Medicaid Breast and Cervical Cancer Screening Initiative of 1990 was a result of this effort, which granted $50 million to the Centers for Disease Control to run a comprehensive mammography and Pap smear screening program for low-income women. This initiative was written into law as the Breast and Cervical Cancer Mortality Prevention Act in 1992 and was recently extended for 5 years by Congress, providing $135 million in funding for 1994 and involving 30 states in the screening of low-income women (Congressional Caucus for Women's Issues, 1993).

The response of individual states to breast cancer screening needs began to accelerate in 1987: 39 states currently require third party coverage for mammography screening at some level; the majority of these states are located in the northeast and southwest regions. Twelve states have legislation relating to breast cancer screening but no policies regarding third party payments; approximately 570,000 Medicaid-eligible women ages 45 to 84 remain uncovered (Boss & Guckes, 1992; Thompson, Kessler, & Boss, 1989).

The 1990 inclusion of routine mammography as a Medicare benefit saves $60,000 to $125,000 in treatment costs for each elderly or disabled woman whose breast cancer is detected early. This important national screening policy has paved the way for breast cancer screening in other federally funded health programs as basic benefits (Oakar, 1992).

Congress recently addressed the need for national standards for mammography certification, funding the Food and Drug Administration in May 1993 to develop accreditation procedures for mammography screening facilities and to conduct annual on-site inspections, guaranteeing the use of proper equipment and certified personnel (Congressional Caucus for Women's Issues, 1993). This was in compliance with the Mammography Quality Standards Act passed by Congress in October 1992 to establish national quality assurance standards for mammography services and radiological equipment.

Are Mammography Screening Policies Sufficient? What About Clinical Breast Exam and Breast Self-Exam?

Although mammography screening appears to reduce breast cancer mortality by 25%, it remains less sensitive in younger women than older women with 10% of cancers palpable but not detectable by mammography (Harris et al., 1992; Kopans, Mayer, & Sadowsky, 1984). Its effectiveness as an early detection tool in women 40 to 49 years old was questioned in a recent overview of Swedish randomized trials demonstrating insignificant reductions in breast cancer mortality during the first 8 years of follow-up for women in this age group who received mammograms. The Canadian National Breast Screening Study also demonstrated few benefits of mammography for 40- to 49-year-olds; however, the screening techniques employed in this study have been called into question ("News," 1992). Mortality reduction was clearly demonstrated in these projects for 50- to 69-year-olds, with a 29% decrease in the Swedish trials (Nystrom et al., 1993).

   Although mammography is more sensitive than breast palpation for cancer detection, the majority of breast cancers are detected by clinical breast exam or breast self-exam (Foster, Worden, Costanza, & Solomon, 1992). The Canadian National Breast Screening Study, with 90,000 women aged 40 to 59, found that competent and well-trained nurse and physician examiners can identify breast cancer 80% of the time, while mammography is accurate 90% of the time (Baines, Miller, & Bassett, 1989). The HIP Study of Greater New York found that, without mammograms, 30% of breast cancers would not have been detected when they were; without clinical exams, 45% would have gone undetected. Together, these two methods accounted for 75% of detections (Shapiro, Venet, Strax, & Venet, 1988).

   The Breast Cancer Detection Demonstration Project with 285,000 women and mammography techniques improved over the HIP study demonstrated 71% mammography sensitivity and 45% clinical breast exam sensitivity. Breast self-exam was most sensitive in 35- to 39-year-olds, who had a 41% tumor discovery rate, and least sensitive in 60- to 74-year-olds, who found 21% of tumors. Screening with clinical breast exam and mammograms was least sensitive for women 35 to 39 years old (60% tumor detection rate) and most sensitive in women 60 to 74 years old (81% detection rate). Mammography was 91% sensitive to breast cancer in 40- to 49-year-olds and 92% effective in 50- to 59-year-olds (Seidman et al., 1987).

   Historic and tumor registry data, observational studies, and randomized trials all suggest that detection of breast cancers at smaller sizes through physical exams can lead to important reduction in mortality. Mammography, clinical breast exam, and breast self-exam are complementary screening modalities (Foster et al., 1992).

   In a review of breast self-exam research from 1989 to 1991, Baines (1992) found strong support for the fact that BSE is associated with reduced tumor size at cancer diagnosis and potential mortality reduction when performed competently and in association with appropriate diagnostic follow-up. A BSE study using women in the state of Vermont as a geographically defined population found that BSE performers had more favorable clinical and pathological stages of disease than nonperformers, and a mortality rate that was 50% of nonperformers (Foster & Costanza, 1984; Foster et al., 1978). In this study,

90% of monthly BSE performers, 82% of less frequent BSE performers, and 54% of nonperformers detected their own cancers.

Although there remains controversy regarding the efficacy of BSE as an early detection technique, and this includes the Vermont study in which there was little difference in survival rates between women performing regular self-exams and those performing infrequent exams, the procedure is associated with heightened body awareness and the perception of increased control over one's health—both important factors in psychological well-being (Foster et al., 1992). BSE is frequently performed by women who have had previous biopsies and a history of benign breast disease, who are well-informed about BSE and screening, who demonstrate self-efficacy in relation to the procedure, and who perceive themselves to be active partners in controlling their own health (Baines, 1992).

Breast Self-Exam and Mammograms: Companions or Adversaries?

While some researchers maintain the viewpoint that breast self-exam "has consumed substantial financial and other resources that now should be diverted to encourage and support mammography," and that our efforts in early detection should "no longer rely on a second-best technique that women have failed to adopt" (Cassileth, 1992, p. 2), it appears prudent to continue investigating the hypothesis that breast self-exam leads to an earlier diagnosis of breast cancer (Grady, 1992).

For example, 10% to 15% of breast cancers are missed by mammography (Dawson & Thompson, 1989). The ability of mammography to detect breast cancer is age dependent; younger women have greater breast tissue density and less breast fat, making X-ray penetration more difficult. The reported rates of false-negative mammograms across women of all ages is 10% to 22%, with even higher rates in younger women according to two studies of litigation involving misdiagnosis of breast cancer (Brenner, 1991; Kern, in press; Physician Insurers Association of America [PIAA], 1990; Potchen, Bisesi, Sierra, & Potchen, 1991).

One study of 45 misdiagnosis cases with women whose mean age was 40 found that more than 75% of the tumors had been initially diagnosed through breast self-exam (BSE). Despite the obvious presence of palpable masses, only 20% of the mammograms were positive for malignancy (Kern, in press). Another study of 273 insurance claims for delayed diagnosis, with women averaging 44 years old, found that, with masses present in 72% of cases, mammography was positive for malignancy in only 32% of the women. The methods of discovering the lesions involved BSE in 70% of cases, clinical breast exam in 23%, and mammography in 4% (PIAA, 1990).

Even though only one third of breast cancers are present in women under 50, 70% of claimants in the PIAA study and 84% of indemnity awards were for women in this age group, leading us to seriously question the effectiveness of mammography in younger women (Brenner, 1992). This becomes particularly significant when we consider that delay in diagnosis of breast cancer is now the second leading cause for negligence lawsuits filed against physicians and the leading cause of dollar awards issued by third party carriers (PIAA, 1990).

Clinical breast exam and breast self-exam are therefore important methods of early detection in younger women, particularly when considering that breast cancer patients ages 35 and younger have the lowest 5-year survival rate of any age group ("News," 1992). These are very important early detection methods when we consider the technical limitations of mammography and compliance with the procedure. The NCI reports that nearly 50% of the eligible women in this country have had at least one mammogram, although compliance with American Cancer Society guidelines falls far short of this figure (NCI Breast Cancer Screening Consortium, 1990). Furthermore, physical exams and breast self-exam appear to be associated with obtaining regular mammograms (Baines, To, & Wall, 1990). As with mammograms, there are quality control issues with physical exams. Women and their physicians must both be urged to practice consistent patterns of coverage and appropriate palpation techniques (Fletcher, O'Malley, & Bunce, 1985; Fletcher, O'Malley, Polgrim, & Gonzalez, 1989; Worden et al., 1990).

Influencing Perceived Control in High-Risk Women

Competent breast screening and early detection are particularly important for women with a family history of breast cancer. Women with a mother or sister history have a twofold overall increased risk of breast cancer, which is greatest for those with mothers diagnosed prior to age 60 (Colditz et al., 1993; Gail et al., 1989). A 40-year-old woman whose sister or mother (prior to age 50) has been diagnosed with breast cancer has a 12% chance of developing the disease before age 70; this risk decreases to 9% when one's mother was older than 60 at diagnosis (Colditz et al., 1993). Research with high-risk women demonstrates that the anxiety and distress they experience in relation to high-risk status reduces their compliance with clinical breast exams and breast self-exam (Kash, Holland, Halper, & Miller, 1992; Royak-Schaler & Benderly, 1992).

Anxiety and perceived lack of control over developing breast cancer increases with the number of women in the family diagnosed with the disease. It is this factor rather than the practices of screening and early detection that produces psychological distress for many high-risk women. Therefore perceived lack of control associated with strong family history correlates with increased anxiety and distress and decreased screening behavior. Demonstration projects with high-risk women conducted at the Strang Cancer Prevention Clinic and the Georgetown Comprehensive Breast Center have shown that high-risk women respond to intervention programs designed to decrease anxiety and maximize cognitive, behavioral, and emotional control (Kash et al., 1992; Royak-Schaler & Benderly, 1992).

Perceived control in relation to health—the belief in one's ability to affect health through personal actions—is critical to the well-being of high-risk women and women with breast cancer. Women who believe in their personal ability to control their health use problem-focused coping and take active roles in breast cancer early detection, diagnosis, treatment, and recovery.

Promoting control in four critical areas was shown to reduce anxiety and promote screening compliance among high-risk participants in the Georgetown Comprehensive Breast Center project. Cognitive control helps to accurately appraise the high-risk situation; behavioral control facilitates regular practice of early detection strategies; information control provides knowledge about risk, the experience of other high-risk women, and methods of early detection and prevention; retrospective control enables understanding of family breast cancer perhaps not effectively dealt with in the past (Royak-Schaler & Benderly, 1992).

A comprehensive approach to breast cancer screening addresses the risks while emphasizing its benefits. Concern regarding anxiety regarding screening produces, the risk of repeated biopsies and misdiagnosis, and the cost of screening programs is offset by the benefits of having the option to use breast-conserving surgery with small tumors, the decreased need for systemic treatment, and reduced anxiety in women with negative results (Nystrom et al., 1993).

Having an Impact on Breast Cancer in the 1990s

Thus the challenge for policymakers, researchers, and practitioners in the 1990s appears to be twofold: first, influencing breast cancer's impact through decreasing its incidence and improving survival rates; second, influencing women's beliefs about ways they can control their risk of breast cancer. Developing a comprehensive National Breast Cancer Screening Program involves addressing the following critical issues:

1. Provider recommendation is the key; women must be sure they need a mammogram or clinical breast exam. On an individual level, physicians are important partners in screening. Most research investigating women's patterns of clinical breast exams and mammograms demonstrates that women rely on their physicians to tell them if they need these procedures and when they should have them (Smith & Haynes, 1992). Convincing recommendations that provide information about the efficacy and value of both regular breast exams and mammograms should be given to all women, regardless of socioeconomic status (Stein, Fox, & Murata, 1991). Physician awareness of socioeconomic differences in screening and survival rates in breast cancer is imperative; it is poverty that underlies observed racial differences (McWhorter, Schatzkin, Horm, & Brown, 1989).

According to a 1989 American Cancer Society survey of physicians, 18% cited cost of mammograms as the reason for not recommending them according to the guidelines' schedule, even though 29% did not know the cost of this procedure (ACS, 1990). Clearly, physicians and consumers alike need to be educated in ways to obtain high-quality mammograms at reasonable cost as well as insurance laws for screening in their states (Stein et al., 1991).

2. Women need to be reminded of annual screening appointments. Educating physicians regarding the need for reminder systems for clinical breast exam and mammograms is important. Currently, a centralized tracking system for screening and follow-up is being tried out in the state of Colorado. Such a system could effectively serve physicians in individual practice settings, helping them comply with mammography screening guidelines and increasing the use of preventive testing by their patients (Smith & Haynes, 1992).

3. Educating health care providers and women consumers alike remains part of the breast cancer challenge for this decade. Widespread teaching of simple and efficient breast self-exam and clinical breast exam procedures will improve screening practices. Education updates that emphasize accuracy, thoroughness, and consistency in breast palpation, coupled with reminders of the companion nature of clinical breast exam, breast self-exams, and mammograms, are essential.

4. Psychosocial barriers to screening for minority women, particularly African American and Hispanic women, must be addressed. These include understanding the need for and efficacy of regular screening, emphasizing the safety of mammography and low levels of radiation exposure, and addressing the anticipated pain and discomfort associated with mammography (Stein et al., 1991).

5. *A comprehensive National Breast Cancer Screening Program necessarily uses techniques that maximize the likelihood of participation by women consumers and their health care providers while addressing the benefits of and barriers to screening.* A coordinated public approach that accounts for survival differences between racial groups as well as differences in health-related beliefs, behaviors, and accessibility to health care is critical (Lauver, 1992). From this approach will emerge national goals and priorities in education, detection, treatment, and research. Nothing less will do.

References

American Cancer Society. (1988). *Cancer facts and figures: 1988.* Atlanta, GA: American Cancer Society.

American Cancer Society. (1990). Survey of physician attitudes and practices in early cancer detection. *Cancer, 40,* 77-101.

American Cancer Society. (1991). *Cancer facts and figures: 1991.* Atlanta, GA: American Cancer Society.

Baines, C. J. (1992). Breast self-examination. *Cancer, 69*(Suppl.), 1942-1946.

Baines, C. J., Miller, A. B., & Bassett, A. A. (1989). Physical examination: Its role as a single screening modality in the Canadian National Breast Screening Study. *Cancer, 63,* 1816-1822.

Baines, C. J., To, T., & Wall, C. (1990). Women's attitudes to screening after participation in the National Breast Screening Study. *Cancer, 65,* 1663-1669.

Baker, L. (1982). Breast cancer detection demonstration project: Five-year summary report. *Cancer, 32,* 194-225.

Boss, L. P., & Guckes, F. H. (1992). Medicaid coverage of screening tests for breast and cervical cancer. *American Journal of Public Health, 82,* 252-253.

Brenner, R. J. (1991). Medicolegal aspects of breast imaging: Variable standards of care relating to different types of practice. *American Journal of Roentgenology, 156,* 719-723.

Brenner, R. J. (1992). Evolving medical-legal concepts for clinicians and imagers in evaluation of breast cancer. *Cancer, 69*(Suppl.), 1950-1953.

Cassileth, B. R. (1992). Breast cancer surveillance: On increasing its effectiveness while reducing its negative psychological effects. *Journal of the National Cancer Institute, 84,* 2-3.

Colditz, G. A., Willett, W. C., Hunter, D. J., Stampfer, M. J., Manson, J. E., Hennekens, C. H., Rosner, B. A., & Speizer, F. E. (1993). Family history, age, and risk of breast cancer: Prospective data from the Nurses' Health Study. *Journal of the American Medical Association, 270,* 338-343.

Congressional Caucus for Women's Issues. (1991). *Update on Women and Family Issues in Congress, 11*(5), 10.

Congressional Caucus for Women's Issues. (1993). *Update on Women and Family Issues in Congress, 13*(5), 4.

Costanza, M. E. (1992). Breast cancer screening in older women: Overview. *Journals of Gerontology, 47* (Special Issue), 1-3.

Dawson, D. A., & Thompson, G. B. (1989). Breast cancer risk factors and screening: United States, 1987 (National Center for Health Statistics). *Vital Health Statistics, 10*(172).

Dodd, G. D. (1992). American Cancer Society guidelines on screening for breast cancer. *Cancer, 69*(Suppl.), 1885-1887.

Fletcher, S. W., O'Malley, M. S., & Bunce, L. A. (1985). Physicians' abilities to detect lumps in silicone breast models. *Journal of the American Medical Association, 253*, 2224-2228.

Fletcher, S. W., O'Malley, M. S., Polgrim, C., & Gonzalez, J. (1989). How do women compare with internal medicine residents in breast lump detection? *Journal of General Internal Medicine, 4*, 277-283.

Foster, R. S., Jr., & Costanza, M. C. (1984). Breast self-examination practices and breast cancer survival. *Cancer, 53*, 999-1005.

Foster, R. S., Jr., Lang, S. P., Costanza, M. C., et al. (1978). Breast self-examination practices and breast cancer stage. *New England Journal of Medicine, 299*, 265-270.

Foster, R. S., Jr., Worden, J. K., Costanza, M. C., & Solomon, L. J. (1992). Clinical breast examination and breast self-examination. *Cancer, 69*(Suppl.), 1992-1998.

Gail, M. H., Brinton, L. A., Byar, D. P., Corle, D. K., Green, S. B. Schairer, C., & Mulvihill, J. J. (1989). Projecting individualized probabilities of developing breast cancer for white females who are being examined annually. *Journal of the National Cancer Institute, 81*, 1879-1886.

Grady, K. E. (1992). The efficacy of breast self-examination. *The Journal of Gerontology, 47* (Special Issue), 69-74.

Harris, J. R., Lippman, M. E., Veronesi, U., & Willett, W. (1992). Breast cancer. *New England Journal of Medicine, 327*, 319-327.

Harris, R. P., Fletcher, S. W., Gonzalez, J. J., et al. (1991). Mammography and age: Are we targeting the wrong women? *Cancer, 19*, 2010-2014.

Kash, K. M., Holland, J. C., Halper, M. S., & Miller, D. G. (1992). Psychological distress and surveillance behaviors of women with a family history of breast cancer. *Journal of the National Cancer Institute, 84*, 24-30.

Kern, K. A. (in press). Medical malpractice involving the delayed diagnosis of breast cancer: A twenty-year civil court review. *Archives of Surgery.*

Kopans, D. B., Mayer, J. E., & Sadowsky, N. (1984). Breast imaging. *New England Journal of Medicine, 310*, 960-967.

Lauver, D. (1992). Psychosocial variables, race, and intention to seek care for breast cancer symptoms. *Nursing Research, 41*, 236-241.

McWhorter, W. P., Schatzkin, A. G., Horm, J. W., & Brown, C. C. (1989). Contribution of socioeconomic status to black/white differences in cancer incidence. *Cancer, 63*, 982-987.

National Cancer Institute. (1978). National Institutes of Health/National Cancer Institute consensus development meeting on breast cancer screening: Issues and recommendations. *Journal of the National Cancer Institute, 60*, 1519-1521.

National Cancer Institute Breast Cancer Screening Consortium. (1990). Screening mammography: A missed clinical opportunity. *Journal of the American Medical Association, 264*, 54-58.

News. (1992). *Journal of the National Cancer Institute, 84*, 832-833.

Nystrom, L., Rutqvist, L. E., Wall, S., Lindgren, A., Lindqvist, M., Ryden, S., Andersson, I., Bjurstam, N., Fagerberg, G., Frisell, J., Tabar, L., & Larsson, L. G. (1993). Breast cancer screening with mammography: Overview of Swedish randomised trials. *The Lancet, 341*, 973-978.

Oakar, M. R. (1992). Legislative effect of the 102nd Congress. *Cancer, 69* (Suppl.), 1954-1956.

Physician Insurers Association of America. (1990). *Breast cancer study.* Lawrenceville, NJ: Author.

Potchen, E. J., Bisesi, M. A., Sierra, A. E., & Potchen, J. E. (1991). Mammography and malpractice. *American Journal of Roentgenology, 156*, 475-480.

Royak-Schaler, R., & Benderly, B. L. (1992). *Challenging the breast cancer legacy: A program of emotional support and medical care for women at risk.* New York: HarperCollins.

Seidman, H., Geib, S. K., Silverbert, E., et al. (1987). Survival experience in the Breast Cancer Detection Demonstration Project. *CA-A Cancer Journal for Clinicians, 37,* 258-290.

Shapiro, S., Venet, W., Strax, P., & Venet, L. (1988). Current results of the breast cancer screening randomized trial: The Health Insurance Plan (HIP) of greater New York study. In N. E. Day & A. B. Miller (Eds.), *Screening for breast cancer.* Toronto: Hans Huber.

Smith, R. A., & Haynes, S. (1992). Barriers to screening for breast cancer. *Cancer, 69,* 1968-1978.

Stein, J. A., Fox, S. A., & Murata, P. J. (1991). The influence of ethnicity, socioeconomic status, and psychological barriers on use of mammography. *Journal of Health and Social Behavior, 32,* 101-113.

Thompson, G. B., Kessler, L. G., & Boss, L. P. (1989). Breast cancer screening legislation in the United States: A commentary. *American Journal of Public Health, 79,* 1541-1543.

U.S. Department of Health and Human Services. (1990). *Healthy people 2000: National health promotion and disease prevention objectives* (Pub. no. [PHS] 91-50212). Washington, DC: Government Printing Office.

Worden, J., Solomon, L., Flynn, B., et al. (1990). A community-wide program in breast self-examination training and maintenance. *Preventive Medicine, 19,* 254-269.

25

Toward a Feminist Methodology in Research on Battered Women

Nanette Silva

Until recently, most research on battered women has been conducted from the point of view of a "social problem" that should be investigated as a criminal justice matter. Ignoring the fact that domestic violence has become the single leading cause of injury to women in the United States (Stark et al., 1981), the research community has been reluctant to apply a "gender lens" to the behavior. A gender lens must be applied to more clearly understand what is missing in priorities, theories, categories, and strategies. Without specifically looking for solutions to women's problems, solutions to all "social problems" are unattainable (Servatius, 1992). The use of a "gender lens" by the research community would mean the further development and use of feminist methodology. Efforts in this direction should not imply a trend toward less elegant methodologies.

Since the early 1970s, the overall women's movement has sought the right for women to control their own bodies, an idea that has naturally extended to a right to control the violence in their lives. As a direct result, telephone hot lines, crisis centers, and eventually battered women's shelters were established. Feminist thought has been inherent in the evolution of the battered women's advocacy community, and a "gender lens" has been applied by activists in the movement. However, to enhance the effectiveness of the direct service programs, there must exist strong data. This establishes the case for support of research activities, yet community activists and practitioners have been resistant to research efforts.

Historically, one of the first obstacles to overcome was to demonstrate to the women's movement that research on battered women could actually be conducted. Significant methodological problems exist, resulting in the conflicts of interest between researchers and service personnel. Ethically, the subjects need protection from possible harm; the abuse may escalate if the perpetrator discovers that the woman has disclosed the violence. Written informed consents must be obtained. Researchers need to promise confidentiality to their subjects, creating a dilemma if a court orders the data released. Approaching subjects for research purposes while they are in a crisis situation may be difficult, as such conditions are not conducive to traditional empirical research. Many shelter personnel do not want their clients placed under the additional stress of answering research questions, as such interventions are generally considered invasive, disruptive, and insensitive to a woman's immediate needs (Finkelhor, Gelles, Hotaling, & Straus, 1983).

On a basic and practical level, the vocabulary used in shelters and other social service agencies is distinct from "scientific" research vocabulary. Social service personnel and researchers work in very different environments, each having its own language, culture, and hierarchical structure. Therefore the wide communication gap that exists between service personnel and researchers in the area of woman battering is not surprising. What is counterintuitive is the communication gap and basic disagreement that exist among members of the research community itself.

Definitions

"Family violence," "spousal abuse," and "marital violence" are not the subjects of this discussion. The behavior to be discussed, specifically, is the battering of women by men. Stark and Flitcraft (1991) distinguish *battering* and *abuse* from the standpoint of health risks, defining *battering* as the physical and psychosocial sequelae of abuse that include a history of injury, often punctuated by sexual assault, general medical complaints, isolation, and psychosocial problems that develop over time. Investigators' analyses of both individuals and couples involved in battering situations have proved insufficient in achieving an academic understanding of a behavior that, despite its prevalence, has quietly been legally and socially sanctioned in most societies throughout history.

For the purpose of this chapter, *feminism* will be defined as the search for an egalitarian balance of power in society, whereby both women and men equally share societal reinforcers, such as employment wages, influence in politics and media, education and subsequent career opportunities and whereby the differences between women and men are not misused. Also, Rich's (1979, p. 78) definition of *patriarchy* will be used, which is any kind of group organization in which men hold dominant power and determine what roles women will play and in which capabilities ascribed to women are generally in the realms of the mystical and aesthetic and exclude the practical (e.g., financial) and political realms.

Incidence and Prevalence

According to some investigators, 3 to 4 million American women are battered annually (Rosenberg, Mercy, & Smith, 1984; Stark et al., 1981). In the United States, a woman is more likely to be assaulted, injured, raped, or killed by a male partner than by any other type of assailant (Browne & Williams, 1987). Battering may be the most common cause of injury to women, accounting for more injuries than automobile accidents, muggings, and rape combined (Stark et al., 1981). Furthermore, the FBI's 1980 Crime Index (FBI, 1986) projected that the actual overall incidence was 10 times more common than official figures indicated. According to the American Medical Association: "Physical and sexual violence against women is a public health problem that has reached epidemic proportions. An estimated 8 to 12 million women in the United States are at risk of being abused by their current or former intimate partners" (Warshaw, Flitcraft, Hadley, McLeer, & Hendricks-Matthews, 1992, p. 1).

Measuring the incidence and prevalence of woman battering is not easy. Great variations in rates are found in the literature, partly because no commonly accepted definition of woman battering exists (Finkelhor, Hotaling, & Yllö, 1988). Further, to measure incidence, onset and duration must be clearly defined. To measure prevalence, a "case" must be clearly defined (Bowen & Sedlak, 1985).

Determining the severity of violent acts is also difficult. Is the damage defined as a slap, a blow, a punch, a kick, or a combination of these? For years, one of the most widely used instruments for measuring intrafamily conflict and violence has been the Conflict Tactics Scale (CTS), developed by Straus and colleagues (Straus, 1979). This instrument is based on the conflict model of society, which assumes that some conflict in human association is inevitable. The CTS rates all "kicks" the same, regardless of whether a man kicks a woman's ribs or she kicks his shins. Likewise, it rates all "slaps" the same, regardless of whether a man weighs 250 pounds or 150 pounds. In addition, the CTS does not measure emotional or sexual abuse. These issues are not handled consistently in the literature. However, Gelles (1987b) has admitted that, with the recent use of large survey research firms that can conduct thousands of telephone interviews, "What we have gained in generalizable, quantitative data, we have lost in terms of understanding the meanings and human side of violence."

History of the Research

Early literature on battered women tended to originate from the psychiatric field, and from it sprang the myth that women's masochism was responsible as well as the idea that the woman provoked the male (Campbell & Humphreys, 1984). The family was viewed as basically nonviolent. Excluding the psychiatric literature, formal research on battered women has been conducted only for the past 17 years. The researcher Murray Straus has stated that woman battering is of interest now because the same social forces that at one time produced "selective inattention" have now created a "social problem" out of behavior that is in no way different than that which previously existed (Gelles, 1987b).

The index of the *Journal of Marriage and the Family* contained no reference to "violence" until 1969 (Schechter, 1982). Woman battering was not officially considered a public health problem until 1985, when Surgeon General Koop sponsored an invitational workshop on violence and public health (Surgeon General's Workshop, 1986).

Studies have been conducted from a variety of ideological perspectives. Researchers differ on how best to measure the behavior. Most research has been sociological, with Gelles and Straus in the forefront, applying traditional patriarchally developed methodologies and describing their approach as a "value-free orientation" (Gelles, 1987b). One of the most controversial arguments regarding the Conflict Tactics Scale and its use, for example, arose from the results of their 1985 National Survey (Straus & Gelles, 1986), which sampled 3,520 individuals via telephone interviews. The results were compared with their 1975 survey, which had used face-to-face interviews. The controversial conclusion was that over the 10 years woman battering had decreased by 27%. Dobash and Dobash (1979, 1984), on the other hand, suggest that research must do more than observe and record the behavior of the individuals or couples and, instead, build hypotheses in a broad socio-historical context, at the same time making objective and measurable the conception of battering. They have provided detailed historical documentation of the aforementioned legal and societal sanctioning of woman battering. Unfortunately, traditionally empirical testing of the model is not practical under commonly accepted methodologies. For example, the independent variable of patriarchy is very difficult to define operationally.

Gelles (1987a) criticizes Dobash and Dobash for what he categorizes as their single-factor explanation. Dobash and Dobash (1988) criticize Gelles's "narrow perspective." Yet, Straus and Gelles (1986) do provide ample documentation of the worldwide societal subordinate status of women, which is consistent with the patriarchal construct of most societies.

Other feminist researchers such as Wardell, Gillespie, and Leffler (1983) and Yllö and Bograd (1988) believe that scientific research, like other areas of society such as government policy, media depictions, and medicinal models, is biased by a sexist, male-dominated framework. Yllö and Bograd argue that a feminist perspective can and must be incorporated into all aspects of society that report, treat, or investigate the battering of women. They believe that data collection, interpretation, and use are political activities. Dobash and Dobash (1988) acknowledge the relationship between social research and political issues and point out that no effective models exist that explain how to develop science within a political context, how to conduct research within a sociopolitical framework, or how to maintain ongoing communication among researchers, community groups, and social service agencies. Too often, the quality of research is compromised by the power and authority of the men who are invested in it. Research conducted from a feminist viewpoint acknowledges this power inequality.

Wardell et al. (1983) state that, "despite its genuinely benevolent intentions, the wife beating literature is riddled with misogyny" (p. 79). Bograd (1984) adds that "objectivity is man's subjectivity rendered unquestionable" (p. 563). Yet, Campbell and Humphreys (1984) point out that Straus does acknowledge the violent and sexist character of society and observes that the family is inherently at high risk for violent interaction because of the large amounts of time family members may spend together, familial assumptions that individual members have the right to try to change each other's behavior, and the involuntary nature of membership. But Schechter (1988) believes that, although violence may be built into the very structure of society and the family system, the problem is not the family but the power relations within it. Stark and Flitcraft (1983) suggest that it is the incongruity between continued male privilege and the concurrent growing opportunities for female independence that render modern family conflict inevitable. Dobash and Dobash (1984) underscore the importance of gender in the analysis of the dynamics of violent events. It is the real or perceived challenges to male possession, authority, and control that ultimately result in acts of violence against women (Dobash & Dobash, 1979). "Family violence" is not evenly distributed and is disproportionately directed toward women. The Bureau of Justice Statistics (1983) indicates that approximately 95% of domestic violence victims are women.

A Feminist Approach

In more recent work, Stark and Flitcraft (1991) and Warshaw (1993) have shifted away from a discussion of the conflicting causal theories to an emphasis on investigating primary and secondary preventive measures. The causes do not need to be understood and agreed upon in order to implement effective prevention programs while simultaneously gathering robust data. According to Campbell and Humphreys (1984), primary prevention should include health promotion interventions at the societal level and identification of women at risk for abuse. Secondary prevention should include early identification of battered women with early intervention, in settings like hospital emergency rooms, thereby yielding more accurate prevalence data on morbidity.

The reframing of woman battering as "gender-based trauma" serves to redefine the issue so that it becomes more than a criminal justice problem. Such reframing was a major catalyst in producing the American Medical Association's 1992 publication for health professionals of protocols for diagnostic and treatment guidelines on domestic violence. Although a sign of progress, implementation of such training must include caveats against old myths and stereotypes. Health care professionals may focus on the solution of keeping the family together, or on the medical symptoms of a woman's physical trauma, or on treating "secondary" problems such as alcohol abuse or depression as the "primary diagnosis" instead of acknowledging the complex interplay of forces (Flitcraft, 1992; Stark, Flitcraft, & Frazier, 1979). In so doing, these professionals avoid the issues of male responsibility for these violent acts.

Feminist research looks at how language defines reality (Bograd, 1984; Yllö & Bograd, 1988). Stark et al. (1981) propose that to ask why individuals hit each other and why millions of women are beaten in their homes is asking two separate questions. Bograd (Yllö & Bograd, 1988) asserts that feminists ask different questions than do traditional researchers. The question, "Why do women stay?" subtly blames the woman for her victimization. The question, "What social factors constrain women from leaving?" does not confer blame on the woman. Likewise, consider the difference between the question, "What did you do to provoke your husband?" which implies, "How did you challenge male authority?" versus the question, "What did you do after your husband hit you?" which asks about her survival behavior.

Gelles (1987a) agrees that, if woman battering is produced by sociocultural norms that tolerate and even approve of violence, effective prevention means changing prevailing cultural norms, including the family's social organization. It means eliminating the values that legitimize violence. Gelles further states that, because stress from factors such as unemployment, poverty, and inadequate medical care can limit the ability of individuals and families to cope with conflict in their homes, a reduction of this stress can reduce the violence.

Recommended Strategies

Definitions and assumptions must be stated and agreed upon to produce data on woman battering that can be used in prevention. The existing empirical knowledge should be consolidated so as to make it clinically useful to practitioners and to the community. The use of a common language and the abandonment of academic rhetoric would diminish the chance for misinterpretations of information.

Validation studies on research methodologies should be conducted. Agreed-upon operational definitions for battering, beating, abuse, and violence need to be developed. Campbell (1992) suggests that feminist theory should distinguish between wife beating, wife battering, and mutual violence (and admit the latter exists) and discriminate more carefully among the various forms of violence against women. Schechter (1988) challenges researchers to document the series of complex steps involved in the cycle of violence. When and why does the woman make the choice to make a life change?

Researchers in the field of woman battering often conduct studies on other forms of violence against women, or on other forms of violence in general. Again, the language becomes cloudy. Is there a categorical language problem? Both the distinctions and the correlations among woman battering, family violence, wife beating, spousal abuse, marital rape, sexual assault, elder abuse, child abuse, youth violence, and street homicide must be addressed by the researchers. A more collaborative approach is needed. More opportunities for open, creative, and noncompetitive dialogue must be arranged. For example, the movement to end violence against women and the gun control movement at times appear to exist on opposite ends of a spectrum. There exists little or no overlap of individuals in the movements, despite the seemingly obvious interconnectedness of the issues.

As no single factor can explain the battering of women by men, more attention likewise needs to be paid to the interconnectedness among correlate behaviors such as battering, substance abuse, depression, homelessness, and risk of HIV infection. To underscore the significance of the "complex interplay" of the behaviors, researchers must form partnerships with the community. However, cooperative and collaborative work takes time. It is seldom objective and detached. The training of a traditional scientific researcher does not usually include course work on collaboration. Of interest, Straus and Gelles concede that Wardell and her coauthors "force us out of certain established and constricting modes of thinking and research" (Finkelhor et al., 1983, p. 30).

The relatively new public health approach to violence prevention may be a vehicle by which to foster communication and collaboration. This model places an emphasis on community intervention and not on a medical "cure." A sample strategy is the implementation of school-based prevention/education programs that incorporate a behavioral social skills training model and that address not only violence but HIV/STD and substance abuse risk reduction behaviors as well. As institutions ranging from the Centers for Disease Control to philanthropic foundations begin to embrace violence prevention as a priority, this provides an excellent opportunity for researchers to form creative collaborations with each other and with other professional communities.

As stated earlier, we must develop methods by which to analyze research messages within a sociopolitical framework. We must keep cognizant of societally ingrained inequalities of power and strive to share societal reinforcers. Despite methodological differences, there does emerge some common ground. Researchers of woman battering all seem to envision a grand change at the policy-making level. To facilitate this, partnerships with each other and with community institutions and organizations should be actively encouraged, pursued, and maintained. Such cooperation can only serve to yield a broader understanding of the complex behavior of woman battering.

References

Bograd, M. (1984). Family systems approaches to wife battering: A feminist critique. *American Journal of Orthopsychiatry, 54*(4), 558-568.

Bowen, G. L., & Sedlak, A. J. (1985). Toward a domestic violence surveillance system: Issues and prospects. *Response to the Victimization of Women and Children, 8*(3), 2-7.

Browne, A., & Williams, K. R. (1987, November 11-14). *Resource availability for women at risk: Its relationship to rates of female perpetrated partner homicide.* Paper presented at the American Society of Criminology Annual Meeting, Montreal, Canada.

Bureau of Justice Statistics. (1983, October). *Report to the nation on crime and justice: The data.* Washington, DC: U.S. Department of Justice, Office of Justice Programs.

Campbell, J. C. (1992). Wife-battering: Cultural contexts versus Western social sciences. In D. Counts, J. Brown, & J. Campbell (Eds.), *Sanctions and sanctuary: Cultural perspectives on the beating of wives.* Boulder, CO: Westview.

Campbell, J. C., & Humphreys, J. H. (1984). *Nursing care of victims of family violence.* Englewood Cliffs, NJ: Reston.

Dobash, R. E., & Dobash, R. P. (1979). *Violence against wives: A case against the patriarchy.* New York: Free Press.

Dobash, R. E., & Dobash, R. P. (1984). The nature and antecedents of violent events. *British Journal of Criminology, 24*(3), 269-288.

Dobash, R. E., & Dobash, R. P. (1988). Research as social action: The struggle for battered women. In K. Yllö & M. Bograd (Eds.), *Feminist perspectives in wife abuse* (pp. 51-74). Newbury Park, CA: Sage.

Federal Bureau of Investigation (FBI). (1986). *Crime in the United States.* Washington, DC: Author.

Finkelhor, D., Gelles, R., Hotaling, G., & Straus, M. (Eds.). (1983). *The dark side of families: Current family violence research.* Beverly Hills, CA: Sage.

Finkelhor, D., Hotaling, G., & Yllö, K. (1988). *Stopping family violence: Research priorities for the coming decade.* Newbury Park, CA: Sage.

Flitcraft, A. (1992). Violence, values, and gender. *Journal of the American Medical Association, 267*(23), 3194-3195.

Gelles, R. (1987a). *Family violence* (2nd ed.). Newbury Park, CA: Sage.

Gelles, R. (1987b). *The violent home.* Newbury Park, CA: Sage.

Rich, A. (1979). *On lies, secrets, and silence.* New York: Norton.

Rosenberg, M. L., Mercy, J. A., & Smith, J. C. (1984). Violence as a public health problem: A new role for CDC and a new alliance with educators. *Educational Horizons, 62*(4), 124-127.

Schechter, S. (1982). *Women and male violence: The visions and struggles of the battered women's movement.* Boston: South End.

Schechter, S. (1988). Building bridges between activists, professionals and researchers. In K. Yllö & M. Bograd (Eds.), *Feminist perspectives on wife abuse* (pp. 299-312). Newbury Park, CA: Sage.

Servatius, M. (1992). *Shortsighted: How Chicago area grantmakers can apply a gender lens to see the connections between social problems and women's needs.* Chicago: Chicago Women in Philanthropy.

Stark, E., & Flitcraft, A. (1983). Social knowledge, social policy and the abuse of women: The case against patriarchial benevolence. In D. Finkelhor, R. Gelles, G. Hotaling, & M. Straus (Eds.), *The dark side of families: Current family violence research* (pp. 330-348). Beverly Hills, CA: Sage.

Stark, E., & Flitcraft, A. (1991). Spouse abuse. In M. Rosenberg & M. Fenley (Eds.), *Violence in America: A public health approach* (pp. 123-155). New York: Oxford University Press.

Stark, E., Flitcraft, A., & Frazier, W. (1979). Medicine and patriarchial violence: The social construction of a "private" event. *International Journal of Health Services, 9*(3), 461-493.

Stark, E., Flitcraft, A., Zuckerman, D., Grey, A., Robison, J., & Frazier, W. (1981). *Wife abuse in the medical setting: An introduction for health personnel.* Rockville, MD: National Clearinghouse on Domestic Violence.

Straus, M. A. (1979). Measuring intrafamily conflict and violence: The Conflict Tactics (CT) Scales. *Journal of Marriage and the Family, 41,* 75-88.

Straus, M. A., & Gelles, R. J. (1986). Societal change and change in family violence from 1975 to 1985 as revealed by two national surveys. *Journal of Marriage and the Family, 48,* 465-479.

Surgeon General's Workshop on Violence. (1986). Recommendations on spouse abuse. *Response to the Victimization of Women and Children, 9*(1), 19-21.

Wardell, L., Gillespie, D., & Leffler, A. (1983). Science and violence against wives. In D. Finkelhor, R. Gelles, G. Hotaling, & M. Straus (Eds.), *The dark side of families: Current family violence research* (pp. 69-84). Beverly Hills, CA: Sage.

Warshaw, C. (1993). Domestic violence: Challenges to medical practice. *Journal of Women's Health, 2*(1), 73-80.

Warshaw, C., Flitcraft, A., Hadley, S., McLeer, S., & Hendricks-Matthews, M. B. (1992). *Diagnostic and treatment guidelines on domestic violence.* Chicago: American Medical Association.

Yllö, K., & Bograd, M. (Eds.). (1988). *Feminist perspectives on wife abuse.* Newbury Park, CA: Sage.

PART VI

Practice Issues

26

Is Care a Remedy?
The Case of Nurse Practitioners[1]

Sue Fisher

Caring, at least since the emergence of the "cult of domesticity" (Cott, 1977), has been gendered. In rapidly changing times, it has played an important role in shoring up the ideology of gender difference. As the informal, unpaid labor that women do to protect and promote the well-being of others, as a routine feature of the domestic economy, as a part of women's everyday life in the family and in the community, caring contributes to the glorification of the home and women's roles in it. There is, in addition, a strong association between caring and taking care of, including taking care of the health of others. Women have long been responsible for providing the domestic conditions necessary both for the maintenance of health and for the recovery from illness (Graham, 1985).

In the social transformation from preindustrial to modern industrial work patterns, women began to turn their usual domestic occupations into paid work (Cott, 1977). Health care was no exception. In her history of American nursing, Reverby (1987) argues that caring for the needs of others for love became, for some, caring for others as paid labor. In the early years, paid nursing was a trade "professed" in the marketplace, learned at home and practiced by older women with no formal training or schooling. When nursing moved out of the home and into the hospital and especially after the Nightingale-based reforms, female character built on the obligation to care contributed to the sacrifice of autonomy on what Reverby refers to as "the alter of altruism." Caring has remained central to nursing. The later separation of

SOURCE: This chapter originally appeared in modified form in *Negotiating at the Margins: Women and the Gendered Discourses of Power and Resistance* edited by Sue Fisher and Kathy Davis. Copyright © 1993 by Rutgers, The State University. Reprinted by permission of Rutgers University Press.

nursing education from nursing service diminished neither the obligation to care nor nursing's position as a woman's occupation. Neither a university education nor the move toward professional autonomy eliminated the cultural identification of nursing with caring.

During the 1960s, when federal policies in the United States were directed toward countering societal inequalities, including inequalities in health care, a new health professional came into being—the nurse practitioner. While nurses had long been subordinate to physicians by custom and law (Melosh, 1982), nurse practitioners sought to establish themselves as fellow professionals. The medical profession has as Freidson (1970) points out "an official approved monopoly to the right to define health and illness and to treat illness"—a right based in the professionals' control over a body of medical knowledge and technical skill and in their freedom from outside control, their professional autonomy. On what grounds, then, could nurse practitioners establish themselves as medical professionals? If nurse practitioners share a body of medical knowledge and technical skills with physicians and if they are positioned in relationship to them as physician extenders, on what could their professional autonomy rest?

Nurse practitioners turned caring from an obligation to a virtue. Operationalizing it as psychosocial skills, patient education, and prevention, caring provided the knowledge and skill they could control and upon which their declaration of professional autonomy could rest. Nurse practitioners claim to offer a system of care that adds caring to curing, and this does not seem to be an empty assertion. There is an ample literature demonstrating that they provide medical care that is comparable with the care provided by primary care physicians—care that is of high quality, efficient, effective, and economical (Diers & Molde, 1979; Sackett, 1974; Shamansky, 1985). In addition, nurse practitioners are generally acclaimed for their psychosocial skills (Lohr & Brooks, 1984). It is this combination of medical and psychosocial skills that differentiates nursing from medical practice and that grounds nurse practitioners' claim for professional autonomy.

Caring, couched in terms of qualities understood as natural—qualities that could jump from the private to the public spheres without threatening the identity of its bearer—has been vital to important transitions for women. Caring, while remaining pivotal to women's identity, took them from the home to nursing in the paid labor force. At a later time when women's participation in the public sphere as nurses working in a secondary labor market was more accepted, caring emerged as central to another battle—the battle nurse practitioners are fighting for professional status. Caring has been at the heart of the campaign to move from being a doctor's handmaiden (Melosh, 1982) to being an autonomous medical practitioner. It grounds the identities of nurse practitioners as women and is foundational to their struggle for professional autonomy. In nurse practitioners' fight, caring provides the basis for both a new political reality—the nurse practitioner as autonomous medical provider—and the basis for a different kind of provider-patient relationship—one that integrates medical and psychosocial skills. However, these claims are problematic.

To pose a system of care as the justification for a different kind of provider-patient relationship, the ground for professional autonomy, and/or the basis for professional identity participates in the reinscription of two convergent sets of social relations. It reinforces a sexual division of labor and women's participation in a secondary labor market as nurses and it fortifies what some refer to as the public patriarchy (Brown, 1981). In addition, it raises questions about whether caring, which has embedded in it some of the deepest dimensions of traditional gender differentiation in our society (Tronto, 1989), could provide a warrant for nursing's claims. These are at one and the same time empirical and theoretical questions.

The Evidence: Caring as Practice

Overwhelmingly, researchers, myself among them, have concentrated on the doctor-patient relationship. We have gathered an impressive array of empirical materials—materials that suggest that the medical relationship is characterized by an asymmetry between provider and patient and by an almost exclusive concern with medical topics to the nearly total exclusion of the social, biographical context of patients' lives (Mishler, 1984; Todd, 1989). This medical relationship rests on a medical model that presents illness as the organic pathology of individual patients. From this perspective, neither non-organic complaints nor the social context of patients' lives fits comfortably. The medical problem to be solved is located in the individual's body—organs malfunction in mechanistic style. Diagnosis identifies the specific etiology—the specific pathological disturbance—and treatment optimally returns the system to its normal state of balance.

The system of care nursing claims to offer challenges this model. Nurse practitioners argue that the problems patients bring to examining rooms cannot be separated from the complex social and psychological lives people lead. A nursing practice that integrates the social psychological and the medical aspects of care blurs the distinction between the medical and the social, the physiological and the psychological.

Given that the delivery of health care is essentially a communication event, this challenge to the medical model implies skills that are linguistically based. To gain access to biographical information, nurse practitioners would have to encourage patients to speak about their lives. Would a nursing practice that adds caring to curing, then, minimize the asymmetry in the provider-patient relationship? In so doing, would it maximize the patient's voice, providing a discourse that adds the social, contextual to the medical found to characterize doctor-patient discourse? And, if so, would caring provide a discourse upon which to redefine the medical model and the clinical practice that flows from it?

These are empirical questions without ready answers. They ask what a nursing practice that adds caring to curing would look like and whether it could provide the bases for a different kind of provider-patient relationship. But while there are studies that evaluate the quality and effectiveness of nursing practice, there is very little systematic information about what nurse practitioners actually do in examining rooms. Without such data, we do not know how caring, or for that matter quality and effectiveness, translate into nursing practice. Nor can we understand what consequences, if any, such translations might have. It is one thing to posit that nurse practitioners offer a system of care, it is quite another to display what this system of care looks like in practice.

The Theoretical Remedy: A Discourse of the Social

At another level, the ways we understand the relationship between provider and patient, the medical and the social, and medicine and society, pose theoretical issues—issues central to three recent sociological studies by Mishler (1984), Silverman (1987), and Waitzkin (1983). While each of these studies focuses on the doctor-patient relationship, the issues they raise are directly applicable to the nurse practitioner-patient relationship.

Mishler (1984) describes the practice of medicine as divided into two separate discourses—the voice of medicine and the voice of the lifeworld. Doctors who are oriented almost exclusively to the technical bioscientific aspects of medicine have the dominant voice. They speak in the voice of medicine, while patients who are subordinate have difficulty getting heard, have difficulty inserting their voices—the voices of the lifeworld. Reformers, like Mishler, challenge the dominance of the medical model and call for a more humanistic, patient-centered medical practice that includes both social psychological and medical aspects of patients' lives.

If patients are treated as whole people rather than sick body parts, if the medical and social, the pathological and the psychological, are valued equally, if the emphasis on diagnosis and treatment is extended to include education and prevention, if patients are recognized as the experts on their own lives, if doctors ask open-ended questions, if they share medical information, if they listen to what patients have to tell them and if they encourage patients to participate, then an asymmetrical relationship could become more equalitarian. Providers, by broadening the medical model, by having a more humanistic attitude, and by minimizing their power and sharing their knowledge, could maximize the patient's voice, her participation in the diagnostic-treatment process and therefore her potential for agency. This recommendation sounds much like the system of care nurse practitioners claim to provide.

Silverman (1987) and Waitzkin (1983) are critical of this remedy to the problems in the medical encounter. Silverman argues that Mishler's call to humanize medical practice by encouraging patients to speak about their lives relies on faulty assumptions. It poses the social in opposition to the medical, assumes that doctors speak in the medical and patients speak in the social voice and that encouraging a "discourse of the social" as an authentic (it speaks the truth) voice is liberating. Calling for, inciting, a discourse of the social, then, could correct the imbalances in the medical relationship. Rather than relying on these polarities, Silverman suggests that we see in the medical consultation a plurality of voices, each interrupting and interpenetrating the other. Doctors and patients can and do speak in both medical and social voices. Speaking in a common language, a field of power forms to govern them both.

Waitzkin (1983) has a very different conception of how power works. Doctors and patients do not speak in a common voice. They do not form a field of power that governs them both. Nor does the voluntary inclusion of a more humanistic discourse of the social resolve the troubles in the medical relationship. Both positions present the medical relationship as if it were independent from the larger social context; both accept the context of patients' lives uncritically.

Because the medical relationship does not occur in a vacuum, larger social contradictions penetrate the purported intimacy of the medical relationship. During medical consultations, doctors routinely do ideological work that reflects and reinforces dominant structural arrangements, especially economic arrangements, encouraging patients' consent to them. Both social and medical discourses, then, are deeply political.

For Waitzkin, the remedy is for socially conscious doctors to engage in ideological work that reveals and resists oppressive structural arrangements. The starting place for social change is a new form of medical practice that redirects patients toward political action. Doctors can *help* patients break the ideological chains that bind them.

Positioned against the background of Mishler's call for a discourse of the social and Silverman's and Waitzkin's very different theoretical stance, I do a detailed empirical analysis of two cases—one with a family practice doctor and one with a nurse practitioner—and interrogate the data to illuminate the interactional and ideological work this communication does. By juxtaposing the ways nurse practitioner-patient and doctor-patient communicate during medical encounters, the evidence garnered may shed light both on empirical questions about what nurse practitioners actually do in examining rooms— about caring as medical practice—and on theoretical questions about the viability of caring as a discourse of the social that remedies the problems in the provider-patient encounter.

Background Context

With the permission of provider and patient, I audio- and videotaped consultations and transcribed the tapes for later analysis. I chose the two cases I am about to discuss for their comparability. Both the doctor, Dr. Aster, and the nurse practitioner, Katherine Heinz,[2] are primary care providers—family medicine and community medicine, respectively. Family practice shares with nursing a commitment to patient-centered holistic medicine that integrates the medical and social psychological. In these cases, then, the stated intention of both the medical and the nursing practices are quite similar.

The patients, Wendy Foster and Prudence Batson, are young women—25 and 27 years old, respectively. Both of them are married, are mothers, and live in an intact nuclear family. While Wendy is a new mother of a first child, Prudence has three small children. They each live out a double day, working and having primary responsibility for child care and housework. Wendy works part time for her husband and Prudence works full time alongside her husband in a factory. Both of them are Caucasian and working to middle class, a fact evidenced in their ability to pay for health care.

Both doctor-patient and nurse practitioner-patient are meeting each other for the first time. In each case, in this initial visit, the patients have sought medical attention with vague and nonspecific complaints. Wendy's presenting complaint is that she felt faint, nauseated, and had nearly passed out. Prudence's primary complaint is fatigue. Complaints of this kind, where no organic pathology is found, are often attributed to psychological rather than physiological distress. Such attributes provide a fertile site for exploring the ways the social is dealt with in medical and nursing encounters.

The Medical Consultation

After the doctor introduces himself and asks what he can do for the patient, the patient presents her complaints. She says:

Well, this morning I nearly passed out and my whole body felt like it was going numb (D: uh huh) in here it goes through this sort of tingle (D: uh huh) I just felt like that all over. Then my arms started hurting and I couldn't open my hands, mostly my left hand but my right hand was doing a little bit but . . . (D: ok, ok) I felt a little bit nauseated but that's passed but I got real feverish//

Here the doctor interrupts to ask medical questions: whether the symptoms began all of a sudden and what the patient had been doing when they began. Once he finds out that the onset had been sudden and that the patient had been feeding her 6-month-old baby breakfast when the symptoms began, he abandons medical questions for social ones[3] and the patient offers no resistance. The doctor does not ask for additional information about nausea and fever. Instead, he asks if there are any other children and if the baby is healthy. Rather than asking open-ended, probing questions to find out what is going on in the patient's life, the doctor locates the problem narrowly in the patient's domestic arrangements. This location then shapes the questions he asks, limiting the exchange of information and leaving the way open for his assumptions to structure subsequent exchanges. These assumptions can be seen from the beginning. The doctor questions whether the baby is healthy, how many children the patient has, and whether anything else is going on, "like having to get your husband off to work or anything." He does not ask how it feels to be a new mother but he does ask whether the baby "was eating all right."

Both the questions and the silences—the questions not asked—do interactional and ideological work. They recirculate dominant cultural assumptions about the identities of doctors and patients and the nature of the medical relationship. An asymmetrical medical relationship with a dominant doctor and a subordinate patient is reinscribed. And, in addition, they justify the traditional nuclear family, which has at its center a *mother* whose very sense of herself as healthy or sick is tied to her domestic responsibilities. By implication, when babies don't feed well, or when a woman is confronted with both a small child and the responsibility of getting a husband off to work, the stress may be too much for her and so she somatizes—she makes herself unwell. The medical interaction, then, is functioning as an ideological forum in which culturally contradictory versions of woman, mother, and family are worked out. As the interaction continues, the ways the medical interview function as an occasion for recirculating hegemonic discourses emerge much more clearly.

During the medical history, the doctor learns that Wendy is breast-feeding her baby (information she tacks onto a question about whether she takes any medication regularly) and that she works part time for her husband—they are both sales representatives. He, then, asks a few more questions about what the baby eats and how well he eats it. The patient seems to hear in these questions both the doctor's search for a social psychological "cause" for her presenting symptoms and a challenge to the way she has accepted her new motherhood role—a challenge that she questions. She asks:

> You think I might have some (laughs) (D: What?). You think I might have some mental problems with (slight pause) the baby?

The patient names what has been implied—that her problems are social psychological in nature and tied to motherhood. In so doing, she challenges both the asymmetry of the medical relationship and the dominant cultural assumptions about women, work, and the nuclear family. A struggle ensues— a struggle in which the patient does not prevail. Rather than answering the question the patient has asked, the doctor responds by making his diagnosis. He says:

> Well I'll just tell you what I'm thinking right now, uh, what you're describing sounds like a classic hyperventilation syndrome, which is, usually happens *when you're upset about something* and you cannot be aware of it but you're breathing too fast, and when you do that you blow off too much carbon dioxide and that makes you feel weak, makes your hands tingle, feel numb and can make you feel dizzy (P: uh huh) uh, but like I say it can happen really without being aware of it or really without being upset but I just wanted to find out if that was anything you were upset about, you know, if something was (P: not) going on.

The patient reads this as a request for information and responds:

> Not really this morning, it's just that well like the last couple of weeks my husband's been out of town opening a new store so I had to fill in more hours (D: more hours) and I think, that's what I thought my headaches were from (P: laughs; D: laughs) because I had so much to do. But this morning I felt nauseated but I just, it was just like dry heaves you know (D: uh huh, uh huh) I never really did get sick so my husband told me to put your head between your legs and breathe slower and I felt better.

Here we have a medical solution to a problem identified as emotional and we have a diagnosis that locates the cause of Wendy's symptoms in her emotions. When you're upset about something, you breathe too fast, blow off too much carbon dioxide, and cause the symptoms you describe. What we do not have is much information about why the patient was upset. We know, because she found a way to squeeze it into the discourse, that she has been feeling tense, that she attributes this tension to the fact that her husband has been away opening a new store, and that she has had so much to do that she has worked more hours. She laughs as if to indicate her discomfort with the explanation she is providing and concludes that the stress of her husband being away and the extra burden of work *may* have produced her tension headaches.

While doctor and patient seem to agree that the cause for her symptoms resides in the social context of her life, their agreement ends here. For Dr. Aster, Wendy's domestic arrangements produce an emotional conflict that causes her to hyperventilate. This description supports a culturally hegemonic view of women as ruled by their emotions and blames the patient for her problem. If she could control her emotions, she would not hyperventilate. Wendy resists this definition of the situation. For her there have been life problems that generated situationally relevant stress and may have produced tension headaches. Her explanation is much less global than the doctor's. It blames the situation, not her inability to control her emotions, providing an alternative to the dominant cultural view of women as ruled by their emotions—an alternative that resists both Dr. Aster's definition of the situation and the asymmetry of the medical relationship.

Moreover, a diagnosis of tension and hyperventilation do not, for Wendy, tell the whole story. She continues by saying: *"But* this morning I felt nauseated." We do not know what the nausea means to her. We do know that she has mentioned it twice, once in her presenting complaint and again now and that she has expanded it here by saying that she had the dry heaves. The doctor does not pick up on this medical topic; rather, he comments on her husband's recommendation to put her head between her knees and breathe more slowly. He says: "That's a good thing to do." The patient tries to interrupt saying "but" and the doctor continues, "that's a real good thing to do."

Both what is attended to and what is not do interactional and ideological work. The medical interaction is functioning as a site to reproduce dominant cultural assumptions. Just as the doctor is refigured as the dominant participant in an asymmetrical medical relationship, the husband is presented as the dominant participant in the family. Both the doctor and the husband/father know what is best for Wendy. While these presentations reinforce dominant cultural assumptions about the identities of doctor and patient, the nature of the medical relationship, and the domestic arrangements of the traditional nuclear family, they do not attend to Wendy's medical complaint—her nausea.

A little later in the consultation, the doctor again reinforces traditional domestic arrangements. He says:

Well, you know, if *this* continues to be a problem, you know, if you have any more episodes then you know you might need to look into ways that *you could limit the amounts of any work that you have to do,* uh and I think that that would be a good place to start.

These are very interesting sequences. Wendy has tentatively linked the stress of her husband's being away more than usual and the *extra* burden of work this produces for her to provide a context that explains her increased tension. These tentative links are transformed. *Wendy's work* becomes the problem. The doctor recommends that, if "this" continues, and the "this" implied is the tension that makes Wendy sick, she "could limit the amount of any work" that she does. These transformations take a social problem— tension—and transform it into a medical one, and take a social contextual issue—the conflict between domestic responsibilities and participation in the labor force—and transform it into both an individual problem and a specific medical etiology. While this is done without determining the meaning of work in this patient's life, it functions to reinforce the doctor's authority to define social reality—a reality that foregrounds one version of domestic life— the traditional one—and in so doing recirculates and reinscribes the doctor's institutional authority and culturally dominant domestic arrangements.

The doctor continues by asking: "Are you and you husband getting along fairly well?" Wendy responds, tacking on what may be the reason for her visit. She says:

> Yeah, fine. Well, see, there is the problem that I'm still getting up with the baby (D: huh) at night, you know, and that wears me out, so I didn't realize, (D: yeah) *I thought I was pregnant again* (P: laughs) (D: laughs) Oh no.

Now the patient's concern with nausea makes more sense. She was afraid that she was pregnant. In fact, this fear, rather than the fact that she works, could account for her tension, her headaches, and her hyperventilation. The doctor responds medically to this new information by saying:

> Well (pause) well, I'll tell you that it is a possibility and I think it's remote (unintelligible) breast-feeding, but since you are here we might as well go ahead and check it, if it's OK with you (P: Yeah) you know just to be safe.

He continues by giving her some information about breast-feeding as a form of contraception and advises her that *after* she has stopped breast-feeding she can come back and talk about birth control with him. This is dubious information at best and especially so as the patient is weaning the baby and is down to one breast-feeding a day. Whether the information the doctor provides is accurate or not, he speaks in the voice of medical authority. This voice reinforces his identity as medical expert and implies that the patient is inappropriately concerned, fortifying the view that she is an overly emotional woman.

Toward the end of the consultation, the doctor asks: "Do you have any questions?" It is in the doctor's responses, here, that the interactional and ideological messages are the strongest. The patient asks:

No, I just didn't realize that that could do to you, a little bit of stress (D: yeah) it just seemed like a little bit to me (D: uh huh) but//

The doctor interrupts her to correct her mistaken impression that she is under just a little bit of stress. He says:

//Well actually it may seem like a little bit to you but to most people I think it'd be a great deal really, being a mother, you know, and a 6-month-old and working too and, you know, breast-feeding. All those are really, that's, those are lots of demands on your body, really. So I'd really try to think about ways that you could try to reduce that.

And the patient responds: "Well, it was, you know, it might just be because I had to work so much these past two weeks."

What you see here is the continuation of their struggle. Doctor and patient have been struggling over the contested meaning of wife, mother, and the nuclear family and in so doing have been struggling over the asymmetrical nature of the medical relationship. But while the patient has resisted, the doctor has prevailed and in the process both his reading of the dominant culture and their identities as doctor and patient interacting in an asymmetrical medical context have been reinforced. For the doctor, Wendy's stress is to be found in the conflicting demands of work and domestic roles—demands that can be eliminated if she does not work. He calls upon common understandings to support his position, saying that *most people* would find being the mother of a 6-month-old, breast-feeding, and working stressful.

Wendy agrees that the situation produces "a little bit of stress," but the problem for her is neither work per se nor the conflict between being a mother, even the mother of a nursing infant, and working. The conflict is to be found in the situationally produced increase in her isolation and responsibility and the iatrogenically produced fear that she is pregnant. Her husband has been away more than usual and responsibilities at work have increased proportionally at a time when she is unable to get an uninterrupted night's sleep and is more tired than she would usually be. In addition, she has gotten bad medical advice. She has been told that she needs birth control only *after* she stops nursing—an impression reinforced in this medical consultation. She is weaning the baby, has felt nauseated, and fears that she is pregnant again. In this context, it is not hard to understand why the fear that she is

pregnant and the thought of another baby could produce the tension headaches and hyperventilation she has described.

Early in this encounter, the doctor identifies Wendy's problem as social
psychological and narrowly locates it in her domestic arrangements. In so
doing, he largely abandons the discussion of medical topics. He does not pursue
Wendy's nausea, even though she mentions it more than once, and he only
does a pregnancy test after Wendy tells him that she thinks she may be pregnant. While Wendy leaves this consultation reassured that she is not pregnant,
she leaves without a prescription for birth control and without accurate
contraceptive information. The treatment that is recommended is for her to
stop working to reduce her stress. While Wendy struggles against Dr. Aster's
definition of the situation, these interactions leave dominant cultural assumptions about the identities of doctors and patients, and the nature of the medical
relationship and of women, work, and the nuclear family, firmly in place.

The Nursing Consultation

The nursing encounter begins with Katherine Heinz, the nurse practitioner,
introducing herself to Prudence Batson, the patient. Provider and patient
then communicate to establish the meaning of the presenting complaint.
Katherine opens this sequence by asking:

K: I see on the little slip that Martha (the receptionist) made out, that, uh, you're
feeling tired a lot

P: Yeah, just tired.

K: When did it start?

P: Um, a few weeks ago. Cause I'm falling asleep early at night. Usually I can
stay awake till 11, 11:30 and it doesn't bother me. And I've been falling
asleep, like almost literally passing out 8, 8:30, 9 o'clock. And I'm sitting
(unintelligible) and it's like I just run out (laughs)

K: Um hm Has this been true every night?

P: Mnn, well, it's almost every night. Just about I get tired, I don't know, I don't
know if it's the job or what?

The consultation opens very much like the last. The nurse practitioner, like
the doctor, encourages the patient to expand on her presenting complaint. Both
patients describe symptoms usually coded as psychosomatic. And the provider
in each case probes to get a little more information. Here the similarity ends.
The doctor provides very little space for the patient to explain what her
symptoms mean in the context of her life and lets both contextual and medical

cues pass unexplored. The nurse practitioner maximizes the space for the patient to explain what her symptoms mean as she pursues cues.[4] In the next exchange, Katherine picks up the patient's cue, "I don't know if it's the job or what?" and uses an open-ended question that she follows with a series of probes. She asks: "Tell me, go back about your job and tell me, fill me in a little bit about what your life is like now."

In response, Prudence describes what she calls a "normal day" and Katherine learns that the patient's day starts at about 5:30 in the morning, that she has total responsibility for domestic arrangements from taking the children to the baby-sitter, to taking care of house and family, and that she also has a job outside the home that involves physically hard labor. When the children go to bed around 8 o'clock, her responsibilities end and that's when she feels tired. While being tired seems easy to understand, she describes her day as follows: "You know, just the normal things that I've always been doing. I don't know, I'm just tired. I don't know if I need vitamins or what?"

Katherine responds: "And then you fall face forward on the floor."

Katherine does not pick up the medical cue—whether the patient needs vitamins. To do so would be to medicalize and individualize a social problem.[5] Instead, she legitimizes the patient's experience, implying that anyone, after putting in a day like the patient describes, would be tired. She then probes, looking for what has changed. She asks what the patient does when she gets home from work at 3:30, whether she cooks dinner and whether she cooks it alone, whether Prudence's husband helps with "the kids, or dinner or any of that," how long she has been working, and whether anything has changed recently. She finds that Prudence's schedule and her domestic responsibilities are essentially unchanged. She also discovers that Prudence works next to her husband during the day and that she has been confronting him at night about taking a more active role at home. She is angry and describes her anger in the following way:

> I'm just getting so mad at him, though, he's, he's not very helpful sometimes, a lot, he well, he is, but sometimes you know, when it comes to cooking, and just being able to walk out of the house and go work on the lawn mower, or the motorcycle or something. It's a lot, it's freedom to him, you know, it's, that's what I look at it as. Because he's got the freedom to just walk out the door and, you know, go talk to his friends or something. I don't have that. I've gotta stop and say (K: sure) somebody's gotta watch these kids you know (K: sure) I just can't leave them all free there or you know I'll come home to a mess. (laughs)

Once again Katherine picks up on the social cues and probes for more information. She asks what's different with Prudence's husband now. As the patient answers, she begins to diagnose herself. She describes herself as "just wanting to stay away" from her husband in the last few weeks and concludes:

> Maybe that's why I'm falling asleep so early (laughs) so I don't even have to listen to him or anything. But he gets mad at me, like at night, sometimes I want to sit there and read a book or something and he gets mad . . .

Again Katherine probes: "What's his anger?"

And Prudence explains: "He thinks his sex life is crazy, he thinks 'why do you want to read books,' when you know it . . ."

Her voice trails off and Katherine finishes her sentence: "when you could be having sex."

In the discussion that follows, Katherine learns that Prudence wants what she describes as her freedom "to go out and do something, not with other men or anything, you know, with my friends," that she feels as if she is suffocating by being with her husband 24 hours a day, that she is trying to change jobs so that she won't have to work next to him and that her husband is critical of her work both in the factory and at home. Both husband and wife are angry—an anger that is being argued out over sex and is perhaps being acted out in Prudence's fatigue.

What has emerged here is a picture of a husband and wife struggling over the changing meaning of being wife/mother, husband/father in an economic climate that makes it increasingly necessary for both husband and wife to be wage earners. While the economic context has changed, the social changes that make domestic duties a shared responsibility develop much more slowly. Prudence has moved into her husband's workplace. She is angry because he resists moving into the domestic arena traditionally seen as her workplace. She is angry because her husband has the "freedom" to be with friends and do things that he enjoys—things like working on his motorcycle. Yet when she wants to be with friends or do things she enjoys, like reading or playing with the children, her husband gets angry. Katherine sympathizes, saying: "I can certainly understand that (P: Yeah) I can tell you that I, and most women I know would not survive well on that kind of atmosphere."

Unlike Dr. Aster, Katherine neither moves rapidly toward diagnostic closure nor does she narrowly locate the patient's presenting complaint in her domestic arrangements. Instead, she repeatedly gives Prudence the opportunity to talk about her life and in so doing to explain her presenting complaint. As the story unfolds, Katherine both elicits social/contextual information and responds to it. In addition, while Dr. Aster consistently reinforces dominant cultural assumptions about women, Katherine does not. She does not tell Prudence that her symptoms are caused by a conflict between her domestic responsibilities and her participation in the paid labor force. She does not intimate that Prudence's problems are the result of her out-of-control emotions, and she does not even imply that Prudence's stress would be reduced if she stopped working and stayed at home. Quite the contrary, Katherine legitimates the reasons for both Prudence's fatigue and her anger.

Katherine, like Dr. Aster, is clearly the dominant interactional partner. She initiates topics for discussion and controls the conversational floor. But where Dr. Aster consistently relates to Wendy in ways that recirculate his authority, Katherine does not. Katherine reinforces her authority; however, at the same time and even in the same interactions, she distances herself from it, minimizing her professional status. While Katherine and Prudence relate to each other as provider and patient, by saying that she and most of the women she knows would not survive well in Prudence's life, Katherine locates herself in a community of women and in so doing positions herself as a woman like Prudence. In so doing, the nurse practitioner both personifies the institutional authority associated with her professional status and works to establish and maintain a gender solidarity based in women's common experiences. Because this is a professional consultation, not a meeting between friends, a certain tension between these discourses seems unavoidable (see Davis, 1988), and where there is tension a struggle often follows.

While it is the patient, not the provider, who makes a diagnosis, pinpointing the problem in the ongoing conflict between husband and wife—a conflict she escapes by going to bed early—it is Katherine who, whether talking as a provider or talking as a woman, asks a series of deeply probing questions about the way this anger is expressed and about possible treatment options. It is Katherine's professional status, a status completely lacking for the patient, that positions her to ask these questions. She begins with a question: "Did you ever think of leaving him?"

And Prudence responds:

Yeah, I thought of it a couple of times. But I don't know, It just gets so . . . I don't know, I want to stay, but . . . you know, I mean we got married when I was 15, you know and it's like I never had other boyfriends. I never . . . I don't know. I've always been a mother, a wife, and a housecleaner. I want to do something else (laughs). You know?

Katherine legitimizes her feelings:

You know that's absolutely understandable. That's, that doesn't (P: Good, laughs) make you a bad person.

Prudence continues:

> Good (laughs) that's one reason I went out and got a job in September cause I couldn't handle it being home all the time, you know, I was, just no adult conversation . . .

Again Katherine legitimizes her actions:

> You know that's a real growth step for you, to realize those needs and then to go take some action, to do something about them. Do you see that as a growth step?

As this line of discussion continues, Katherine learns that Prudence's father left her mother some time back and that after the first year her mother's life got much better. She admits that at some level she thinks the same could happen to her, except:

> I want to know what I'm going to do with three kids, a car payment, the rent. You know, I . . . no way I can cut it on my own with, you know, just one salary. Forget it. There's no way.

A little later Katherine concludes: "So it's economic?"
And Prudence agrees: "Yeah."
This is a particularly interesting sequence. Katherine solicits information about the social biographical context of Prudence's life. What emerges is a complex picture of a woman who both reinscribes and resists the dominant discourses about being a wife, mother, and worker. On the one hand, Prudence describes her identity and financial security in traditional terms. She explains that, while she has thought about divorce, she wants to stay. She was married at 15, has never had any other boyfriends, and has "always been a mother, a wife, and a housecleaner." In addition, she presents herself as unable to afford ending her marriage. She explains that one salary is not enough to cover car payments, rent, and the needs of three children.

While the reality Prudence depicts is all too familiar to many of us, her characterization reinscribes the dominant discourse, which reinforces the traditional nuclear family and women's roles in it. At the same time, when Prudence delineates her reasons for getting a job in the paid labor force, her portrayal is oppositional. She claims that she wants to work because she feels suffocated, because she wants adult conversation. In the dominant cultural discourse that foregrounds women's domestic responsibilities, work may be an economic necessity but it should not provide an opportunity for the pursuit of self-interest, the "selfish" pursuit of individual interests.

Prudence describes marriage and motherhood as the source of both her definition of self and her economic stability. While Katherine does not explicitly challenge the traditional reasons Prudence gives for not leaving her marriage, when the opportunity presents itself she supports Prudence in views that are far from traditional. She affirms that it is a significant growth step for Prudence to realize that her needs are unmet and take the necessary steps to meet her needs. Here Katherine's support circulates an alternative discourse as she legitimates the pursuit of Prudence's self-interest.

The picture of Prudence's life that is emerging here is a distressing one. Prudence is angry and frustrated. These emotions are being expressed in a physical symptom, fatigue. Katherine has explored the possible treatment options of a divorce and of therapy and neither seems feasible. Prudence doesn't want, and cannot afford, to end her marriage, and therapy is not an option either. She explains that her husband refuses to go, doesn't want her to go, and "knows every move she makes." These potential treatment options now seem closed; however, Katherine raises the topic of divorce once again and a struggle ensues. First she asks, "Are you pretty clear that if the economics of the situation were different you would leave?" and Prudence responds by explaining that she is *not* at all sure. Later:

K: How long can you keep this up?

P: I don't know because I am getting sick and tired of going to sleep early. It's been a long time.

K: I suspect that's not the only way you're showing your anger. I suspect that other parts of your body are closing down as well. It's just not as easy for you to see. I'm really concerned that this kind of strain over time will have a really negative effect on you. I absolutely understand that the economics of the situation . . . so that's why I was asking if the economics of the situation were taken care of, if that was out of the question, would you leave?

P: I don't know, I, I thought about it, but if it came right down to it, I don't know if I could.

K: Not right now anyway.

P: Yeah, probably not, not right now. I've been thinking about it. And it's getting more and more serious in my own mind, you know. At first, it's like, you know just playing around with the idea. But it's getting more and more concrete as the time goes on. I just . . .

This is a telling series of exchanges. Although Katherine has recirculated the institutional authority associated with her professional status, she has assiduously refrained from imposing either her medical expertise or her definition of the situation. In addition, she has consistently avoided closure and resisted the temptation to make a medical diagnosis. Instead, whether speaking as a medical provider or as a woman, she has supported Prudence. Yet, after divorce and therapy are rejected as possible treatments, Katherine's approach seems to change.

In this exchange, the nurse practitioner switches from a social to a medical register. In so doing, she brings all of the authority associated with her professional role to bear as she presses her definition of the situation—albeit an alternative one. First she asks Prudence how long she can continue to live in an untenable situation. Next she tells her that being tired and falling asleep early are not the only ways she is showing her anger: "other parts of her body are closing down as well." The image here is both unpleasant and frightening. Katherine continues by expressing her concern that the stress Prudence lives with "will over time have a really negative effect."

Speaking as a medical provider, these messages take the form of a diagnosis and a treatment recommendation. As such, they carry a heavy load of cultural baggage. Even as they resist dominant cultural assumptions about women, work, and the nuclear family, they rely on and recirculate dominant assumptions about the identities of providers and patients and about the asymmetrical nature of the medical encounter. Prudence resists both the oppositional message about her life and the traditional message about the nature of the provider-patient relationship and, at least for the moment, she prevails.

It is hard to know if Katherine's next questions pick up Prudence's frustration or her own, but in either case she does not avoid the emotions associated with the patient's presenting complaint as Dr. Aster has. Instead, she probes and in doing so she provides a site for Prudence to speak about her life. Hearing that Prudence feels trapped and suffocated, Katherine asks her to consider what she does with that anger. Is she taking it out on her children in the form of child abuse? Is she taking it out on herself in the form of depression? Is she considering suicide? Hearing that husband and wife are struggling over the contested meaning of wife/mother, husband/father in today's society and that both of them are very angry, she asks whether Prudence's husband is acting his anger out by battering her. These are unusual questions for a medical encounter. It is much more common for providers to overlook these deeply troubling issues.[6]

With these questions asked and answered, Katherine seems able to accept Prudence's definition of the situation. After exploring both the possibility of divorce and the possibility of therapy and finding these options blocked, Katherine relies on her status as a medical expert to suggest that Prudence find a friend or two she can talk to so she can "unload some of the feelings." She impresses on Prudence that long-term stress and repressed anger over time can produce physical symptoms. She advises that she continue to try to change her job so that she is no longer working next to her husband. She urges Prudence to take up running again. Both changing jobs and exercising would reduce her stress. Running would also provide a positive outlet for her anger and help with her depression.

Talking with friends, exercise, and changing jobs are the treatment recommendations agreed upon *after* nurse practitioner and patient have struggled over divorce and therapy. Each recommendation has caused prior trouble in Prudence's marriage. Her husband pouts and punishes her because he sees them as an expression of her independence. Katherine points out that, if she is damned if she does and damned if she does not, then she might as well do what is good for her and talking with friends, exercising, and changing jobs would be good for her. Here the provider is offering an alternative discourse, one that in its alternativeness holds the potential to challenge more dominant discourses. While her earlier oppositional recommendation—divorce—was not successful, Prudence agrees to this compromise.

Caring as Practice Revisited

Throughout the consultation, Katherine has encouraged/incited Prudence to speak about her life, to add the social contextual to the medical so characteristic of the provider-patient relationship. While this is just the kind of discourse of the social that Mishler (1984) has recommended and many of us would prefer in our own health care, neither the medical model nor the asymmetry usually associated with the provider-patient relationship have disappeared. In the medical and the nursing consultations, Katherine and Dr. Aster both rely on and recirculate the medical model. To reach a diagnosis and recommend treatment, they search for the *cause* of the patient's presenting complaint, search for a specific etiology, but do so quite differently.

In the medical encounter, the doctor consistently recirculates dominant cultural assumptions about the identities of doctor and patient and the nature of the medical relationship. From this position of institutional authority, Dr. Aster does not ask open-ended, probing questions to determine what Wendy's presenting complaint means in the context of her life. Instead, he diagnoses Wendy's problem as social psychological *rather* than medical in nature and narrowly locates the social in the patient's domestic arrangements. Without inquiring about the meaning of work in her life, work becomes the problem. *Working,* and the out-of-control emotions it produces, causes Wendy to hyperventilate, and hyperventilation explains her presenting complaint of dizziness. Both the diagnosis and the recommendation for treatment recirculate hegemonic assumptions about women, work, and the nuclear family.

It seems the doctor is operating from a two-place logic here. Either the presenting complaint has a medical basis or it does not. Either Wendy's problem is located in her body or in her psyche. Either Wendy is a wife and mother or she is a worker in the paid labor force. This logic, when combined with the persistent revivication of his institutional authority, has both medical and social consequences. Once Wendy's presenting complaint is identified as social psychological, Dr. Aster abandons the medical in favor of the social. He does only a cursory physical examination and he misses Wendy's medical cues about nausea. In the end a social problem, tension, resulting from a situation-specific conflict between Wendy's domestic responsibilities and her participation in the paid labor force, is transformed into a specific medical etiology and this etiology becomes the basis of the treatment recommendation to stop working and stay at home with her child.

At first glance, the nursing encounter looks quite different. The nurse practitioner does not move rapidly toward diagnostic closure. She neither abandons medical topics for social psychological ones nor narrowly locates the presenting complaint in Prudence's domestic arrangements. Instead, she persistently asks open-ended probing questions that maximize the space for Prudence to explain what her presenting complaint means in the context of her life. What emerges is a richly textured narrative in which the patient, not the provider, locates her presenting complaint in her domestic arrangements and diagnoses herself. Provider and patient agree that Prudence is living in an untenable situation, one that makes her legitimately angry. This anger is making her tired now and has the potential to make her sick later; however, while they agree on the diagnosis, they disagree about the proposed treatment recommendation of divorce.

The two-place logic that characterized the medical encounter seems to be entirely lacking in the nursing encounter, which is more multilayered, complex, and fluid. For Katherine, the medical and the social interrupt and interpenetrate each other. In addition, Katherine neither simply reflects nor unambiguously negates the institutional authority usually associated with medical providers. Instead, she relates to Prudence in ways that both foreground the institutional authority associated with her professional status *and* highlight her distance from it. Moreover, she and Katherine do not associate *only* as provider and patient. They also relate to each other as women, and it is from this position that Katherine legitimates Prudence's anger. Finally, although Katherine consistently promotes an alternative discourse about women, she supports Prudence whether she is circulating traditional or alternative discourses.

While in each case the patient resists the provider's definition of the situation and a struggle ensues, the outcomes are quite dissimilar. Where Wendy struggles with Dr. Aster's definition, the doctor systematically prevails. By contrast, Prudence struggles both with herself and with Katherine. While the struggle with herself may be inconclusive, the struggle with Katherine has not been.

Katherine uses both her status as a medical provider and her location as a woman like Prudence to push for her definition of the situation, yet at first she is not successful. Prudence retains control and remains ambivalent about a divorce. Where Dr. Aster sticks to his definition of the situation notwithstanding Wendy's resistance, Katherine does not. After asking deeply probing questions about whether anger is acted out in domestic violence, she accepts Prudence's definition of the situation and recommends talking with friends, changing jobs, and running as ways to treat her presenting complaint. Prudence accepts Katherine's recommendation and in so doing accepts the oppositional message that, because her husband pouts in any case, she may as well do what is good for her.

These differences in the medical and nursing encounters are not insignificant. The disparity between a discourse that reinscribes hegemonic assumptions about women and one that offers oppositional alternatives is meaningful. The potential to establish a solidarity based in gender, to legitimate the patient's feelings, and to support her oppositional understanding is useful. The distinction between a medical consultation that consistently reinscribes the asymmetrical nature of the provider-patient relationship and a nursing encounter that both recirculates and resists this asymmetry is notable. And the dissimilarity between the two-place logic that characterizes the doctor-patient encounter and the more multilayered, complex nature of the nurse practitioner-patient consultation is also important.

These differences are most evident when patients contest the provider's definition of the situation and a struggle ensues. While in both the medical and the nursing encounter, providers and patients struggle, the outcomes are quite different. Where Wendy and Dr. Aster never reach agreement on what caused her presenting complaint or how to treat it, Katherine and Prudence reach a compromise agreement.

Despite these differences, there are striking similarities in the way Katherine is communicating with Prudence and the way Dr. Aster is talking with Wendy. It is the provider who is interactionally dominant, controlling the topic under discussion and access to the conversational floor. It is the provider's location in the institution of medicine that positions him or her, providing a site from which to access institutional resources. Patients have no similar access. And it is the provider who calls his or her status into play and speaks as a medical expert or, in the case of the nurse practitioner, distances from this status. While providers and patients struggle over contested concepts— concepts that need translation—in the end, it is the provider's definition that prevails. Wendy never successfully challenges Dr. Aster's recommendation that she stop working, and Prudence finally accepts Katherine's compromise recommendation that she stand up to her husband. Their perspectives are quite different; nevertheless, doctor and nurse practitioner each define the correct way to deal with problems in the patient's life and in so doing neither one is a neutral objective provider of medical care. In each case the ways doctor and nurse practitioner communicate with patients is thoroughly ideological and deeply political.

Notwithstanding the differences in the medical and the nursing encounters, empirical support is far from clear for the claim that nurse practitioners offer a system of care that, while maximizing the patient's voice, minimizes the asymmetry in the provider-patient relationship. While Katherine certainly makes space for Prudence's voice, while she actively solicits information about the social context of her life, this shift in focus in no way diminishes her control.

Caring as a Discourse
of the Social Revisited

The system of care that nurse practitioners claim to provide is much like the discourse of the social that Mishler (1984) and other reformers call for. For these reformers, the problems in the provider-patient encounter result because providers do not probe beneath the surface of the provider-patient relationship to gain access to biographical information, do not lay bare the socioemotional context of the patient's symptoms. But while Katherine *does* all that is recommended, these practices are not liberatory. By itself, social talk has not "disappeared" power or humanized medical practice.

Furthermore, by dichotomizing the voice of medicine and the voice of the lifeworld and declaring that the social is to be found in the lifeworld, reformers direct our attention away from the very issues that arise in these transcripts. As Silverman (1987) points out, the distinction Mishler makes between the lifeworld and medicine is itself problematic. He argues that the social and the medical are not oppositional voices. These voices "interrupt and interpenetrate each other" (Silverman & Torode, 1980). Moreover, for Silverman, this distinction ignores "the place of medical discourse in modern societies and, indeed, the ways it has entered our own account of ourselves" (Silverman, 1987, p. 198).

Silverman points us in the right direction by arguing that providers do not speak solely in the medical voice and patients cannot speak the truth about their lives in authentic social voices and in so doing liberate themselves. However, his claim that medical discourse has become part of our cultural understanding only makes part of the argument. Although there is little doubt that the language of medicine has entered our own accounts of ourselves, in both the doctor and the nurse practitioner-patient consultations, a social/ cultural discourse about women, work, and the nuclear family is brought into the medical setting, where it interrupts and interpenetrates a presumable medical discourse.[7] Silverman fails to specify how the social is already incorporated into medical practice, how the provider draws the social into what is presumably medical discourse, and how the social becomes a site for struggle. These failures obscure how thoroughly ideological and political social topics are.

It also seems quite apparent that the distinction between the lifeworld and medicine ignores the relationship between voices. However, Silverman's claims—that both doctor and patient can speak in either voice, that the medical and the social interrupt and interpenetrate each other, and that in each case the discourse is shaped in this process—relies on a particular, and not uncontested, understanding of power. Drawing from Foucault (1979, 1981), Silverman argues that power is neither something that can be possessed nor something that operates from above through constraint and repression. It is "capillary," circulating everywhere and in everyone. It operates in everyday social practices at the lowest rather than the topmost extremities of the social body and works as much through encouraging as repressing speech.

If, as Silverman claims, doctors and patients are "compelled to speak to one another in a common language around which a field of power forms to govern them both" (Arney & Bergen, 1983, quoted in Silverman, 1987, p. 198), then medical domination no longer provides an appropriate model for understanding either the medical relationship or the challenges to it. It follows, then, that neither medical providers nor social scientists can engineer new forms of practice and/or new forms of discourse. Change can come only through practical struggles. Quoting Foucault (1981, pp. 12-13), Silverman concludes, "The problem is one for the subject who acts" (Silverman, 1987, p. 203).

Once again Silverman seems to have pointed us in the right direction. Certainly, it seems that power can work as much through encouraging as repressing speech. No doubt, the medical relationship is a site for struggle—a struggle that does not disappear if the patient is encouraged to talk about her life. But an important question remains unanswered: Does agreement, here, imply total reliance on a notion of power as productive? If the social provides a site to reinscribe and/or resist hegemonic discourses—a site for struggle—do we theoretically have to reject any concept of medical domination and instead accept a shared capacity for action?

From Silverman's perspective, the answer to these questions is a resounding yes. However, it is hard to reconcile his arguments about medical domination, his conception of the subject, and his notion of power with the consultations just discussed. If one looks at the nurse practitioner-patient consultation and discounts the nurse practitioner's interactional dominance, then power—at least the power to disseminate hegemonic and alternative discourses about women—may circulate everywhere and in everyone. But this look may be deceptive. While Prudence is caught between hegemonic and alternative discourses about women, Katherine is not. She consistently supports Prudence's resistance and persistently pushes oppositional understandings about women, work, and the nuclear family, and in the end she prevails. Is the nurse practitioner, then, the subject who acts and, if so, what ramifications would this have for Silverman's claims?

If one looks at the doctor-patient consultation, a shared capacity for action and the notion of power as productive are even harder to support. Throughout the medical encounter, Dr. Aster tenaciously reinscribes one version of reality. He foregrounds the traditional nuclear family with a woman who is defined by her domestic responsibilities and with men, whether doctor or husband, who know what's best for her. Wendy does not passively accept this definition of the situation; she resolutely resists, but she does not prevail. Even though she struggles, the doctor's representation of the dominant order prevails. If this is not medical domination, is it produced by a subject/patient who fails to struggle sufficiently?

It seems clear that, while doctor and patient and nurse practitioner and patient may speak a common language, a field of power does not seem to form to govern them both. However, from a Foucauldian perspective, questions about institutional authority, about dominance and subordination, are inappropriate. Fraser (1989a), for example, argues that, with a conception of power as productive, uneliminable, and therefore normatively neutral, and on the basis of analyses that are descriptive, it is neither possible nor desirable to specify "who is dominating or subjugating whom and who is resisting or submitting to whom." Nor from this perspective can we justify a "preference for a commitment to one side as opposed to another" (Fraser, 1989a, p. 29).[8]

There is an additional problem that Fraser does not address. If patients are engaged in a practical struggle, where does this resistance come from? Because Silverman is relying on a Foucauldian conception of power, resistance is not merely an expression of some preexisting structural or symbolic order. This leaves him without a conception of society, without any notion of power as other than productive—as domination or as constraint. But as Hall (1986) points out, without a conceptualization of society, it is impossible to assess how strong the power is, how strong the resistance is, or the changing balance between them. Here is where structural criticism confronts Foucauldian analysis.

It is just this relationship between society and the practice of medicine that is central to a structural criticism. Waitzkin (1983), for example, argues that medical discourse does not exist in a vacuum. It reflects and reinforces broader social relations. When patients talk about troubles in their lives during medical consultations, doctors have an opportunity to do ideological work. Using the symbolic trappings of scientific medicine, they can encourage patients' consent to behaviors that are consistent with traditional or alternative expectations and in so doing reproduce or undermine material conditions, especially economic conditions. If doctors analyze the social roots of suffering, if they avoid medicalizing nonmedical problems, and if they stimulate patients to become actively engaged in organized resistance, then they can become socially conscious agents of change.

Waitzkin, like Silverman, seems to point us in the right direction—albeit a different one. It seems quite apparent that ideological work is being done in these consultations and done differently by doctor and nurse practitioner. It is not too hard to see how Dr. Aster functions as an agent of social control, guiding Wendy toward more traditional behavior. It is more difficult to see how he could simultaneously become an agent for social change and encourage her to engage in organized political activity.

It is also hard to see the nurse practitioner as an agent of either social control or social change. Katherine consistently provides oppositional readings of Prudence's life; therefore she is certainly not functioning as an agent of social control. While it could be argued that she is functioning as an agent of social change, there is a theoretical problem here. As Silverman's position suggests, to see Katherine as an agent of change implies that she has discovered the *truth* about society and is speaking this truth in an authentic voice as she encourages Prudence to become actively engaged in political activities. Putting this problem aside for a moment, neither the medical nor the nursing encounters can be read, as Waitzkin suggests, in primarily economic terms.

One thing seems clear here. Whether coded as a system of care that adds caring to curing or as a discourse of the social, neither the medical model nor the asymmetry associated with the provider-patient relationship have disappeared and this is so even in the nursing encounter where the patient is encouraged to speak about her life. This finding leaves little support for either the claim that what differentiates nursing from medical practice is a system of care or the argument that a discourse of the social would remedy the problems so characteristic of medical practice. Neither nursing's claim nor Mishler's recommendation are sufficient to resolve empirical questions about caring as medical practice or theoretical issues about the relationship between provider and patient, the medical and the social, and/or medicine and society. And while Waitzkin and Silverman point us in the right direction, they each leave important issues unaddressed.

Nevertheless, the medical and the nursing encounters are different in significant ways. The medical encounter is simpler and it insistently reinscribes hegemonic understandings about the nature of the medical relationship, the status of providers and patients, and the identity of women. The nursing encounter, by contrast, is more multilayered, complex, and fluid, and in this context women, work, and the nuclear family are consistently represented in ways that contest hegemonic understandings. How are we to understand these differences?

A Somewhat Different Perspective

Hall (1986) argues that ideology is not reducible to its economic determinants. It is "a social process in thought" that enables us to represent to ourselves and others the way the system works, why it functions as it does. From this perspective, the differences just discussed are cast in another light. Clearly woman is not just a preexisting identity and the roles assigned to her a preexisting reality. Women, work, and the nuclear family are contested categories. The institutions of medicine and nursing—institutions that were constituted historically as gendered professions—provide different sites for their translation—different sites for the production of knowledge about gender, for the fixing of identity, for the differentiation of men from women, doctors from nurses.

Historically, it is widely recognized that doctors gained their professional dominance in the nineteenth century by competing in a loosely organized field of medical providers—a field not dominated by any one group (Starr, 1982; Stevens, 1966). "Regular" doctors tied by class, race, and gender to powerful men in foundations and government gained control. They gained a state-supported monopoly to practice medicine. Their ascendancy was more of a social and political victory than it was a medical one—a victory in which medicine was constituted as a gendered profession.

Nursing has no similar history. It evolved in the context of a medical monopoly and as a woman's occupation it had few ties to the powerful in society. In addition, while united by gender, from its inception nursing has been stratified by race, class, and status. This history leaves nursing without the political clout and internal cohesion of the medical profession. It also places nurses in a different position economically. The medical profession gains from its location in a capitalist economy as doctors predominantly provide medical care in a fee-for-service system. Nurses rarely practice autonomously, rarely gain economically. They are usually salaried employees—a position doctors encourage and hospitals and insurance companies reinforce. While this arrangement may place less time pressure on their practice as time for them does not mean money—an apparent benefit—it is tied to a distributive injustice—nurses are underpaid especially in relation to doctors.

But, perhaps most important, caring, whether as an obligation or a virtue, played a pivotal role in this history. It has contributed to the glorification of the home, to women's movement into the paid labor force, to the emergence of nursing as a woman's occupation, and to nurse practitioners' battle for professional autonomy. Represented as a natural quality of women, it has functioned to shore up the ideology of gender difference, to bifurcate reality into separate, but unequal, spheres. The notion that women care, but men reason, reinscribes a gender hierarchy and a sexual division of labor. In other words, a discourse of caring has played a central role in the constitution of nursing as a gendered profession.

Doctor and nurse practitioner are professionals whose identities are produced by their location in a gendered profession. It is their position as social actors and as members of a gendered professional group that provides a different relationship to the system of knowledge called medicine, that provides the basis for an institutionalized pattern of interpretation.[9] Providers and patients represent how the system works to themselves and to their patients. They speak social structure (Molotch & Boden, 1985). In so doing, they provide very different institutionalized patterns of interpretation—patterns of interpretation that constitute women patients as objects of knowledge or subjects who act differently, interpretations that clarify the meaning of maleness and femaleness.

Notes

1. Another version, with another title, has been published (Fisher, 1991). While both versions primarily discuss the same data, in this chapter caring is a much more central category of the analysis. In addition, my understanding of the data has evolved and my reading of them has expanded. In the earlier reading I was content to see the differences in the ways doctor-patient and nurse practitioner-patient recirculated and/or resisted dominant discourse about women, work, and the nuclear family. While this interest remains central to my task here, I now see the provider-patient relationship as more multilayered, complex, and contested than I did before. In this chapter I suggest that women, work, and the nuclear family are concepts that require translation, that translation is a contested process, and that the medical and nursing encounters provide different sites for it.

2. The names used are fictitious to protect the anonymity of providers and patients.

3. It is interesting and telling that from this time on in the interaction the doctor defines the patient's symptoms as social psychological. Once defined in this way, he abandons the medical altogether.

4. While the nurse practitioner does not pursue every medical symptom as it is presented, she does a thorough physical examination. By contrast, the doctor neither pursues medical cues nor does a thorough physical examination. His physical examination, like his medical history, is cursory at best.

5. In the prior encounter, I criticized the doctor for not pursuing the patient's medical symptom, nausea. Here I seem to be praising the nurse practitioner for a similar lack of attention

to a medical cue. How can I account for this apparent discrepancy? Nausea and a need for vitamins are not equivalent. Nausea is a symptom, a clue in the search for a differential diagnosis. Vitamins are a treatment recommendation. Dr. Aster might have gotten medically relevant information by pursuing Wendy's nausea. There is no similar gain in exploring whether Prudence needs vitamins. At this point in the consultation, Katherine does not have enough information to discuss their potential benefits.

     6. And Katherine does not stop here. In the sections of the transcript I am not discussing here, she does not let the identification of a social psychological problem block the discussion of medical topics or the performance of a complete physical examination. While doing the exam, she asks about birth control. If Prudence feels backed against the wall, another pregnancy might tip a precarious balance.

     7. Whether provider and patient can both speak in the medical voice is an open empirical question that will be dealt with in a subsequent work; however, prior work suggests that at least for doctors and patients there is not a shared capacity for medical talk. Patients' ability to enter the domain marked as medical varies by gender and is probably influenced by other factors as well—factors such as race, class, and status (see Fisher & Groce, 1990).

     8. Fraser (1989) goes on to question whether, if subjects are described as resisting, this implies a normative standard. I agree with her that it does and will address this topic in greater detail in the larger project from which this chapter is drawn: *Caring Gone Public: The Case of Nurse Practitioners* (Fisher, in press).

     9. I am indebted to Nancy Fraser (1989) for this insight. While she is talking about social work and I am talking about medicine, her thinking has influenced mine.

References

Arney, W., & Bergen, B. (1983). The chronic patient. *Sociology of Health and Illness, 5*(1), 1-24.

Brown, C. (1981). Mothers, fathers and children: From private to public patriarchy. In L. Sargent (Ed.), *Women and revolution* (pp. 239-268). Boston: South End.

Cott, N. F. (1977). *The bonds of womanhood.* New Haven, CT: Yale University Press.

Davis, K. (1988). *Power under the microscope.* Rotterdam: Foris.

Diers, D., & Molde, S. (1979). Some conceptual and methodological issues in nurse practitioner research. *Nursing and Health, 2,* 73-84.

Fisher, S. (1991). A discourse of the social: Medical talk/power talk/oppositional talk. *Discourse and Society, 2*(2), 157-182.

Fisher, S. (in press). *Caring gone public: The case of nurse practitioners.* New Brunswick, NJ: Rutgers University Press.

Fisher, S., & Groce, S. (1990). Accounting practices in medical interviews. *Language in Society, 19,* 225-250.

Foucault, M. (1979). *The history of sexuality* (Vol. 1). London: Allen Lane.

Foucault, M. (1981). Questions of method. *Ideology and Consciousness, 8,* 3-14.

Fraser, N. (1989a). Foucault on modern power: Empirical insights and normative confusions. In N. Fraser (Ed.), *Unruly practices: Power discourse and gender in contemporary social theory* (pp. 17-34). Minneapolis: University of Minnesota Press.

Fraser, N. (1989b). Women, welfare and the politics of need interpretation. In N. Fraser (Ed.), *Unruly practices: Power discourse and gender in contemporary social theory* (pp. 144-160). Minneapolis: University of Minnesota Press.

Freidson, E. (1970). *Profession of medicine.* New York: Dodd Mead.

Graham, H. (1985). Providers, negotiators and mediators: Women as the hidden carers. In E. Lewin & V. Olesen (Eds.), *Women, health and healing* (pp. 25-52). New York: Tavistock.

Hall, S. (1986). The problem of ideology—Marxism without guarantees. *The Journal of Communications Inquiry, 10*(2), 29-43.

Lohr, K. N., & Brooks, R. H. (1984). Quality assurance in medicine. *American Behavioral Scientist, 27,* 583.

Melosh, B. (1982). *The physician's hand.* Philadelphia: Temple University Press.

Mishler, E. G. (1984). *The discourse of medicine: Dialectics of medical interviews.* Norwood, NJ: Ablex.

Molotch, H., & Boden, D. (1985). Talking social structure: Discourse, domination and the Watergate hearings. *American Sociological Review, 50*(30), 273-288.

Reverby, S. M. (1987). *Ordered to care: The dilemma of American nursing.* Cambridge: Cambridge University Press.

Sackett, D. L. (1974). The Burlington randomized trial of the nurse practitioner: Health outcomes of patients. *Annals of Internal Medicine, 80*(2), 137-142.

Shamansky, S. L. (1985). Nurse practitioner and primary care research: Promises and pitfalls. In H. Werley & J. Fitzpatric (Eds.), *Annual review of nursing research* (Vol. 3). New York: Springer.

Silverman, D. (1987). *Communication and medical practice: Social relations in the clinic.* London: Sage.

Silverman, D., & Torode, B. (1980). *The material world: Theories of language and its limits.* London: Routledge.

Starr, P. (1982). *The social transformation of American medicine.* New York: Basic Books.

Stevens, R. (1966). *Medical practice in modern England: The impact of specialization and state medicine.* New Haven, CT: Yale University Press.

Todd, A. D. (1989). *Intimate adversaries: Cultural conflicts between doctors and women patients.* Philadelphia: University of Pennsylvania Press.

Tronto, J. C. (1989). Women and caring: What can feminists learn about morality from caring. In A. M. Jaggar & S. R. Bordo (Eds.), *Gender/body/knowledge: Feminist reconstructions of being and knowing* (pp. 172-187). New Brunswick, NJ: Rutgers University Press.

Waitzkin, H. B. (1983). *The second sickness: Contradictions in capitalist health care.* New York: Free Press.

27

Reframing Women's Weight:
Does Thin Equal Healthy?

Joan C. Chrisler

Since the description of the calorie and the manufacture of household scales in the 1800s, Americans have been obsessed with body weight (Schwartz, 1986). At first the emphasis was on diets to help the thin gain weight to improve their health, but by the 1920s the focus had shifted, and dieting to lose weight became fashionable. Thinness had been associated with tuberculosis, which was a major cause of death in the 1800s (Bennett & Gurin, 1982); by the 1920s physicians had made considerable progress in curing TB and other infectious diseases (Rothblum, 1992a). Oscar Rogers, a physician working for the Metropolitan Life Insurance Company, reviewed a sample of the company's records in 1901 and reported that those who were substantially *above* or *below* their "ideal weights" had higher than average mortality rates (Bennett & Gurin, 1982). Later, Louis Dublin, a statistician employed by Met Life, pronounced obesity "America's No. 1 Health Problem," and his views were published widely in both medical and popular literature (Bennett & Gurin, 1982, p. 133).

By the time the U.S. Metropolitan Life Insurance Company tables of ideal weights were constructed in 1959 (by Dublin, who was already convinced that weight was a health risk), Americans had believed that thinness equals health for nearly 40 years (Rothblum, 1990). In the 1960s obstetricians regularly advised pregnant women to keep to a strict diet to gain no more than 20 pounds, advice later rejected after it was determined to affect fetal growth adversely (Freedman, 1986). Fashion-conscious women in the 1960s tried to emulate the model Twiggy, who weighed less than 100 lbs. The body weight of Miss America contestants was found to decrease significantly from 1959 to 1979, and since 1970 there has been a trend for the winners to be among the thinnest contestants (Garner, Garfinkel, Schwartz, & Thompson, 1980).

A glance at the illustrations in women's magazines over recent decades will make the same point (Logue, 1991). Women have been told in many ways that thinness equals not only health but social acceptability.

Feminists in the Fat Liberation Movement (see Brown & Rothblum, 1989; Mayer, 1981; Schoenfielder & Wieser, 1983) have pointed out that fat oppression is one of the last remaining acceptable forms of prejudice; they have been working against size discrimination and toward size acceptance since the 1970s. Research results support the need for such work. Children as young as age 6 describe silhouettes of the obese as "lazy," "stupid," and "cheats" (Staffieri, 1967). Obese women have experienced discrimination in various areas, including college admissions (Canning & Mayer, 1966), hiring and promotion (Larkin & Pines, 1979; Rothblum, Miller, & Gorbutt, 1988), and apartment rentals (Karris, 1977). Even nutritionists (Maiman, Wang, Becker, Finlay, & Simonson, 1979), physicians (Maddox & Liederman, 1969), medical students (Breytspraak, McGee, Conger, Whatley, & Moore, 1977), and psychotherapists (Brown, 1989; Young & Powell, 1985) to whom obese women are likely to turn for help have been found to exhibit fat phobia and to express negative attitudes toward their obese patients. In a review of the research on the social stigma of obesity, Rothblum (1992b) concluded that the dieting industry combined with Western attitudes toward weight and attractiveness causes more pain and problems for women than for men.

Weight and Health

Nurse-psychotherapist Donna Ciliska (1990) remembers being trained to recommend weight loss to any patients who weighed even 5 or 10 lbs above average, regardless of whether they had a health problem. Such advice was considered preventive medicine and for the patient's own good. Her informal surveys of primary care clinicians suggest that this remains standard practice. This was certainly true in the mid-1980s when I worked for a weight loss program that required a physician's referral. Clients well within the Met Life "guidelines" were routinely recommended to our program (Chrisler, 1989). Advertisements for the diet industry, which regularly grosses $30 billion per year (Stoffel, 1989), feature health care practitioners who urge people they've never examined to lose weight to "look better, feel better."

Is this sound medical advice? Or are health care practitioners, like the general public, so accepting of the idea that thin equals healthy that we cannot evaluate the data in a disinterested manner? Certainly massive obesity affects the quality of life, and perhaps the length of life, through emotional stress, ease of mobility, and circulatory and respiratory functioning (Ciliska, 1990). Yet, there is a debate in the literature about the extent of the risk involved for those who are less than 100% above average weight (Ciliska, 1990). Keys (1980) has concluded that, if weight is connected to poor health, it is likely to be at the extreme *high* and *low* ends of the continuum. It is unknown how much weight one must carry to experience a negative influence on health but is almost certain that many of those dieting to improve their health need not do so.

Obesity has been correlated with a variety of health problems, including cardiovascular disease, hypertension, diabetes, arthritis, gall bladder disease, and some cancers (Fitzgerald, 1981; Rodin, 1990). Recent evidence suggests that the connection of obesity to some of these disorders may be due not to the amount of fat but to its location in the body. Abdominally localized fat (sometimes referred to as the android pattern or apple shape) appears to significantly increase the risk of cardiovascular disease, diabetes, hypertension, and cancer (see Rodin, 1990, for a review of this literature). This pattern of fat localization is more common in men than in women, who are more likely to have fat located in the thighs and buttocks (the gynoid pattern or pear shape; Rodin, 1990). Although these data suggest that more men than women might benefit from weight loss, women far outnumber men in weight loss programs. Furthermore, women whose weight is localized in the thighs and buttocks are more dissatisfied with their bodies and more likely to be disordered eaters than those whose weight is abdominally localized (Radke-Sharpe, Whitney-Saltiel, & Rodin, 1990).

It is important to note that, although *obesity* is a medical term, it cannot be objectively defined. Many researchers refer to the Met Life tables, which were not normed on a multicultural sample (most purchasers of life insurance are white, middle-class males), and assume that the average person does not gain additional weight after age 25 (Rothblum, 1990). A study (Young, Blondin, Tensuan, & Fryer, 1963) of a large sample of midlife and older women found an increase in body fat after age 40, and women tend to gain weight at each of the reproductive milestones: menarche, pregnancy, and menopause (Rodin, Silberstein, & Striegel-Moore, 1985). Although men tend to achieve their maximum weights in their twenties and thirties, women are leaner earlier in life and gain weight as they age (Rothblum, 1990). Other measures of obesity include skin fold thickness and eyeball analysis, both of which are obviously subject to value judgments, and body mass index (weight in kilograms/ square of height in meters), which was originally developed for use in cross-cultural studies but is still compared to an ideal standard (Fitzgerald, 1981; Rothblum, 1990).

Furthermore, the evidence that obesity is related to poor health is not as solid as it might seem due to common design flaws in the studies (Rothblum, 1990). First, there is no control for dieting among the obese subjects despite the evidence that dieting itself can lead to health risks (Brownell, 1988;

Ernsberger, 1985). Given the societal pressure to lose weight, it is likely that many of the obese subjects were dieting at the time of the studies. Second, there is generally no control for socioeconomic status despite the fact that members of lower socioeconomic classes tend to weigh more than members of higher socioeconomic classes (Bowen, Tomoyasu, & Cauce, 1991; Goldblatt, Moore, & Stunkard, 1965). The more affluent subjects are likely to be better educated and to receive better medical care than the less affluent subjects, which results in a serious confounding of variables (Rothblum, 1990). Third, cigarette smoking (Jeffrey, 1992; Simopoulos & Van Itallie, 1984), which is linked to many of the same diseases as obesity, and which many women use as an appetite suppressor, is rarely analyzed separately from weight. It has been suggested that obesity and smoking are more likely to be linked in the lower socioeconomic classes than in the higher ones (Andres, 1980). Fourth, many of these studies were done with all male subjects (see Andres, 1980; Brunzell, 1984; Jeffrey, 1992, for reviews). It is difficult to say whether these results can be generalized to women, particularly given the new findings about the importance of fat localization. Finally, it must be noted that not every study finds links between weight and mortality or disease and that experts such as Ancel Keys (Keys et al., 1972), Elizabeth Barrett-Connor (1985), and Reubin Andres (1980) have asserted that the evidence is inconclusive or negative, especially as it relates to cardiovascular disease.

Dieting and Health

Dieting should not be considered a risk-free activity. Dieting has resulted in inadequate nutrition, fatigue, weakness, irritability, depression, social withdrawal, loss of sexual desire, and sudden death from cardiac arrhythmias (Ciliska, 1990). Animal studies suggest that hypertension may be a result of dieting. Ernsberger and Haskew (1987) repeatedly starved their subjects to lose at least 20% of their body weight, then refed them. The animals developed high blood pressure and cardiovascular disease. Elevated free fatty acid levels that are characteristic of the obese have been found to correlate with chronic restrained eating in both obese and average weight individuals (Hibscher & Herman, 1977), which suggests that disordered eating rather than body weight is responsible for the elevation.

Chronic restrained eating has been linked to overwhelming hunger, weakened control over food intake, heightened responsiveness to external hunger cues (Herman & Polivy, 1980), and infertility (Allison, Kalucy, Gilchrist, & Jones, 1988) and may be related to cigarette smoking and a risk factor for bulimia. Surveys indicate that at least 80% of young women in treatment for bulimia were attempting to lose weight when they experienced their first binge-purge episode (Fairburn & Cooper, 1982; Pyle, Mitchell, & Eckert, 1981). The high relapse rate (over 90% of dieters regain the weight they lost and then some) has led many chronic dieters to weight loss techniques (e.g., liquid protein, amphetamines, stomach stapling, jaw wiring, and gastric balloons) that are more dangerous than maintaining their original weight (Chrisler, 1989).

Furthermore, dieting appears to be a cause of weight gain as well as weight loss. It is a well-established fact that severely restricting food intake causes a decrease in metabolic rate, which results in calorie conservation (Apfelbaum, 1976). The longer the diet, the longer it takes the body to return to the prediet metabolic rate (Even & Nicolaidis, 1981), which makes it easier to gain weight after a period of dieting. Repeated cycles of dieting may serve to disregulate the system to such an extent that weight loss goals cannot be reached (Rodin et al., 1985). A well-designed experiment (Brownell, Greenwood, Stellar, & Shrager, 1986) that compared a group of rats on a high-fat diet with a group that experienced two cycles of food restraint and refeeding found that during the second restriction phase the weight loss occurred at half the rate and the regain at three times the rate of the first cycle. By the end of the study, the "dieting" rats had a fourfold increase in metabolic efficiency compared with the rats on the high-fat diet. Furthermore, it appears that weight cycling stresses the cardiovascular system and may increase the chance that the regained weight is distributed to the upper body in the android pattern (Brownell et al., 1986; Rodin, Radke-Sharpe, Rebuffe-Scrive, & Greenwood, 1990). We don't even know if weight loss actually improves medical conditions because dropout and relapse rates are so high that few studies have been carried out (Ciliska, 1990).

Clinical Implications

In recent years there has been increased interest in studying the physiology of weight; the impact of genetics, metabolism, thermogenesis, and the theoretical set-point have been described (see Garner & Wooley, 1991, for a review of the literature). Such information makes it clear that obesity is much more than a failure of willpower and explains why it is so difficult to maintain weight loss. Because it is neither feminist nor therapeutic to encourage clients to attempt the impossible (Chrisler, 1989), some feminist therapists have argued against referring clients to weight loss clinics (e.g., Brown, 1985; Chrisler, 1993; Wooley & Wooley, 1984). The unwillingness of the medical/psychological establishment and the general public to accept the findings of the research on the physiology of weight and their willingness to dismiss the suggestion that fat is not necessarily detrimental to health is testament to the morality our culture has assigned to weight and the strength of fat phobia in our society (Chrisler, 1989). We must ask ourselves why there are no empirical studies on the personality, attitudes, health, and coping strategies of well-adjusted obese people (Wooley & Wooley, 1984) and why, despite the high rates of anorexia nervosa and bulimia in our society, we are not developing "thinness prevention projects" (Bowen et al., 1991).

Diets don't work, and programs based on education, insight, or behavioral self-management are of limited value. Clinicians can provide lasting help to only a small minority of their patients (Wooley & Wooley, 1984). Repeated failures cause psychological distress and add to the pain of the social stigma of obesity. Categorizing obesity as a disease state or syndrome may further stress medical patients and contribute to their ill health (Fitzgerald, 1981). Encouraging people who have made many previous attempts to lose weight to try again is contributing to unhealthy weight cycling (Goldrick & Foreyt, 1991) and violates the caregivers' code to "do no harm." Given the high failure rate of weight loss programs, ethicist Andrew Lustig (1991) has suggested that obesity treatment should properly be described as "research" rather than "therapy," and informed consent, which reflects the probability of harm and low possibility of benefits, should be obtained.

Health care practitioners should be cautious about referring women to weight loss programs until we know that weight loss will improve their health and until there are effective ways for them to lose weight. Until that time, women with weight concerns can be better helped by being encouraged to develop self-acceptance, eat healthy foods, increase physical fitness, and avoid unhealthy weight cycling. See Chrisler (1993), Ciliska (1990), Garner and Wooley (1991), Leonard (1988), and Tenzer (1989) for therapeutic suggestions. Women with weight concerns can also be referred to politically active groups such as Ample Opportunity or the National Association to Advance Fat Acceptance (NAAFA); here they will be able to help themselves and others by working against fat oppression.

References

Allison, A., Kalucy, R., Gilchrist, P., & Jones, W. (1988). Weight preoccupation among infertile women. *International Journal of Eating Disorders, 7,* 743-748.

Andres, R. (1980). Effect of obesity on total mortality. *International Journal of Obesity, 4,* 381-386.

Apfelbaum, M. (1976). The effects of very restrictive high protein diets. *Clinics in Endocrinology and Metabolism, 5,* 417-430.

Barrett-Connor, E. (1985). Obesity, atherosclerosis, and coronary heart disease. *Annals of Internal Medicine, 103,* 1010-1019.

Bennett, W., & Gurin, J. (1982). *The dieter's dilemma.* New York: Basic Books.

Bowen, D. J., Tomoyasu, N., & Cauce, A. M. (1991). The triple threat: A discussion of gender, class, and race differences in weight. *Women & Health, 17*(4), 123-143.

Breytspraak, L. M., McGee, J., Conger, J. C., Whatley, J. L., & Moore, J. T. (1977). Sensitizing medical students to impression formation processes in the patient interview. *Journal of Medical Education, 52,* 47-54.

Brown, L. S. (1985). Women, weight, and power: Feminist theoretical and therapeutic issues. *Women & Therapy, 4*(1), 61-71.

Brown, L. S. (1989). Fat oppressive attitudes and the feminist therapist: Directions for change. *Women & Therapy, 8*(3), 19-30.

Brown, L. S., & Rothblum, E. D. (Eds.). (1989). *Fat oppression and psychotherapy: A feminist perspective.* New York: Haworth.

Brownell, K. (1988, January). Yo-yo dieting. *Psychology Today,* pp. 20-23.

Brownell, K. D., Greenwood, M. R., Stellar, E., & Shrager, E. E. (1986). The effects of repeated cycles of weight loss and regain in rats. *Physiology & Behavior, 38,* 459-464.

Brunzell, J. D. (1984). Are all obese patients at risk for cardiovascular disease? *International Journal of Obesity, 8,* 571-578.

Canning, H., & Mayer, J. (1966). Obesity: An influence on high school performance. *Journal of Clinical Nutrition, 20,* 352-354.

Chrisler, J. C. (1989). Should feminist therapists do weight loss counseling? *Women & Therapy, 8*(3), 31-37.

Chrisler, J. C. (1993). Feminist perspectives on weight loss therapy. *Journal of Training and Practice in Professional Psychology, 7*(1), 35-48.

Ciliska, D. (1990). *Beyond dieting: Psychoeducational interventions for chronically obese women—a non-dieting approach.* New York: Brunner/Mazel.

Ernsberger, P. (1985). The death of dieting. *American Health, 4,* 29-33.

Ernsberger, P., & Haskew, P. (1987). Health implications of obesity: An alternative view. *Journal of Obesity and Weight Regulation, 6,* 58-137.

Even, P., & Nicolaidis, S. (1981). Changes in efficiency of ingestants are a major factor of regulation of energy balance. In L. A. Cioffi, W. P. James, & T. B. Van Itallie (Eds.), *The body weight regulatory system: Normal and disturbed mechanisms* (pp. 115-123). New York: Raven.

Fairburn, C. G., & Cooper, P. J. (1982). Self-induced vomiting and bulimia nervosa: An undetected problem. *British Medical Journal, 284,* 1153-1155.

Fitzgerald, F. (1981). The problem of obesity. *Annual Review of Medicine, 32,* 221-231.

Freedman, R. (1986). *Beauty bound.* Lexington, MA: D. C. Heath.

Garner, D. M., Garfinkel, P. E., Schwartz, D., & Thompson, M. (1980). Cultural expectations of thinness in women. *Psychological Reports, 47,* 483-491.

Garner, D. M., & Wooley, S. C. (1991). Confronting the failure of behavioral and dietary treatments for obesity. *Clinical Psychology Review, 11,* 729-780.

Goldblatt, J. T., Moore, M. E., & Stunkard, A. J. (1965). Social factors in obesity. *Journal of the American Medical Association, 192,* 1039-1044.

Goldrick, C. K., & Foreyt, J. P. (1991). Why treatments for obesity don't last. *Journal of the American Dietetic Association, 91,* 1243-1247.

Herman, C. P., & Polivy, J. (1980). Restrained eating. In A. J. Stunkard (Ed.), *Obesity* (pp. 208-224). Toronto: W. B. Saunders.

Hibscher, J. A., & Herman, C. P. (1977). Obesity, dieting, and the expression of "obese" characteristics. *Journal of Comparative and Physiological Psychology, 91,* 374-380.

Jeffrey, R. W. (1992). Is obesity a risk factor for cardiovascular disease? *Annals of Behavioral Medicine, 14,* 109-112.

Karris, L. (1977). Prejudice against obese renters. *Journal of Social Psychology, 101,* 159-160.

Keys, A. (1980). Overweight, obesity, coronary heart disease, and mortality. *Nutrition Review, 38,* 297-307.

Keys, A., et al. (1972). Coronary heart disease: Overweight and obesity as risk factors. *Annals of Internal Medicine, 77,* 15-27.

Larkin, J., & Pines, H. (1979). No fat person need apply. *Sociology of Work and Occupations, 6,* 312-327.

Leonard, P. J. (1988). A group approach for women with self-worth issues due to chronic dieting for weight reduction. *Journal of Counseling and Human Service Professions, 3*(1), 15-24.

Logue, A. W. (1991). *The psychology of eating and drinking: An introduction.* New York: Freeman.

Lustig, A. (1991). Weight loss programs: Failing to meet ethical standards? *Journal of the American Dietetic Association, 91,* 1252-1254.

Maddox, G., & Liederman, V. (1969). Overweight as a social disability with medical implications. *Journal of Medical Education, 44,* 214-220.

Maiman, L. A., Wang, V. L., Becker, M. H., Finlay, J., & Simonson, M. (1979). Attitudes toward obesity and the obese among professionals. *Journal of the American Dietetic Association, 74,* 331-335.

Mayer, V. (1981). Why liberated eating? *Women: A Journal of Liberation, 7,* 32-38.

Pyle, R. L., Mitchell, J. E., & Eckert, E. D. (1981). Bulimia: A report of 34 cases. *Journal of Clinical Psychiatry, 42,* 60-64.

Radke-Sharpe, N., Whitney-Saltiel, D., & Rodin, J. (1990). Fat distribution as a risk factor for weight and eating concerns. *International Journal of Eating Disorders, 9,* 27-36.

Rodin, J. (1990). Determinants of body fat localization and its implications for health. *Annals of Behavioral Medicine, 14,* 275-281.

Rodin, J., Radke-Sharpe, N., Rebuffe-Scrive, M., & Greenwood, M. R. (1990). Weight cycling and fat distribution. *International Journal of Obesity, 14,* 303-310.

Rodin, J., Silberstein, L., & Striegel-Moore, R. (1985). Women and weight: A normative discontent. In T. B. Sonderegger (Ed.), *Nebraska Symposium on Motivation: Psychology and gender* (pp. 267-304). Lincoln: University of Nebraska Press.

Rothblum, E. D. (1990). Women and weight: Fad and fiction. *Journal of Psychology, 124,* 5-24.

Rothblum, E. D. (1992a). Women and weight: An international perspective. In U. P. Gielen, L. L. Adler, & N. A. Milgram (Eds.), *Psychology in international perspective* (pp. 271-280). Amsterdam: Swets & Zeitlinger.

Rothblum, E. D. (1992b). The stigma of women's weight: Social and economic realities. *Feminism & Psychology, 2*(1), 61-73.

Rothblum, E. D., Miller, C., & Gorbutt, B. (1988). Stereotypes of obese female job applicants. *International Journal of Eating Disorders, 7,* 277-283.

Schoenfielder, L., & Wieser, B. (Eds.). (1983). *Shadow on a tightrope: Writings by women on fat oppression.* San Francisco: Spinsters/Aunt Lute.

Schwartz, H. (1986). *Never satisfied: A cultural history of diets, fantasies, and fat.* New York: Free Press.

Simopoulos, A. P., & Van Itallie, T. B. (1984). Body weight, health, and longevity. *Annals of Internal Medicine, 100,* 285-295.

Staffieri, J. R. (1967). A study of social stereotypes of body image in children. *Journal of Personality and Social Psychology, 7,* 101-104.

Stoffel, J. (1989, November 26). What's new in weight control? A market mushrooms as motivations change. *The New York Times,* p. C17.

Tenzer, S. (1989). Fat Acceptance Therapy (FAT): A non-dieting group approach to physical wellness, insight, and self-acceptance. *Women & Therapy, 8*(3), 39-47.

Wooley, S. C., & Wooley, O. W. (1984). Should obesity be treated at all? In A. J. Stunkard & E. Stellar (Eds.), *Eating and its disorders* (pp. 185-192). New York: Raven.

Young, C. M., Blondin, J., Tensuan, R., & Fryer, J. H. (1963). Body composition studies of older women, thirty-seventy years of age. *Annals of the New York Academy of Sciences, 110,* 589-607.

Young, L. M., & Powell, B. (1985). The effects of obesity on the clinical judgments of mental health professionals. *Journal of Health and Social Behavior, 26,* 233-246.

28

Lesbian Health Issues:
An Overview

Ann Pollinger Haas

The biggest issue in lesbian health is that health care practitioners know so little about it. As in the general society, lesbians are a virtually invisible segment of health services consumers and are not identified as a subgroup in clinical reporting or in mainstream health research. Perhaps more disturbing, lesbians have remained quite solidly locked behind the closet door within the women's health movement (Stern, 1992).

For most health care providers, as for most women (including many lesbians), "lesbian health" prompts the question of whether and how the health issues of lesbians differ from those of other women. The aim of this chapter is to address this question first through examining what is currently known about the health status, problems, needs, and concerns of lesbians. Following this, strategies are identified and suggestions made about ways in which women's health care providers can better serve this unrecognized minority among their clientele.

Background

Prior to the late 1970s, lesbians were rarely mentioned within medical literature, with the notable exception of psychiatric treatises and case reports, which invariably depicted sexual relationships among women as pathological and self-destructive (Berg, 1958; Caprio, 1954; Saghir, Robins, Walbran, & Gentry, 1970; Wilbur, 1965; Wolff, 1971). Around 1980 papers began appearing in the literature of medical disciplines other than psychiatry (Owen, 1980; Whyte & Capaldini, 1980), that urged practitioners toward greater sensitivity in dealing with homosexual patients. These made few distinctions, however, between the health status or needs of lesbians and gay men.

In 1976 a survey of gynecologists was conducted that provided the first empirical evidence of lesbians' invisibility within medical practice (Good, 1976). Among the 110 respondents to the survey, fully half said they had never treated a woman they knew or thought to be a lesbian; not a single physician could identify more than six lesbians in their practice.

This study was followed shortly by the first articulation of specific lesbian health concerns (O'Donnell, 1978; O'Donnell, Leoffler, Pollock, & Saunders, 1979; Santa Cruz Women's Health Collective, 1977) and the first systematic attempts to study lesbian health and health care experiences. Over the last decade and a half, a considerable amount of research has been done in this area, much of it emanating from the discipline of nursing. The bulk of the studies conducted to date have been surveys (Bradford & Ryan, 1988; Buenting, 1992; Cochran & Mays, 1988; Dardick & Grady, 1980; Deevy, 1990; Harvey, Carr, & Bernheine, 1989; Hitchcock & Wilson, 1992; Johnson, Guenther, Laube, & Keettel, 1981; Johnson, Smith, & Guenther, 1987a; Lucas, 1992; Olesker & Walsh, 1984; Parowski, 1987; Reagan, 1981; Robertson, 1992; Saunders, Tupac, & MacCulloch, 1988; Smith, Johnson, & Guenther, 1985; Stevens & Hall, 1988; Trippet & Bain, 1992; Zeidenstein, 1990), focused primarily on lesbians' experiences with health care professionals.

Only a small number of these surveys have attempted to assess the actual status of lesbian health. These include a survey of 117 lesbians recruited through lesbian organizations in the Iowa City area by Johnson and her colleagues (1981), a survey by some of the same authors (Johnson et al., 1987a; Smith et al., 1985) of 1,921 geographically diverse lesbians attending women's music festivals in the Midwest and New England in 1980, and a national survey of 1,917 lesbians conducted in the mid-1980s by Bradford and Ryan (1988) and sponsored by the National Lesbian and Gay Health Foundation. An even smaller number of lesbian health studies have involved physical examinations (Robertson & Schecter, 1981) or reviews of medical records (Degan & Waitkavicz, 1982).

While reporting extensive descriptive data, virtually all studies of lesbian health have suffered from significant methodological weaknesses that have limited the generalizability of their findings and resulted in sometimes considerable variations in their conclusions. Of primary importance is the fact that they have relied almost exclusively on samples of self-identified lesbians, typically volunteers recruited from among individuals engaged in lesbian social organizations or activities. Respondents have been overwhelmingly white, middle-class, under the age of 40, well educated, and, on the whole, relatively open regarding disclosure of their lesbianism. Survey findings thus provide extremely limited information about lesbians who are poor, old, from minority backgrounds, and not at all open about their sexual orientation.

A second weakness is that studies of lesbian health have generally not obtained data from comparable heterosexual women, making it difficult to draw conclusions about differences between the two groups. In some cases, notably the Bradford and Ryan survey (1988), attempts have been made to draw comparisons from general women's health surveys, but these have been limited by variations in the wording of questions and by the presumed inclusion of unspecified numbers of lesbians within the figures reported for women in general.

Third, studies have not used a consistent definition of what constitutes a lesbian for the purposes of health research. In determining their samples, most researchers have used measures based on Kinsey's original scale (Kinsey, Pomeroy, Martin, & Gebbard, 1953), with extremes ranging from "exclusively lesbian" to "exclusively heterosexual." There has been considerable variation, however, in whether the scale has been used to measure specific sexual activity as opposed to general sexual orientation and whether the samples have been limited to those who describe themselves as "exclusively lesbian." Moreover, the use of the word *lesbian* in these measures may have excluded some appropriate subjects who do not identify with this label.

Of final concern is the fact that most findings about lesbians' actual health status that have been reported have been based solely on self-report data and have not been validated through either physical examination or medical records. In spite of these methodological weaknesses and inconsistencies, a number of conclusions are suggested from the accumulated research on lesbian health. These are summarized below under the key categories that have been investigated.

Lesbians' Interactions With Health Care Professionals

In virtually all surveys reported to date, substantial numbers of lesbians have described hostile, intimidating, and humiliating experiences with health care providers. In some cases, these appear to reflect the blatantly homophobic ideas and attitudes that have been documented among significant numbers of nurses and physicians (Douglas, Kalman, & Kalman, 1985; Gerbert, Maguire, Bleeker, Coates, & McPhee, 1991; Mathews, Booth, Turner, & Kessler, 1986; Randall, 1989; Young, 1988), in particular physicians in the specialties of obstetrics/gynecology, family practice, and surgery.

The most common manifestation of bias among health professionals is the routine presumption of heterosexuality, which lesbians in all studies have identified as the biggest barrier to obtaining quality health care. In an excellent review of the literature on lesbians' health care experiences, Stevens (1992) notes that lesbians have overwhelmingly described their providers as presuming they had male sexual partners and as providing little opportunity to learn otherwise. In addition to making lesbians feel invisible, this presumption has been reported to lead providers to misdiagnose conditions, ask insensitive questions, offer irrelevant information, and provide inadequate treatment to lesbians. Although lesbians clearly feel more comfortable and less vulnerable with female health care providers, most studies have found that female providers are not significantly more likely to specifically inquire about sexual orientation and activity.

Although a large majority of lesbians in all surveys say they would like to be able to disclose their lesbian status to their health care provider, at least half express clear reluctance to do so out of fear of being humiliated or rejected or having their care compromised. Some lesbians say they would refuse to disclose their lesbianism even if asked directly or if they believed their condition to be related to their sexual activity (Dardick & Grady, 1980). Among those who have been open, reported responses include voyeuristic curiosity, shock, withdrawal, physical roughness, insults, and breaches of confidentiality (Stevens, 1992).

Not a surprise, such negative experiences lead many lesbians away from mainstream health services and discourage them from obtaining routine, preventive care. Almost 60%, for example, have been found to seek gynecological care only when a specific problem occurred (Smith et al., 1985), and almost a third describe their usual health care provider as "myself" (Bradford & Ryan, 1988). Studies have also reported a tendency among lesbians to delay seeking medical help and to turn to lesbian friends for advice and help rather than to health professionals (Deevy, 1990; Reagan, 1981; Stevens & Hall, 1988; Zeidenstein, 1990).

Researchers reporting these findings have noted their disturbing implications for the timely detection and treatment of health problems among lesbians. In addition, the lack of trust and comfort so many lesbians experience in their relationships with health care professionals may have negative implications in terms of lesbians' compliance with medical advice as well as their physiological and psychological responses to the treatments they receive.

An additional factor that has been found through several surveys to limit lesbians' interactions with health care providers is financial. For a complex of reasons, lesbians generally have been found to earn incomes considerably below what would be expected given their education, and to report widespread financial concerns (Bradford & Ryan, 1988). In addition, up to 50% in some surveys report having no, or very limited, health insurance coverage.

Physical Health Status of Lesbians

In spite of the fact that considerable numbers of lesbians report infrequent and unsatisfying health care experiences, studies have reported a generally positive picture of their overall health status (Bradford & Ryan, 1988; Johnson et al., 1981). Further, research to date has not identified any health problems specifically linked to female homosexual activity (Johnson et al., 1981). At the same time, a number of health problems and issues have been identified for which lesbian status is particularly relevant to diagnosis, manifestation, or treatment.

Cancer

Although no population-based studies of cancer risk in lesbians have been conducted, a recent review of lesbian survey findings regarding known risk factors for breast cancer has concluded that lesbians have a one-in-three lifetime risk of developing that disease, two to three times the risk for heterosexual women ("Lesbians Found," 1993; Roan, 1993). Relying in particular upon Bradford and Ryan's survey data, the reviewer—epidemiologist Suzanne Haynes of the National Cancer Institute—cited as primary risk factors the lack of childbearing among approximately 70% of lesbians and the avoidance of regular gynecological screening by up to 60%. Added to Haynes's calculation of lesbian susceptibility to breast cancer were the more controversial factors of excessive weight, reported by about a third of lesbians over 50; regular cigarette smoking by about 40%; and heavy alcohol use by more than 20%. Although each of these factors needs to be much more systematically studied and better comparative figures obtained for nonlesbian women, Haynes's as yet unpublished findings suggest the need for greater awareness of lesbians' breast cancer risks among both physicians and consumers, as well as for making screening procedures more accessible and attractive to this population.

There is some indication that lesbians may also be at a slightly higher risk for ovarian and endometrial cancers, both of which have been reported to occur more frequently in women who have not given birth. An added risk factor for ovarian and uterine cancer among lesbians is the lack of use of oral contraceptives, which appear to provide some protective benefit (White & Levinson, 1993).

Cervical cancer, on the other hand, appears to be less common among lesbians than among heterosexual women, given the primary risk factors of early age of first coitus with a man and heterosexually transmitted diseases, in particular human papillomavirus (HPV) (White & Levinson, 1993). One study (Robertson & Schecter, 1981), which screened 148 asymptomatic women who had been sexually active exclusively with women for the prior 6 months, reported abnormal Pap smears for fewer than 3%, as compared with an esti- mated 12% for women generally. Surveys of lesbians, however, have tended to report a somewhat higher frequency of abnormal Pap tests, ranging around 11% (Johnson et al., 1981).

At least in part, the differences in these figures appear to be associated with differences in the subjects' past and current levels of heterosexual contact. The risk of cervical cancer is likely to be rare in lesbians without a history of sex with male partners, and it has been recommended that such women be given Pap smear screenings only every 3 years (White & Levinson, 1993). Lesbians with significant past or current heterosexual activity may well vary little from heterosexual women in regard to cervical cancer risk, and it is recommended that these women be screened annually or more frequently, as warranted by individual risk factors.

Sexually Transmitted Diseases

All studies that have investigated sexually transmitted diseases (STDs) in lesbians have reported very low incidences of syphilis, cervical gonorrhea, herpes simplex virus, pelvic inflammatory disease, venereal warts, and chlamydia, all attributed to lesbians' lack of sexual activity with men (Degan & Waitkavicz, 1982; Johnson et al., 1981; Johnson et al., 1987a; Robertson & Schecter, 1981). These findings have led to the recommendation that routine screening for STDs not be undertaken for lesbians in the absence of specific risk factors, notably recent heterosexual contact (White & Levinson, 1993).

Where herpes and venereal warts caused by HPV are diagnosed in lesbians, however, the possibility of transmission to a female sexual partner must be considered, and in such cases, researchers have recommended that female partners should be evaluated and treated as indicated (Robertson & Schecter, 1981). Likewise, several studies have revealed frequent vaginitis in lesbians, some forms of which (e.g., vaginal candidiasis, Trichomonas vaginitis) have been found in women who are sexually active only with other women and may be transmitted between women through hand-genital contact (Degan & Waitkavicz, 1982). Moreover, although the pathogenesis of nonspecific vaginitis, or bacterial vaginosis, has not been conclusively documented, it is likely that the various organisms responsible for this condition may also be transmitted between women (White & Levinson, 1993). When lesbians are diagnosed with any of these common forms of vaginitis, most researchers have recommended that physicians inquire about symptoms in partners and provide evaluation and treatment as indicated.

Data from the Centers for Disease Control (CDC) indicate that lesbians are not at notable risk for transmission of AIDS, specifically as a result of sexual activity with other women (Chu, Buehler, Fleming, & Berkelman, 1990; White & Levinson, 1993). As of mid-1991, the CDC reported a total of 164 cases of AIDS in lesbians (White & Levinson, 1993), almost 95% of whom were intravenous drug users.

A small number of cases of female-to-female transmission of HIV have been reported (Marmor et al., 1986; Monzon & Capellan, 1987; Sabatini, Patel, & Hirschman, 1984), although not conclusively verified. Nonetheless, vaginal secretions and menstrual blood are potentially infectious, and it is possible that oral and vaginal mucus membrane exposure to these secretions may lead to HIV transmission (Chu et al., 1990). Additionally, it has been reported that HIV has been cultured from cervical and vaginal secretions and cervical biopsies performed at various stages of the menstrual cycle (White & Levinson, 1993).

These findings suggest that, while the likelihood of transmission of HIV through lesbian sexual activity appears low, lesbians should be advised to avoid contact with blood and vaginal secretions of sexual partners who have not tested negative for HIV. The use of dental dams (latex squares) or other latex products such as gloves or condoms are suggested for oral-genital contact with women whose HIV status is unknown, along with latex gloves for the hands and condoms on sexual toys (White & Levinson, 1993).

An additional risk for transmission of HIV to lesbians exists through artificial insemination, particularly with fresh semen from donors who, because of delays in seroconversion, test negative upon donation but later are diagnosed as HIV positive (White & Levinson, 1993). To avoid such possibility, lesbians attempting artificial insemination should be advised to use only frozen sperm from donors who are free of risk factors for HIV and who have tested negative for the virus both at the time of donation and at least 6 months later.

Reproduction

Several studies have produced the consistent finding that slightly less than one third of lesbians surveyed have borne children, most commonly through previous heterosexual marriage. In addition, as many as 70% of those who do not currently have children say they would like to. A later analysis of the 1980 survey data obtained by Johnson and her colleagues (1987b) revealed that approximately 30% of the latter group of lesbians had attempted artificial insemination, and there is evidence that increasing numbers of younger lesbians are using this procedure in the hope of having a child (Harvey et al., 1989; Zeidenstein, 1990).

Despite the fact that there is no evidence that children raised by lesbians are at risk for psychosocial problems to any greater degree than those raised by heterosexuals (Green, 1982; Kirkpatrick, 1987), some lesbians have reported opposition on the part of physicians to their attempts to conceive through artificial insemination (Harvey et al., 1989). In part, this likely reflects the general tendency among U.S. physicians to inseminate only married women (Curie-Cohen, Lattrell, & Shapiro, 1979; White & Levinson, 1993), although it is clear that many physicians have particular difficulty with insemination of lesbians (Fletcher & Magnuson, 1985). Possibly because of a lack of medical support, lesbians who have attempted artificial insemination report relatively low success rates. Johnson et al. (1987b), for example, found that fewer than 40% of lesbians who had tried the procedure actually conceived, compared with a reported conception rate of over 60% among lesbians who sought to become pregnant through intercourse with a man.

Only about half of childbearing lesbians have reported seeking obstetrical care from a physician, while the remainder have used alternative care, in particular midwives (Harvey et al., 1989; Zeidenstein, 1990). Those in the latter group have reported generally higher levels of support from and satisfaction with their provider compared with those who selected physicians (Harvey et al., 1989).

Health providers who have studied the childbearing experiences of lesbians (Harvey et al., 1989; Olesker & Walsh, 1984; White & Levinson, 1993; Wismont & Reame, 1989; Zeidenstein, 1990) have noted that pregnant lesbians frequently encounter a lack of acceptance and support from their families, and have urged particular sensitivity in working with these patients and their female partners. In addition, health care providers have been urged to be mindful of the complex legal and custody implications of lesbian pregnancies and to support pregnant lesbians and their partners to seek appropriate legal protections (Harvey et al., 1989).

Menopause and Aging

Relatively few researchers have addressed the unique health care concerns or problems of older lesbians. The one study that has specifically looked at the health behaviors of lesbians over the age of 50 (Deevy, 1990) attributed some of their invisibility to their marked reluctance to disclose lesbian identity in health care situations. A very large majority of the 78 lesbians surveyed in this study described the health care environment as unsafe and untrustworthy and said they would be unwilling to be open about their lesbianism to any health care provider. Relatedly, many older lesbians were found to minimize their contacts with the health care system at precisely the time when issues related to aging may increase their need for health care services and information.

Given the lack of clinical data and the lack of comparable survey data for older heterosexual women, few conclusions can be drawn about whether older lesbians experience significantly more or different health care problems or concerns. Bradford and Ryan (1991) have reported that about a third of their survey respondents over the age of 40 wanted more information on the topics of menopause and aging, presumably because of their reluctance to discuss these topics with health care providers.

As was noted earlier, there is some evidence that women who have not used oral contraception or borne children may be at greater risk for endometriosis as well as uterine and ovarian cancers, conditions that commonly require hysterectomy. Thus it is possible that lesbians may be more likely than heterosexual women to experience this surgery and the surgical menopause that follows.

Like women generally, lesbians appear to experience a wide gamut of physiological and psychological reactions to hysterectomy as well as to natural menopause (Morgan, 1991). These commonly include vaginal dryness and atrophy and reduced resiliency in the pelvic tissue, which may reduce the intensity of arousal and orgasm. Although health care practitioners often fail to provide their female patients with adequate information about how their sexual activity might be altered to accommodate these bodily changes, this is a vastly greater problem for lesbians, whose sexuality has been virtually ignored by mainstream health care practice (Morgan, 1991).

Another finding having important implications for the health care of older lesbians is that a substantial number, almost 30% over the age of 40, are living alone, nearly double the number of women in the general population (Bradford & Ryan, 1991). This, together with the fact that large percentages of older lesbians appear to be hiding their lesbianism from most or all of their family members, straight friends, and coworkers, suggests that this group may be vulnerable to isolation and a lack of support in times of illness. Given these factors, their alienation from the health care system becomes even more problematic.

Mental Health Issues Among Lesbians

A considerable emphasis in the surveys conducted to date has been placed on identifying the psychological status and problems of lesbians. Although no evidence has been found for the notion that lesbians as a whole have a greater tendency toward mental health problems than heterosexual women (Bell & Weinberg, 1978), recent studies have pointed to a high level of stress among lesbians of all ages (Bradford & Ryan, 1988; Gillow & Davis, 1987) and particularly among those in the older age groups (Bradford & Ryan, 1991). Stress among lesbians has been linked to numerous sources, most commonly including negative societal attitudes toward homosexuality, which causes most lesbians to live with at least some degree of deception; difficulties in intimate relationships emanating in particular from a lack of family and institutional support; fears or actual experiences of antilesbian violence or abuse; and financial insecurity. Bradford and Ryan (1988, 1991), who have provided the fullest investigation of lesbians' mental health concerns of any survey, found that about two thirds of their respondents reported levels of stress severe enough to affect some aspect of their health. Commonly reported stress-related illnesses among lesbians include ulcers, allergies, and hypertension.

Evidence has also been found that most lesbians have more limited social support networks involving family, coworkers, and religious organizations than do heterosexual women (Bradford & Ryan, 1991; Gillow & Davis, 1987; White & Levinson, 1993). Although survey results show that many lesbians derive extensive support from networks of lesbian friends and social organizations, such coping strategies are likely to be much less available to those who keep their lesbianism hidden or who live in areas of the country where an open lesbian presence does not exist. A large proportion of lesbians, perhaps as high as three quarters, have sought mental health care at some point, but dissatisfaction with counselors and therapists appears widespread (Bradford & Ryan, 1988).

Common manifestations of the increased stress faced by lesbians are serious depression, reported by about a third of lesbians; alcohol abuse, also reported in about a third; and suicidal ideation or attempts, each reported in about 20% (Bradford & Ryan, 1988). Estimates of both alcohol problems and suicide among lesbians have varied widely, and it is likely that some studies have overestimated their frequency by using samples drawn disproportionately from gay bars. Where these problems are diagnosed in lesbians, however, it is essential that their linkages to the patient's lesbianism be specifically explored and dealt with in the course of treatment (Weinstein, 1992).

An issue closely linked to both relationship stress and substance use is physical violence between lesbian partners, reported to occur in perhaps as many as a third of women's relationships (Renzetti, 1988; Schilit, Lie, & Montagne, 1990). Until quite recently, this problem has been largely repressed among lesbians themselves and remains virtually unrecognized by shelters and other organizations working with battered women (Renzetti, 1988). In addition, lesbians have quite commonly reported physical and sexual abuse from present or former husbands or other relatives. It has been recommended that health care providers be alert to symptoms of lesbian abuse and be prepared to make appropriate referrals for support (White & Levinson, 1993).

Legal and Partnership Issues
Related to Lesbian Health

Of considerable importance and interest to lesbians are issues concerning their own and their partners' rights in the event of illness or disability. Half of all respondents to the Bradford and Ryan survey (1988) expressed a need to know more about their legal rights related to health, and the apprehension that rights might be violated within the mainstream health care system appears to be widespread among lesbians (Simkin, 1991). Very few, however, have reported taking specific measures to protect their interests in the event of illness or incapacity, through such measures as executing a durable power of attorney, naming a conservator or health proxy, or signing a living will.

Although these procedures offer important sources of control to all persons, for lesbians and gay men they are essential. In cases where no power of attorney or nomination of conservator has been made by the individual while competent, courts have proven to be largely unsympathetic to the claims of lesbian or gay lovers or friends and have most often appointed a parent or sibling to take control of the incapacitated person's affairs (Hunter, Michaelson, & Stoddard, 1992).

Another very difficult problem faced by lesbians who are seriously ill or hospitalized is the exclusion of their partners from participating in decision making regarding medical treatment, receiving information about the ill person's medical status from care providers, or visiting in the intensive care unit (Simkin, 1991). At the time that a serious illness or condition is diagnosed, lesbians are likely to be particularly reluctant to risk any compromising of care that might follow from disclosing their lesbianism. Thus, unless the care provider specifically asks whether the patient wishes to involve any other person in her treatment, the existence of the partner is likely to remain unknown. This not only alienates the patient from the provider but deprives her of the opportunity to integrate the partner's emotional and practical support into the treatment.

Strategies for Improving
Lesbian Health and Health Care

The picture of lesbian health that emerges from the accumulated research literature suggests room for significant improvement in the delivery of care to this minority population. Although they share many of the same screening, prevention, and treatment needs as heterosexual women, lesbians appear to be less likely to have these needs met. And, in the face of lesbians' unique problems and concerns, the mainstream medical system remains largely uninformed and disinterested and far too often provides care that is discriminatory and offensive (Denenberg, 1992).

On an organizational level, there is much that advocates for women's health can do to bring lesbian issues into the mainstream of the women's health agenda as well as into the consciousness of women's health practitioners: speaking out on behalf of the needs and concerns of lesbians, along with those of other minorities; taking a proactive approach to encourage the inclusion of lesbian health issues in the publications, conferences, and workshops of professional groups and organizations; publicly identifying and working to change the systems of health care education and delivery that perpetuate homophobic attitudes and practices; lobbying for identification of sexual orientation in all government-sponsored research on women's health and for support of much-needed research on the key health problems of lesbians, particularly cancer and stress; and disseminating the results of lesbian health research among women's health care providers.

Regarding the critical area of research, pilot efforts are needed to explore solutions to the unique methodological problems involved in studying the diverse lesbian population whose parameters are largely unknown and in which key segments are not readily identifiable. This includes the development of strategies to identify and recruit appropriate comparison groups of heterosexual women. Women's health care advocates can play an effective role by encouraging and facilitating broad-based awareness and discussion of these methodological issues among both researchers and funding agencies.

There is also much that can be done on the level of the individual practitioner to improve the status of lesbian health care. First and most basic, women's health care practitioners must themselves become knowledgeable about lesbians' needs and concerns through availing themselves of the considerable literature in this area and networking with the several different groups and organizations that are actively working for lesbian health on both the national and the local levels. Resources listed at the end of this chapter provide a point of departure; much more can be learned by inviting and listening to the stories and experiences of individual lesbian patients.

Given that all women's health care providers will inevitably be working with lesbians, specific efforts should be made to ensure that one's practice is welcoming and respectful of women of all sexual orientations. It is difficult to escape the conclusion that adequate care cannot be provided to any women whose sexual orientation and activity remains hidden, and special efforts must be made to create an atmosphere of safety and respect that encourages lesbian patients to accurately disclose this information. Much can be conveyed to patients by the presence in the waiting room of educational materials that specifically mention sexual orientation or that directly address issues related to lesbian health. Routine office forms should be reviewed for heterosexist presumptions in questions about marital status or use of birth control. The inclusion of phrases such as *living with a spouse/sexual partner* in place of simply *married* signals the practitioner's openness toward the patient's sexual orientation and relationship status and provides much more useful information than what is obtained when lesbians in committed relationships are forced into the categories of "single" or "divorced."

The health history should include specific, neutrally worded questions on sexual activity (i e., "Are you sexually active with men, with women, or both?"). Patients indicating current relationships only with women should be asked about past heterosexual activity.

Women who relate sexually with women vary widely in their identification with such sexual orientation labels as *lesbian, gay, homosexual,* or *bisexual,* and it is generally best to avoid using these terms in initial inquiries. Other terms to avoid are sexual *preference* or *lifestyle choice,* which many lesbians feel misrepresent their sexual identity and trivialize their relationships. The key to building rapport with lesbian patients is to express interest in their *lives* rather than simply their "lifestyles."

When patients disclose lesbian sexual activity, it is important to discuss the issue of whether or not they wish such information to be documented in the chart. This may be of particular concern in a clinic setting where the patient may be seen by a number of different practitioners or where review of the record by third parties may be of consequence. Although some practitioners use a code to remind them of the patient's sexual orientation, this too should be done only with the patient's knowledge and consent.

Once an initial relationship of respect and concern has been established with the lesbian patient, an effective partnership can be developed around the mutual goal of discovering and learning about the complex ways in which lesbianism affects health status and the health care experience. Most lesbians do not demand that their care providers be "experts" on lesbian health. Like all patients, they do expect that those from whom they seek help be attentive to and willing to learn about their particular problems, needs, and concerns.

Much needs to be done to persuade lesbians that they can be "out," safe, and well cared for within the U.S. health care system. Clearly, it is time for practitioners, educators, researchers, and policymakers to recognize and address the factors that have limited lesbians' access to medical care, fostered and maintained their invisibility as patients, and denied them appropriate treatment.

Resources

Books and Articles

General Introduction to Lesbian Health

Lesbian health: What are the issues? (1992). *Health Care of Women International, 13.* This special issue contains 12 articles on various aspects of lesbian health. Especially helpful is P. E. Stevens, Lesbian health care research: A review of the literature from 1970 to 1990 (pp. 91-120).

Primary Health Care

White, J., & Levinson, W. (1993). Primary care of lesbian patients. *Journal of General Internal Medicine, 8,* 41-47.

Denenberg, R. (1992, Spring). Invisible women: Lesbians and health care. *Health/PAC Bulletin,* pp. 14-21.

Johnson, S. R., & Palermo, J. L. (1984). Gynecologic care for the lesbian. *Clinical Obstetrics and Gynecology, 27,* 724-731.

These articles present excellent summaries of the major issues involved in lesbian health care, each written from the viewpoint of the practitioner and containing valuable references.

Breast Cancer

Butler, S., & Rosenblum, B. (1991). *Cancer in two voices.* San Francisco: Spinsters Book Co.—details the personal experience of breast cancer from the perspective of a lesbian patient and her partner.

Addictions/Clinical Dependency

Weinstein, D. L. (Ed.). (1992). *Lesbians and gay men: Chemical dependency treatment issues.* New York: Harrington Park—contains 10 articles dealing with a variety of approaches to treating chemically addicted lesbians and gay men.

Mental Health

Boston Lesbian Psychologies Collective. (1987). *Lesbian psychologies.* Urbana: University of Illinois Press—an excellent series of articles dealing with different aspects of lesbian mental health.

Organizations

Mautner Project for Lesbians with Cancer, P.O. Box 90437, Washington, D.C. 20090: (202) 332-5536
Chicago Lesbian Community Cancer Project, P.O. Box 90437, Chicago, IL 60646: (312) 763-2951
Women's Cancer Resource Center, 3023 Shattuck Avenue, Berkeley, CA 94705: (415) 548-9272
Women's Community Cancer Project, c/o The Women's Center, 46 Pleasant Street, Cambridge, MA 02139: (617) 354-9888
Lesbian AIDS Project, 129 West 20th Street, New York, NY 10011: (212) 807-6664
National Gay and Lesbian Crisis Line: (800) 221-7044
Pride Institute (residential treatment center for lesbian/gay chemical dependency), Eden Prairee, MENTAL: (800) 547-7433
Center for Research and Gay Education in Sexuality (CERES), Psychology Bldg., Rm. 503, San Francisco State University, San Francisco, CA 94132: (415) 338-1137
Lesbian Rights Project, 1370 Mission St., 4th fl., San Francisco, CA 94103: (415) 621-0505

References

Bell, A. P., & Weinberg, M. S. (1978). *Homosexualities: A study of diversity among men and women.* New York: Simon & Schuster.

Berg, C. (Ed.). (1958). *The problem of homosexuality.* New York: Citadel.

Bradford, J., & Ryan, C. (1988). *The national health care survey: Final report.* Washington, DC: National Lesbian and Gay Health Foundation.

Bradford, J., & Ryan, C. (1991). Who we are: Health concerns of middle-aged lesbians. In B. Sang, J. Warshow, & A. J. Smith (Eds.), *Lesbians at midlife: The creative transition* (pp. 147-163). San Francisco: Spinsters Book Co.

Buenting, J. A. (1992). Health life-styles of lesbian and heterosexual women. *Health Care of Women International, 13,* 165-171.

Caprio, F. S. (1954). *Female homosexuality: A psychodynamic study of lesbianism.* New York: Citadel.

Chu, S. Y., Buehler, J. W., Fleming, P. L., & Berkelman, R. L. (1990). Epidemiology of reported cases of AIDS in lesbians, United States, 1980-90. *American Journal of Public Health, 80,* 1380-1381.

Cochran, S. D., & Mays, V. M. (1988). Disclosure of sexual preference to physicians by black lesbian and bisexual women. *Western Journal of Medicine, 149,* 616-619.

Curie-Cohen, M., Lattrell, L., & Shapiro, S. (1979). Current practice of artificial insemination by donor in the United States. *New England Journal of Medicine, 300,* 585.

Dardick, L., & Grady, K. E. (1980). Openness between gay persons and health professionals. *Annals of Internal Medicine, 93,* 115-119.

Deevy, S. (1990). Older lesbian women: An invisible minority. *Journal of Gerontological Nursing, 16,* 35-39.

Degan, K., & Waitkavicz, H. J. (1982, May). Lesbian health issues. *British Journal of Sexual Medicine,* pp. 40-47.

Denenberg, R. (1992, Spring). Invisible women: Lesbians and health care. *Health/PAC Bulletin,* pp. 14-21.

Douglas, C. J., Kalman, C. M., & Kalman, T. P. (1985). Homophobia among physicians and nurses: An empirical study. *Hospital and Community Psychiatry, 36,* 1309-1311.

Fletcher, J. C., & Magnuson, W. G. (1985). Artificial insemination in lesbians: Ethical considerations. *Archives of Internal Medicine, 145,* 419-420.

Gerbert, B., Maguire, B. T., Bleeker, T., Coates, T. H., & McPhee, S. J. (1991). Primary care physicians and AIDS: Attitudinal and structural barriers to care. *Journal of the American Medical Association, 266,* 2837-2842.

Gillow, K. E., & Davis, L. L. (1987). Lesbian stress and coping methods. *Journal of Psychosocial Nursing, 25,* 28-32.

Good, R. S. (1976). The gynecologist and the lesbian. *Clinical Obstetrics and Gynecology, 19,* 473-483.

Green, R. (1982). The best interests of the child with a lesbian mother. *Bulletin of the American Academy of Psychiatry & Law, 10,* 7-15.

Harvey, S. M., Carr, C., & Bernheine, S. (1989). Lesbian mothers: Health care experiences. *Journal of Nurse-Midwifery, 34,* 115-119.

Hitchcock, J. M., & Wilson, H. S. (1992). Personal risking: Lesbian self-disclosure of sexual orientation to professional health care providers. *Nursing Research, 41,* 178-183.

Hunter, N. D., Michaelson, S. E., & Stoddard, T. B. (1992). *The rights of lesbians and gay men: The basic ACLU guide to a gay person's rights* (3rd ed.). Carbondale: Southern Illinois University Press.

Johnson, S. R., Guenther, S. M., Laube, D. W., & Keettel, W. C. (1981). Factors influencing lesbian gynecological care: A preliminary study. *American Journal of Obstetrics & Gynecology, 140,* 20-28.

Johnson, S. R., Smith, E. M., & Guenther, S. M. (1987a). Comparison of gynecologic health care problems between lesbians and bisexual women. *Journal of Reproductive Medicine, 32,* 805-811.

Johnson, S. R., Smith, E. M., & Guenther, S. M. (1987b). Parenting desires among bisexual women and lesbians. *Journal of Reproductive Medicine, 32,* 198-200.

Kinsey, A. C., Pomeroy, W., Martin, C. E., & Gebbard, P. E. (1953). *Sexual behavior in the human female.* New York: W. B. Saunders.

Kirkpatrick, M. (1987). Clinical implications of lesbian mother studies. *Journal of Homosexuality, 14,* 201-211.

Lesbians found at greater risk of breast cancer. (1993, February 15). *Cancer Weekly,* p. 3.

Lucas, V. A. (1992). An investigation of health care preferences of the lesbian population. *Health Care of Women International, 13,* 221-228.

Marmor, M., Weiss, L. R., Lyden, M., et al. (1986). Possible female-to-female transmission of human immunodeficiency virus [Letter]. *Annals of Internal Medicine, 165,* 969.

Mathews, W. C., Booth, M. W., Turner, J. D., & Kessler, L. (1986). Physicians' attitudes toward homosexuality: Survey of a California county medical society. *Western Journal of Medicine, 144,* 106-110.

Monzon, O. T., & Capellan, J. M. B. (1987). Female-to-female transmission of HIV [Letter]. *Lancet, 2,* 40-41.

Morgan, S. (1991). Menopause, hysterectomy and sexuality. In B. Sang, J. Warshow, & A. J. Smith (Eds.), *Lesbians at midlife: The creative transition* (pp. 173-179). San Francisco: Spinsters Book Co.

O'Donnell, M. (1978). Lesbian health care: Issues and literature. *Science of People, 10,* 8-19.

O'Donnell, M., Leoffler, V., Pollock, K., & Saunders, Z. (1979). *Lesbian health matters!* Santa Cruz, CA: Santa Cruz Women's Health Center.

Olesker, E., & Walsh, L. V. (1984). Childbearing among lesbians: Are we meeting their needs? *Nurse-Midwife, 29,* 322-329.

Owen, W. E., Jr. (1980). The clinical approach to the homosexual patient. *Annals of Internal Medicine, 93,* 90-92.

Parowski, P. A. (1987). Health care delivery and the concerns of gay and lesbian adolescents. *Journals of Adolescent Health Care, 8,* 188-192.

Randall, C. E. (1989). Lesbian phobia among BSN educators: A survey. *Journal of Nursing Education, 28,* 302-306.

Reagan, P. (1981). The interaction of health professionals and their lesbian clients. *Patient Counselling and Health Education, 3,* 21-25.

Renzetti, C. (1988). Violence in lesbian relationships: A preliminary analysis of causal factors. *Journal of Interpersonal Violence, 3,* 381-399.

Roan, S. (1993, March 23). Cancer and the "invisible population." *Los Angeles Times,* p. 1.

Robertson, M. M. (1992). Lesbians as an invisible minority in the health services arena. *Health Care of Women International, 13,* 155-163.

Robertson, P., & Schecter, J. (1981). Failure to identify venereal disease in lesbian population. *Sexually Transmitted Diseases, 8,* 75-76.

Sabatini, M. T., Patel, K., & Hirschman, R. (1984). Kaposi's sarcoma and T-cell lymphoma in an immunodeficient woman: A case report. *AIDS Research, 1,* 135-137.

Saghir, M. J., Robins, E., Walbran, E., & Gentry, K. (1970). Homosexuality: IV. Psychiatric disorders and disability in the female homosexual. *American Journal of Psychiatry, 127,* 147-154.

Santa Cruz Women's Health Collective. (1977). *Lesbian health care: Issues and bibliography.* Santa Cruz, CA: Santa Cruz Women's Health Center.

Saunders, J. M., Tupac, J. D., & MacCulloch, D. (1988). *A lesbian profile: A survey of 1000 lesbians.* West Hollywood: Southern California Women for Understanding.

Schilit, R., Lie, G., & Montagne, M. (1990). Substance use as a correlate of violence in intimate lesbian relationships. *Journal of Homosexuality, 19,* 151-165.

Simkin, R. J. (1991). Lesbians face unique health care problems. *Canadian Medical Association Journal, 145,* 1620-1623.

Smith, E. M., Johnson, S. R., & Guenther, S. M. (1985). Health care attitudes and experiences during gynecological care among lesbians and bisexuals. *American Journal of Public Health, 75,* 1085-1087.

Stern, P. N. (1992). Helping sisters. *Health Care of Women International, 13,* v-vi.

Stevens, P. E. (1992). Lesbian health care research: A review of literature from 1970 to 1990. *Health Care of Women International, 13,* 91-120.

Stevens, P. E., & Hall, J. M. (1988). Stigma, health beliefs, and experiences with health care in lesbian women. *Image: Journal of Nursing Scholarship, 20,* 69-73.

Trippet, S. E., & Bain, J. (1992). Reasons American lesbians fail to seek traditional health care. *Health Care of Women International, 13,* 145-153.

Weinstein, D. L. (Ed.). (1992). *Lesbians and gay men: Chemical dependency treatment issues.* New York: Harrington Park.

White, J., & Levinson, W. (1993). Primary care of lesbian patients. *Journal of General Internal Medicine, 8,* 41-47.

Whyte, J., & Capaldini, L. (1980). Treating the lesbian or gay patient. *Delaware Medical Journal, 52,* 271-280.

Wilbur, C. B. (1965). Clinical aspects of female homosexuality. In J. Marmor (Ed.), *Sexual inversion: The multiple roots of homosexuality* (pp. 268-281). New York: Basic Books.

Wismont, J. M., & Reame, N. E. (1989). The lesbian childbearing experience: Assessing developmental tasks. *Image: Journal of Nursing Scholarship, 21,* 137-141.

Wolff, C. (1971). *Love between women.* New York: Harper & Row.

Young, E. W. (1988). Nurses' attitudes toward homosexuality: Analysis of change in AIDS
    workshops. *Journal of Continuing Education in Nursing, 19,* 9-12.
Zeidenstein, L. (1990). Gynecological and childbearing needs of lesbians. *Journal of Nurse-Mid-
    wifery, 35,* 10-18.

29

Health Services for Women
With Disabilities: Barriers and Portals

Carol J. Gill
Kristi L. Kirschner
Judith Panko Reis

Women with disabilities—members of two large and frequently neglected communities[1]—often get the worst of both worlds. As women, they may experience economic deprivation, abridged choices, and discrimination in many settings, including health service facilities. As people with disabilities, they deal with blocked access to schools, jobs, relationships, leadership power, transportation, and the built environment. Both women and people with disabilities have experienced repeated violations of their rights to self-determination in a historically paternalistic society. Furthermore, both communities have been neglected in medical research, professional training, health policy, and the development of health service delivery.

It has been argued that women with disabilities are one of the most isolated and invisible minority groups in this country. Although strides in medical care have enhanced tremendously the support and stabilization of life in emergency rooms and intensive care units, cracks in the health service system have become increasingly apparent in the chronic phase—the long period of "living with a disability" when most people can no longer be considered "sick." As the focus shifts from "fixing" a problem to preventing complications and augmenting a person's choices and functioning, women and their needs virtually disappear through the cracks in the system.

A quiet revolution, however, has begun to surface across the United States. Drawing strength and strategy from two movements—feminism and disability rights—disabled women are uniting and speaking out about their health needs and experiences as well as their entitlement to better treatment. From Los Angeles to Boston, grassroots groups are forming to reframe the health agenda of women with disabilities based on a new understanding of disability as a sociopolitical phenomenon.

Reframing Disability

The notion of disability as individual tragedy or deficiency has been under attack for the past decade by disability scholars and activists alike. They assert that the *traditional medical model* of disability distorts reality by emphasizing one facet of the disability experience—the medical—while neglecting the more crucial social components. They argue that much of what we know as disability is culturally derived, particularly the limitations we associate with disability. These proponents of the new *sociopolitical model* of disability argue that disability is not contained within a person but derives, instead, from the interaction between that person and society (Hahn, 1985). Heartily embracing this perspective, people with disabilities increasingly speak of overcoming not their physical, sensory, or cognitive limitations but job discrimination, disability bigotry, and thoughtlessly inaccessible structures. Like women, they point out that the negative images assigned to them are social fabrications—stereotypes—not natural facts of biology. From this perspective, being disabled no more renders a person tragic, weak, or dependent than being a woman makes a person innately passive, low achieving, or domestic!

In their writings, group discussions, and presentations to health service providers, women with disabilities—consumers and professionals—have been recalling their health care experiences and outlining the barriers they encounter in seeking adequate services. In these efforts, they have been identifying as a social minority community and using the new social model of disability to map out their health agenda. Working with physicians and allied health professionals whom they trust to understand their needs, they are identifying the major issues they want addressed. The following section summarizes those issues.

Major Barriers

Barriers in medicine. Women with disabilities experience, along with all other women, medicine's long-standing failure to include them in research and the full range of service delivery. With other disabled people, moreover, they share a legacy of dehumanization and infantilization in medical treatment settings, resulting in their being denied information and choices that most nondisabled Americans expect as entitlements. Within medicine, the needs of chronically disabled people have been traditionally sequestered in the specialty known as physical medicine and rehabilitation. Some disability activists have criticized this strict compartmentalization as evidence that many doctors avoid those whom they cannot cure, thus rejecting disability as an integral part of life.

Even within rehabilitation medicine, problems for women continue. Because this specialty historically developed to address the needs of injured male workers and soldiers returning from World War II, attention to women's issues has been emerging gradually. Another problem has been oversimplification. Any new programs designed to respond to the needs of disabled women must negotiate the complexity of disabilities, which can vary considerably from progressive to static, congenital to acquired, extensive to mild, and so on. Treating disability as a unitary concept is inherently fallacious.

It is also a mistake, though, to assume that a disability makes a woman so different that she requires separate "special" services. Women with disabilities are, after all, women, with basically the same constellation of health care problems as nondisabled women. It is also true, however, that nuances of a particular medical issue, such as osteoporosis, may be affected by disability-related alterations in structure or function of an organ system. Understanding the interaction of disability and women's health issues becomes extremely important in determining the best action in the context of the total person. Unfortunately, research on gender and disability interactions is in its infancy, leaving physicians the dangerous task of prescribing treatments for disabled women based on extrapolations from data gathered on disabled men or nondisabled women.

Access. One of the most difficult barriers to adequate health services for all people with disabilities is the first step: getting there and getting in. Access barriers may be physical (e.g., examining tables too high for transferring from a wheelchair, lack of Braille signage in a clinic) or programmatic (e.g., inflexible appointments that fail to accommodate transportation difficulties, lack of staff to assist in the examining room). Communication barriers may prevent women who are deaf, blind, or learning disabled from receiving information in an alternative format they can process. Because most disabled women in our country are unemployed and unmarried, economic factors also severely limit their access to health care resources (Fine & Asch, 1988, p. 10).

Consequences of blocked access can be dire. At one clinic, two women wheelchair users in 1 year reported that they had been rejected for mammography because they could not stand up at the machine. Both ended up with mastectomies when cancer had progressed to the palpable stage. Although most access problems are remediable, these barriers have prevented countless women from receiving services in neighborhood health settings.

Privacy and autonomy. As women with disabilities begin to share their health service experiences, they are piecing together an often poignant and horrifying history of violated privacy and autonomy. Recently, several have written independently about the outrage they call "public stripping"—the humiliation of being forced, as a child or adolescent, to disrobe for educational display in front of large groups or clinical photographers (Blumberg, 1990; McKeen, 1992). Others report continuing incidents of forced sterilization, involuntary abortion, concealed contraception, and other procedures initiated against their will and without adequate information. It is still a disabled woman's common experience to have decisions made about her body without her permission by physicians, officials, and family members whom society recognizes as the "experts" and "caretakers" in her life.

Violence and abuse. Reflecting disabled women's invisibility and devaluation, they have been overlooked, for the most part, in studies and services addressing abuse. Available scattered data and anecdotal evidence indicate, however, that abuse is the rule rather than the exception in the lives of disabled girls and women, much of it perpetrated by family members, personal assistants, and employees of institutions who, knowing their victims "need" them, count on the power differential to keep their crime unreported or disbelieved by others (Bellone & Waxman, n.d.). Furthermore, violent attack is one of the ways in which many women acquire their disabilities in the first place, introducing them to a loop of increased risk of further abuse as disabled women. Because the complex realities of assault against disabled women have never been studied, programs teaching such women self-defense often rely on adapting techniques used successfully by nondisabled women. Unfortunately, this is a "best guess" strategy with untested utility and safety.

Mental health. Feminist mental health professionals and activists have been speaking out for some time about the ravages of sexism on self-esteem. For women with disabilities, the combined assault of sexism and ableism (disability prejudice) can be crushing. From every quarter—even friends and family—women with disabilities receive discounting messages telling them they cannot do what is required in this society to be acceptable women: attract a worthy man, produce children, make a home, remain slim and beautiful, and (if all else fails) be capable of a "successful" career. Disabled women who often attempt these life tasks in their own resourceful style are reminded that theirs is not the "right way."

Carrying this stigma, women with disabilities in our country experience low marriage rates and a high incidence of separation and abandonment (Fine & Asch, 1988, p. 10). Isolation is the central fact of life for many women with disabilities. Another fact of life is stress. Disabled women's struggles for housing, money, transportation, personal assistance services, and expensive disability technology are exhausting, physically and emotionally. When stress "burnout" occurs, however, disabled women have few available resources for mental health services that are accessible, affordable, and informed by an understanding of the disability lifestyle. Alone, socially devalued, exhausted, and cut off from adequate mental health services, women with disabilities are prime candidates for depression. In this context, it is alarming to note that a significant proportion of the persons recently spotlighted for physician-assisted suicides were disabled and chronically ill women.

Reproductive health. Most women must guard the right to delay or terminate pregnancy; disabled women still struggle for the right to experience sexuality and motherhood at all. Barbara Waxman, a disability rights activist and policy analyst on disabled women's health, theorizes that society degenderizes women with disabilities because of primitive fears that "damaged women" produce "damaged offspring," literally and symbolically (Waxman, in press). The fear of genetically transmitted defects as well as the distrust of disabled women's capacity to nurture "healthy" babies leads to a denial of disabled women's sexuality and restrictions on their parenting options that are, according to Waxman, eugenic in intent.

Responding to this eugenics threat to choice, some disabled women activists have started challenging current practices of prenatal screening and abortion. While continuing to uphold any woman's individual right to make her own decisions about completing a pregnancy, they condemn societal pressures on women not to bear anything but physically perfect babies, as well as the lack of public support for women who raise children with disabilities. Some activists also question the growing acceptance of "eugenic abortion" for preventing births simply on the basis of disability (a practice they compare with abortion used for gender selection). They point out that many health professionals, acting on their own disability prejudice, fail to offer prospective parents complete and balanced information and support for electing to have a disabled child.

Contraceptive choices may also be particularly difficult for women with disabilities because the interaction of disability and reproductive health variables has never been adequately researched. For example, contraceptives containing estrogen may increase the risk of blood clots in women with increased propensity to develop deep venous thrombosis from paralysis and immobility. Progesterone-only agents have an unknown long-term effect on osteoporosis—a hazard already present in many women with muscle weakness, paralysis, or a history of prolonged bed rest. Any option that could increase the risk of osteoporosis is particularly difficult for women who cannot use traditional treatments for bone loss. For example, a physically disabled woman may be unable to perform weight-bearing exercise to enhance bone density. Similarly, women with neurogenic bladders who may already have an increased risk for developing kidney and bladder stones could be at further risk on calcium supplementation. On the other hand, barrier method contraceptives, such as the diaphragm or cervical cap, can involve hand dexterity, which may be difficult for some women. Adaptive techniques for managing such methods should be carefully and creatively explored.

Open, frank, and respectful discussions about sexuality and fertility potential should be a routine part of health care for all women. If a woman desires to be sexually active, a variety of birth control options should be made available to her. Protection against sexually transmitted diseases should be reviewed. Decisions concerning pregnancy should involve a discussion of health risks, preventive health care measures, and wonderful possibilities.

Unfortunately, this has been anything but routine for most women with disabilities. They commonly complain of feeling dehumanized in medical settings—seen as diagnostic categories instead of total persons or women. They report that few physicians discuss sexuality during exams (Beckmann, Gittler, Barzansky, & Beckmann, 1989) and are, in fact, unreceptive to the women's questions about subjects such as orgasm, fertility, sexual positioning, breast size, cosmetic concerns, and weight gain. This can be devastating to women who struggle against social stigma to feel confident and attractive. It can also be life threatening when doctors overlook sexually transmitted disease and other reproductive health problems because they feel a woman's disability is "overwhelming enough without looking for other problems."[2]

Policy issues. Women with disabilities have been speaking out against public policies that overmedicalize and restrict their lives. They denounce welfare rules that cut funding for expensive therapy, adaptive equipment, and personal assistance when a person with a disability tries to go to work. Added to the considerable barriers of sexism and disability discrimination already experienced by disabled women seeking jobs, such policies can effectively prevent them from pursuing careers and advancing in life.

Women with disabilities are prominent in supporting a more equitable health insurance system. Many call for a system that does not ration services based on diagnosis or quality-of-life judgments—both of which, they feel, are biased against people with disabilities and chronic illnesses as well as older people. They also call for the inclusion in any national health care system funding for personal assistance services so persons with disabilities across the country could choose to live in their own homes with dignified consumer-controlled assistance instead of being forced into the costly nursing home industry.

A problem related to personal assistance is that, in some states, child care is expressly excluded from the list of "activities of daily living" for which a disabled adult can get help. Funds may be allocated for such tasks as housecleaning, driving, meal preparation, even gardening, but not for tasks as simple as helping a disabled mother warm her child's dinner or aiding her in positioning her infant for breast-feeding. Without such assistance, disabled women who were unable to afford private help have lost custody of their children when the state argued they were unfit parents (Gill, 1992; Mathews, 1991; McKnight, 1991).[3] Significantly, this problem only affects disabled mothers who have children without disabilities. When the child is disabled, most states provide child care.

The Future of Disabled Women's Health

Opening portals. The passage of the Americans with Disabilities Act in 1990 mandated sweeping antidiscrimination changes in services, accommodations, communications, and transportation. Many women with physical, sensory, and mental disabilities are hopeful that the new law will integrate them into community services that have been inaccessible, including health settings.

Although several pioneering community projects have been developed by women with disabilities over the past two decades, there has been a detectable upsurge in the last few years of efforts on several fronts: groups for support and consciousness-raising regarding the sociopolitical issues confronting disabled women, projects on parenting with a disability, mentoring programs for disabled girls, publications, research, and health service delivery. More than ever, women with disabilities are recognizing and acting on the importance of organizing collectively to demand inclusion in planned and existing health services. They are asserting their role as the authentic experts regarding their own lives and are demanding more decision-making authority in the programs that serve their needs, or should. They are also claiming a power that has long been denied them: acknowledgment and fair compensation for their skills and work. Consequently, they are pursuing paying jobs and positions of leadership in, among others, the organizations that provide their services.

A new model for disabled women's health. The authors have been involved for the past 3 years in the development of a new comprehensive program to address disabled women's health needs and concerns. It rests on a dynamic relationship between consumers and hospital service providers that challenges traditional health professional-patient models in the United

States. In place of the "expert versus problem" approach, our program—the Health Resource Center for Women with Disabilities (HRCWD) at the Rehabilitation Institute of Chicago—recognizes the value of problem-solving abilities inherent in community groups. The center fosters community participation in creating and executing a plan that will empower women to get their medical and psychosocial health needs met rather than encouraging institutional dependency (McKnight, 1991). Self-determination for women with disabilities is, in fact, the guiding philosophy. It is manifest on three levels:

1. Through their presence on an advisory board, women with disabilities (some of whom, themselves, are professionals in the community) are active in determining the center's structure for health service delivery.

2. Whenever possible, women with disabilities are hired to provide and monitor services.

3. Each woman who seeks information or services at the center is encouraged to make her own decisions. To support individual self-determination, all efforts are expended to provide consumers with the fullest range of information and options possible.

The center not only provides accessible medical services from gynecologists and rehabilitation physicians, it also contains an education/resource component and a research program. Priority setting for the latter two components is guided by community input, and disabled women professionals are employed to coordinate them. Rehabilitation hospital staff assist as needed with education and research as well as fund-raising.

The balanced collaboration between hospital staff and community representatives that drives our center is, we believe, its most innovative and unique feature. It is a flexible, creative arrangement that, like a living organism, continues to evolve and adapt. It has required a good deal of openness on both parts—hospital personnel have had to move beyond traditional medical views of disability to work with a community that rejects medical domination; community representatives have had to trust medical professionals to respect their goal of self-determination.

Although many of the community women ideally would like to see these services offered in the "mainstream" community, others prefer to remain in the rehabilitation setting where physicians understand their disability-related needs and hazards. A practical consideration is that services to women are already being provided in rehabilitation, so it makes sense for the community to monitor those services. Rehabilitation is, after all, the place where many women with disabilities first learn about disability, sexuality, and their own bodies. Moreover, our rehabilitation facility is part of a larger university-hospital network, allowing us to maintain educational and service contacts with "mainstream" institutions. For example, several gynecologists who work in our OB/GYN clinic are from a hospital for women where a section of the library will soon be dedicated to publications on disabled women's health. Still, the dream remains for most of the community women that the services they are helping to provide at the center will one day, due to their continuing efforts, be available in integrated neighborhood settings. At that point, disabled women in the Chicago area will finally have a viable choice based on their own preferences and sense of comfort.

Conclusion

Of great frustration to women with disabilities has been the reluctance of many women's right groups to include them and recognize their issues as women's issues (Klein, 1992). In truth, the sociopolitical reality of being "disabled, female, and proud"—a motto of the Boston Project on Women and Disability—contains themes of struggle familiar to many in the women's movement. The successes of the DisAbled Women's Network (DAWN) of Canada in allying with feminist organizations there prove that women with disabilities can become another welcome facet in women's valued diversity. In this context, we are pleased to have the opportunity of contributing this chapter and seeing the health concerns of disabled women take their rightful place in a book that reframes the health issues of all women.

Notes

1. The text of the Americans with Disabilities Act cites the number of Americans with physical, sensory, and mental impairments and chronic illnesses that substantially limit life activities as 43 million.

2. This is a comment heard by one of the authors from a resident physician explaining why he deliberately ignored complaints of pelvic discomfort from a woman with cerebral palsy.

3. For further information about *Resourceful Woman*, the newsletter published by the Health Resource Center for Women with Disabilities at the Rehabilitation Institute of Chicago, please write to 345 E. Superior Street, Suite 681, Chicago, IL 60611 or call (312) 908-4744.

References

Beckmann, D. R. B., Gittler, M., Barzansky, B. M., & Beckmann, C. A. (1989). Gynecologic health care of women with disabilities. *Obstetrics and Gynecology, 74,* 75-79.

Bellone, E., & Waxman, B. F. (n.d.). *Sexual assault and women with disabilities: An overview* (monograph). Los Angeles: Planned Parenthood.

Blumberg, L. (1990, January/February). Public stripping. *Disability Rag*, pp. 18-20.

Fine, M., & Asch, A. (Eds.). (1988). *Women with disabilities: Essays in psychology, culture, and politics*. Philadelphia: Temple University Press.

Gill, C. (1992). A grieving mother shares her story. *Resourceful Woman, 1*(1), 2.

Hahn, H. (1985). Disability policy and the problem of discrimination. *American Behavioral Scientist, 28,* 293-318.

Klein, B. S. (1992, November/December). We are who you are: Feminism and disability. *Ms.,* pp. 70-74.

Mathews, J. (1992). *A mother's touch: The Tiffany Callo story*. New York: Holt.

McKeen, D. G. (1992, July/August). Such a good little patient. *Disability Rag*, p. 43.

McKnight, J. L. (1991, Spring/Summer). Services are bad for people. *Organizing*, pp. 41-44.

Waxman, B. F. (in press). Up against eugenics: Disabled women's challenge to receive reproductive health services. *Sexuality and Disability*.

30

Factors Related to Secondary Prevention Behaviors for Breast Cancer

Diane Lauver

Secondary prevention efforts are crucial for better control of breast cancer. Although the incidence of breast cancer remains high, the mortality rates secondary to breast cancer have been relatively stable, and primary prevention efforts are limited (Kessler, Feuer, & Brown, 1991). Secondary prevention involves asymptomatic screening for disease detection of abnormality as well as differential diagnosis. Secondary prevention for breast cancer includes mammography, clinical breast examination, breast self-examination, client recognition of and care seeking for a symptom, as well as clinician detection and diagnosis. This chapter focuses on seeking asymptomatic mammograms and evaluations for breast symptoms because these are two behaviors important to breast cancer control over which women have some control.

Background

Breast cancer is a concern for all women. Overall, Caucasian women develop breast cancer more often than women of color (Boring, Squires, & Tong, 1991). However, women of color with breast cancer often have higher stages on diagnosis (Briele et al., 1990; Richardson et al., 1992), higher death rates (Farley & Flannery, 1989), and, specifically, lower 5-year survival rates (Boring, Squires, & Tong, 1993). Differences in socioeconomic status may, in part, explain racial differences in survival (Bassett & Kreiger, 1986; Freeman, 1989). Women of lower socioeconomic status may have more advanced disease and lower survival rates because they lack affordable and accessible health care or because of their particular beliefs and norms about secondary prevention

(Freeman & Waisfe, 1989; Richardson et al., 1992; Stein, Fox, & Murata, 1991; Vernon, Tilley, Neale, & Steinfelt, 1985).

A theory of care-seeking behavior can guide understanding of women's secondary prevention for breast cancer (Lauver, 1992a; Triandis, 1980). Psychosocial variables and facilitating conditions are proposed to influence care-seeking behavior. The psychosocial variables are affect, beliefs and values about outcomes, norms, and habits. Applied to secondary prevention, *affect* refers to feelings associated with secondary prevention. *Beliefs* are the expected likelihood of outcomes of prevention; *values* are the perceived importance of those outcomes. Whereas *personal norms* reflect what one believes is acceptable regarding secondary prevention, *social norms* reflect what others (e.g., friends and family or health practitioners) believe about it. *Habit* refers to how one usually behaves regarding secondary prevention. *Facilitators* are external, objective conditions that enable one to engage in secondary prevention, such as having transportation or health insurance.

Discussion

Affective factors may influence some women's seeking of mammography. Fear of results and embarrassment are barriers to mammography for some women (e.g., about 9%-12%; Gregorio, Kegeles, Parker, & Benn, 1990; Lantz, Remington, & Soref, 1990). In one study, anxiety about mammography was associated with less mammography use when examined alone but not when examined with other variables (Lerman, Rimer, Trock, Balshem, & Engstrom, 1990). Embarrassment may be an issue for less acculturated Latinas regarding mammography use (Stein et al., 1991).

Affect—such as fear of cancer, anxiety, or denial—has been related to delayed care seeking among some women with breast cancer (Green & Roberts, 1974; Magarey, Todd, & Blizard, 1977; Worden & Weisman, 1975). In contrast, anxiety and strong emotional responses have been associated with greater intention to seek care promptly for breast symptoms and actually doing so among other women (Cameron & Hinton, 1968; Lauver & Chang, 1991; Timko, 1987). In two studies, anxiety did not explain delay directly when examined with other variables, but anxiety explained delay conditionally, based on having an identified health practitioner for routine health concerns. Among women without an identified practitioner, greater anxiety was associated with less delay; among women with an identified practitioner, anxiety was not associated with delay. Women who lacked an identified practitioner and who had little anxiety about care seeking delayed longer than other women, perhaps because they had less understanding of breast symptom management and of using the health care system (Lauver, 1993; Lauver & Ho, 1993).

Women's beliefs about mammography are critical to their use of it. One major reason for not using mammography is that women do not perceive the need for it if they do not have symptoms (National Cancer Institute [NCI] Breast Screening Consortium, 1990; Smith & Haynes, 1992). Beliefs about the benefits of mammography (i.e., early detection) have been associated with greater mammography use (Burack & Liang, 1989; Montano & Taplin, 1991). Older women are more likely to doubt the need for and benefit of mammography (Rimer, Ross, Cristinzio, & King, 1992; Taplin & Montano, 1993). Some women (e.g., 26%) have concerns about radiation exposure with mammography (Lantz et al., 1990; Stein et al., 1991; Zapka, Costanza, Stoddard, & Green, 1990).

Beliefs about outcomes of care seeking (e.g., beliefs about effective treatments) have been associated with care seeking for cancer symptoms (American Cancer Society, 1986; Bransfield, Hankey, & Wesley, 1989; Green & Roberts, 1974). In one study, beliefs about having to learn about treatment options and having lengthy appointments were associated with more delay in care seeking for breast symptoms. Perhaps the expectation of having to make treatment decisions was overwhelming to these women who were not well educated, overall. However, generalized beliefs of optimism were associated with less delay in care seeking among women of low socioeconomic status (Lauver, 1993).

Social norms, including recommendations from health practitioners, are critical to mammography use. One major reason for use of mammography, particularly among older women, is physician recommendations for the test (NCI Consortium, 1990; Rimer, Ross, et al., 1992; Smith & Haynes, 1992). This underscores the importance of discussion between women and practitioners about the need and timing of mammography. Also, encouragement from friends and family promotes mammography use (Montano & Taplin, 1991; Zapka, Stoddard, Costanza, & Greene, 1989). Sometimes, having had a friend or family member with breast cancer fosters asymptomatic mammography use (Glanz et al., 1992; Rimer, Resch, et al., 1992).

Personal and social norms may promote prompt care seeking for breast symptoms (Lauver & Ho, 1993). Social norms may promote greater intentions to seek care promptly for breast symptoms (Timko, 1987). Also, women who discuss their breast symptoms with friends or family may seek care more promptly (Coates et al., 1992).

Habits, such as having engaged in prior breast cancer screening, sometimes have been associated with mammography use (Burack & Liang, 1989; Johnson & Murata, 1988; Vernon, Laville, & Jackson, 1990). Also, habits of having sought regular checkups or symptomatic care have been associated with prompt care seeking for breast cancer symptoms (Coates et al., 1992; Samet, Hunt, Lerchen, & Goodwin, 1988).

In addition, facilitators (e.g., system-related factors) are important to secondary preventive behaviors. Having financial coverage for mammography can promote its use, especially among Latinas and African Americans of lower socioeconomic status (Burack & Liang, 1989; Gregorio et al., 1990; Lerman et al., 1990; Stein et al., 1991). Access to care may depend, in part, on socioeconomic resources. The type of health care insurance one has can influence mammography use; those with HMO coverage tend to use it more (Johnson & Murata, 1988; Zapka, Stoddard, Maul, & Costanza, 1991). Income has been associated with greater use of mammography (Smith & Haynes, 1992) and higher socioeconomic status has been associated with prompt care seeking for symptoms (Coates et al., 1992).

Accessibility to health services is important to both screening and symptomatic care seeking (Coates et al., 1992). When mobile mammography vans have been provided, women use these services (Baines, To, & Wall, 1990; Richardson, 1990; U.S. Department of Health and Human Services, 1991). However, services that are geographically close to women are not necessarily those that are covered financially; financial coverage may be limited to certain sites.

Coordinated and continuous care can be important to secondary prevention. Having an identified health practitioner or regular source of care is associated consistently with greater breast screening and preventive care seeking (NCI Consortium, 1990; Smith & Haynes, 1992). Furthermore, women have reported that sensitive staff at mammography sites support mammography use (Baines et al., 1990). Similarly, some women have identified that one outcome of seeking care for a breast cancer symptom would be dealing with insensitive physicians (Lauver & Angerame, 1993). The dissatisfaction with the medical care system of African Americans partially explains inadequate use of the system (Blendon, Aiken, Freeman, & Corey, 1989).

Clinical variables, such as presence and type of breast symptom, and history of prior related problems, sometimes have been associated with greater mammography use (Rimer, Resch, et al., 1992; Zapka et al., 1991). For some women, discomfort or pain is a barrier to mammography (Baines et al., 1990; Zapka et al., 1990). Although most women do not have pain with mammography, anticipation of pain can inhibit its use, especially among some Latina and African American women (Stein et al., 1991). Family history has been associated with greater mammography use only infrequently (Smith & Haynes, 1992; Vernon et al., 1990; Zapka et al., 1991). Women with breast lumps seek care more promptly than those with other breast symptoms (Coates et al., 1992; Funch, 1988). However, personal history and family history of breast disease (benign or malignant) have not been related to care seeking for breast symptoms (Lauver, 1993; Lauver & Ho, 1993).

Regarding demographic factors, certain subgroups of women are under-represented among women screened. Although older women are at greater risk for developing breast cancer, they are less likely to get referrals for or use mammography than younger women (Coll, O'Connor, Crabtree, & Besdine, 1989; Smith & Haynes, 1992). Although African Americans have poorer survival rates with breast cancer, they are less likely to get referrals for or use mammograms than Caucasians (Gemson, Elinson, & Messeri, 1988; Smith & Haynes, 1992). Although women of low socioeconomic status may need more assistance in dealing with the health care system, they get fewer referrals for and have less use of mammograms (Coll et al., 1989; NCI Consortium, 1990; Smith & Haynes, 1992).

Some researchers have proposed that women's care-seeking behaviors differ between racial groups. In some studies, Caucasians have sought care more promptly than African Americans, after controlling for socioeconomic factors (Lauver & Ho, 1993; Richardson et al., 1992; Vernon et al., 1985). However, in a large national study, Caucasians sought care slightly earlier than African Americans, but this difference was of borderline statistical significance and questionable clinical significance (Coates et al., 1992). Also, in a midwestern sample of largely urban women of lower socioeconomic status, there were no differences in care seeking between Caucasians and African Americans (Lauver, 1993).

One may wonder whether explanatory variables of care seeking are conditional on race (Lauver, 1992b). In two studies of care seeking for breast symptoms, the influence of affect, beliefs, norms, habits, and facilitators was not conditional on race. Also, there were no differences between Caucasians and African Americans in their anxiety, beliefs, and habits about care seeking. Findings in the two studies were contradictory regarding differences between racial groups in norms and having an identified practitioner (Lauver, 1993; Lauver & Ho, 1993). Thus Caucasian and African Americans in these samples were similar in terms of their anxiety, beliefs and values, and habits relevant to care seeking and in how these variables influenced care seeking.

Recommendations

To promote secondary prevention behaviors for breast cancer, affective factors can be discussed, appreciating that women have feelings about such behaviors. However, clinicians and journalists can recognize that anxiety about mammography or cancer usually does not inhibit breast screening behaviors, and they could stop perpetuating the myth that anxiety is a major barrier to breast screening.

To increase positive beliefs about cancer screening, educational efforts can strengthen women's beliefs about the need for asymptomatic mammography, especially among older women (Rimer, Ross, et al., 1992; Smith & Haynes, 1992), and about the worth of early intervention with breast symptoms, especially among lower socioeconomic African Americans (Burack & Liang, 1989). To increase women's knowledge about secondary prevention, materials must be culturally sensitive and any written text must be written at lower reading levels.

Creative informational interventions regarding secondary prevention can be designed and tested using both written and videotaped messages. Messages could emphasize the potential gains of screening, such as having peace of mind; women have identified confirmation of normality as one reason for seeking breast screening (Lauver & Angerame, 1993). Audiovisual presentations could be available in non-health care settings such as hairdressers' salons. Nurses have designed an educational program about early detection with culturally appropriate information for local ethnic groups. This information was presented in local black churches and also translated from English into two other languages (McCoy, Nielsen, Chitwood, Zavertnik, & Khoury, 1991).

Regarding norms and secondary prevention, increased discussion between clinicians and clients is needed. Clinicians should initiate discussion about the reason for asymptomatic breast screening with all female clients (NCI Consortium, 1990; Smith & Haynes, 1992). During discussion, clinicians could address women's concerns and correct any misperceptions. Also, women's groups could set aside time to discuss contemporary issues about breast screening. Lay health educators have been used successfully to share preventive information and serve as advocates for Native American women in the health care system (Brownstein, Cheal, Ackermann, Bassford, & Campos-Outcalt, 1992).

More rigorous research is needed to test specific interventions to promote secondary prevention. Experts believe that research on practical interventions to increase early cancer detection should be linked with theory-guided research (Burish, 1991; Schecter, 1991). Researchers could examine what interventions are most effective and how such interventions influence behavior. These interventions must be studied in different age and ethnic groups and in varied settings (Baquet & Ringen, 1987).

To increase facilitators for secondary prevention, women could establish a relationship with an identified practitioner for coordinated care, and health care institutions could develop policies to support such care. Also, institutional policies should support equitable reimbursement for all cost-effective health care practitioners who can conduct cancer screening. For example, nurse practitioners are competent, cost-effective practitioners. Further, institutional policies can provide incentives for use of managed care (i.e., an organized system of delivery of services with a set of practitioners and a focus on cost-effectiveness; American Nurses Association [ANA], 1991). Prevention efforts can be coordinated best when women relate to one practitioner or seek care within one system. Recommendations for improving clinicians' efforts in early cancer detection are summarized elsewhere (Lauver, 1992b).

To increase access, institutional policies should support decentralized, community-based sites to provide secondary prevention services (ANA, 1991). Screening can be offered at work sites or in inner-city or rural clinics (Glanz et al., 1992; Renneker, 1991). Community groups as well as Medicaid and Medicare offices could be information and referral sites for comprehensive health care (Baquet & Ringen, 1987). Practical information such as directions to the clinics, bus routes, and parking could be included. Clinical services can be offered during non-working hours to increase use.

To increase affordability for secondary prevention, long- and short-term solutions are needed. In the long run, women can lobby for a national health coverage program to guarantee basic health services, including prevention and early detection, for all Americans (ANA, 1991). Such services are cost-effective, politically popular, and thus might be maintained (Miller, 1987).

In the short run, women can lobby for extensions of employer health insurance and Medicaid eligibility, providing coverage to more individuals. Also, expansion of services covered by both worker and Medicaid plans could be authorized (Miller, 1987; Schramm, 1991). Women can lobby for passage of national legislation such as the Breast and Cervical Cancer Mortality Prevention Act of 1990 (which provided funds to focus secondary prevention efforts on low-income groups and women of color), for bills in the Women's Health Equity Act to authorize coverage for cancer screening for Medicaid-eligible women, and for legislation to assure coverage for mammography by third party insurance (Lauver, 1992b).

Despite the attention given to breast cancer, more efforts are needed to improve secondary prevention of the disease. In educational interventions, beliefs about the need for mammography without primary symptoms and the benefits of early detection should be addressed. Women can identify a practitioner for their coordinated care. Practitioners must address the need for mammography and specifically recommend it for women over 50. Also, they can encourage women to seek prompt evaluations for breast changes and to overcome concerns about dealing with insensitive practitioners or bothering a practitioner "unnecessarily" (Lauver & Angerame, 1993; Timko, 1987). Women's groups can establish norms that foster early detection; they can offer emotional and tangible support for friends as they go through breast screening or evaluation. Finally, women can lobby for long- and short-term changes in our health care system to provide financial coverage for secondary prevention for *all* women.

References

American Cancer Society. (1986). *Cancer in the economically disadvantaged*. Prepared by the Subcommittee on Cancer in the Economically Disadvantaged, New York.

American Nurses Association. (1991). *Nursing's agenda for health care reform* (Report No. PR-3 220M). Kansas City, MO: American Nurses Association.

Baines, C., To, T., & Wall, C. (1990). Women's attitudes to screening after participation in the national breast screening study. *Cancer, 65*, 1663-1669.

Baquet, C., & Ringen, K. (1987). Health policy: Gaps in access, delivery, and utilization of the Pap smear in the United States. *The Milbank Quarterly, 65*, 322-347.

Bassett, M., & Kreiger, M. (1986). Social class and black-white differences in breast cancer survival. *American Journal of Public Health, 76*, 1400-1403.

Blendon, R., Aiken, L., Freeman, H., & Corey, C. R. (1989). Access to medical care for black and white Americans: A matter of continuing concern. *Journal of the American Medical Association, 261*, 278-281.

Boring, C., Squires, T., & Tong, T. (1991). Cancer statistics, 1991. *Ca: A Cancer Journal for Clinicians, 41*, 19-36.

Boring, C., Squires, T., & Tong, T. (1993). Cancer statistics, 1993. *Ca: A Cancer Journal for Clinicians, 43*, 7-26.

Bransfield, D., Hankey, B., & Wesley, M. (1989, October). *Sociodemographic variables associated with patient delay among black/white breast cancer patients*. Paper presented at the American Public Health Association, Chicago.

Briele, H., Walker, M., Wild, L., Wood, D., Greager, J., Schneebaum, S., Silva-Lopez, E., Han, M., Gunter, T., & DasGupta, T. (1990). Results of treatment of stage I-III breast cancer in black Americans: The Cook County Hospital experience, 1973-1987. *Cancer, 65*, 1062-1071.

Brownstein, J., Cheal, N., Ackermann, S., Bassford, T., & Campos-Outcalt, D. (1992). Breast and cervical cancer screening in minority populations: A model for using lay health educators. *Journal of Cancer Education, 7*, 321-326.

Burack, R., & Liang, J. (1989). Acceptance and completion of mammography by older black women. *American Journal of Public Health, 79*, 721-726.

Burish, T. (1991). Behavioral and psychosocial cancer research: Building on the past, preparing for the future. *Cancer, 67*(3 Suppl.), 865-867.

Cameron, A., & Hinton, J. (1968). Delay in seeking treatment for mammary tumors. *Cancer, 21*, 1121-1126.

Coates, R., Bransfield, D., Wesley, M., Hankey, B., Eley, J., Greenberg, R., Flanders, D., Hunter, C., Edwards, B., Forman, M., Chen, V., Reynolds, P., Boyd, P., Austin, D., Muss, H., & Blacklow, R. (1992). Black/White Cancer Survival Study Group: Differences between black and white women with breast cancer in time from symptom recognition to medical consultation. *Journal of the National Cancer Institute, 84*, 938-950.

Coll, P., O'Connor, P., Crabtree, B., & Besdine, R. (1989). Effects of age, education, and physician advice on utilization of screening mammography. *Journal of the American Geriatrics Society, 37*, 957-962.

Farley, T., & Flannery, J. (1989). Late-stage diagnosis of breast cancer in women of lower socioeconomic status: Public health implications. *American Journal of Public Health, 79*, 1508-1512.

Freeman, H. (1989). Cancer in the economically disadvantaged. *Cancer, 64*(July Suppl.), 324-334.

Freeman, H., & Waisfe, T. (1989). Cancer of the breast in poor black women. *Cancer, 63*, 2562-2569.

Funch, D. (1988). Predictors and consequences of symptom reporting behaviors in colorectal cancer patients. *Medical Care, 26,* 1000-1008.

Gemson, D., Elinson, J., & Messeri, P. (1988). Differences in physician prevention practice patterns for white and minority patients. *Journal of Community Health, 13*(1), 53-64.

Glanz, K., Resch, N., Lerman, C., Blake, A., Gorchov, P., & Rimer, B. (1992). Factors associated with adherence to breast cancer screening among working women. *Journal of Occupational Medicine, 34,* 1071-1078.

Green, L., & Roberts, B. (1974). The research literature on why women delay in seeking medical care for breast symptoms. *Health Education Monographs, 2,* 129-177.

Gregorio, D., Kegeles, S., Parker, C., & Benn, S. (1990). Encouraging screening mammograms: Results of the 1988 Connecticut breast cancer detection campaign. *Connecticut Medicine, 54*(7), 370-373.

Johnson, R., & Murata, P. (1988). Demographic, clinical, and financial factors relating to the completion rate of screening mammography. *Cancer Detection and Prevention, 11,* 259-266.

Kessler, L., Feuer, E., & Brown, M. (1991). Projections of the breast cancer burden to U.S. women: 1990-2000. *Preventive Medicine, 20,* 170-182.

Lantz, P., Remington, P., & Soref, M. (1990). Self-reported barriers to mammography: Implications for physicals. *Wisconsin Medical Journal, 89,* 604-606.

Lauver, D. (1992a). A theory of care-seeking behavior. *Image, 24,* 265-271.

Lauver, D. (1992b). Addressing infrequent cancer screening among women. *Nursing Outlook, 40,* 207-212.

Lauver, D. (1993). *Care-seeking behavior with breast cancer symptoms in Caucasian and African-American women.* Manuscript submitted for publication.

Lauver, D., & Angerame, M. (1993). Women's expectations about seeking care for a breast cancer symptom. *Oncology Nursing Forum, 20,* 519-525.

Lauver, D., & Chang, A. (1991). Testing theoretical explanations of intentions to seek care for a breast cancer symptom. *Journal of Applied Social Psychology, 21,* 1440-1458.

Lauver, D., & Ho, C. (1993). Explaining delay in care seeking for breast cancer symptoms. *Journal of Applied Social Psychology, 23,* 1806-1825.

Lerman, C., Rimer, B., Trock, B., Balshem, A., & Engstrom, P. (1990). Factors associated with repeat adherence to breast cancer screening. *Preventive Medicine, 19,* 279-290.

Magarey, C., Todd, P., & Blizard, P. (1977). Psychosocial factors influencing delay and breast self-examination in women with symptoms of breast cancer. *Social Science and Medicine, 11,* 229-232.

McCoy, C., Nielsen, B., Chitwood, D., Zavertnik, J., & Khoury, E. (1991). Increasing the cancer screening of the medically underserved in south Florida. *Cancer, 67,* 1808-1813.

Miller, S. (1987). Race in the health of America. *Milbank Quarterly, 65,* 500-531.

Montano, D., & Taplin, S. (1991). A test of an expanded theory of reasoned action to predict mammography participation. *Social Science and Medicine, 32,* 733-741.

NCI Breast Cancer Screening Consortium. (1990). Screening mammography: A missed clinical opportunity? *Journal of the American Medical Association, 264,* 54-58.

Renneker, M. (1991). An inner city cancer prevention clinic: Design, methods, and early results. *Cancer, 67*(Suppl.), 1802-1807.

Richardson, A. (1990). Factors likely to affect participation in mammographic screening. *New Zealand Medical Journal, 103*(887), 155-156.

Richardson, J., Langholz, B., Bernstein, L., Burciaga, C., Danley, K., & Ross, R. (1992). Stage and delay in breast cancer diagnosis by race, socioeconomic status, age and year. *British Journal of Cancer, 65,* 922-926.

Rimer, B., Resch, N., King, E., Ross, E., Lerman, C., Boyce, A., Kessler, H., & Engstrom, P. (1992). Multistrategy health education program to increase mammography use among women ages 65 and older. *Public Health Reports, 107*, 369-380.

Rimer, B., Ross, E., Cristinzio, C., & King, E. (1992). Older women's participation in breast screening. *The Journals of Gerontology, 47* (Special Issue), 85-91.

Samet, J., Hunt, W., Lerchen, M., & Goodwin, J. (1988). Delay in seeking care for cancer symptoms: A population-based study of elderly New Mexicans. *Journal of the National Cancer Institute, 80*, 432-438.

Schecter, C. (1991, November). *Public education plan for the national strategic plan for early detection and control of breast and cervical cancer.* Paper presented at the annual APHA meeting, Atlanta, GA.

Schramm, C. (1991). Health care financing for all Americans. *Journal of the American Medical Association, 265*, 3296-3299.

Smith, R., & Haynes, S. (1992). Barriers to screening for breast cancer. *Cancer, 69*, 1968-1978.

Stein, J., Fox, S., & Murata, P. (1991). The influence of ethnicity, socioeconomic status, and psychological barriers on use of mammography. *Journal of Health and Social Behavior, 32*, 101-113.

Taplin, S., & Montano, D. (1993). Attitudes, age, and participation in mammographic screening: A prospective analysis. *Journal of the American Board of Family Practice, 6*, 13-23.

Timko, C. (1987). Seeking medical care for a breast cancer symptom: Determinants of intentions to engage in prompt or delay behavior. *Health Psychology, 6*, 305-328.

Triandis, H. (1980). Values, attitudes and interpersonal behavior. In M. M. Page (Ed.), *1979 Nebraska Symposium on Motivation* (pp. 195-259). Lincoln: University of Nebraska Press.

U.S. Department of Health and Human Services Public Health Service. (1991). Increasing breast cancer screening among the medically underserved: Dade County, Florida, September 1987-March 1991. *Morbidity and Mortality Weekly Report, 40*, 261-263.

Vernon, S., Laville, E., & Jackson, G. (1990). Participation in breast cancer screening programs: A review. *Social Science Medicine, 30*, 1107-1118.

Vernon, S., Tilley, B., Neale, A., & Steinfeldt, L. (1985). Ethnicity, survival, and delay in seeking treatment for symptoms of breast cancer. *Cancer, 55*, 1563-1571.

Worden, J., & Weisman, A. (1975). Psychosocial components of lagtime in cancer diagnosis. *Journal of Psychosomatic Research, 19*, 69-79.

Zapka, J., Costanza, M., Stoddard, A., & Green, H. (1990). Breast cancer screening perceptions and experience of primary care physicians, radiologists and women. *Progress in Clinical and Biological Research, 339*, 253-257.

Zapka, J., Stoddard, A., Costanza, M., & Greene, H. (1989). Breast cancer screening by mammography: Utilization and associated factors. *American Journal of Public Health, 79*, 1499-1502.

Zapka, J., Stoddard, A., Maul, L., & Costanza, M. (1991). Interval adherence to mammography screening guidelines. *Medical Care, 29*, 697-707.

31

Tension and Paradox in Framing Interstitial Cystitis

Denise C. Webster

Perhaps the most pressing question facing us in health care is whether we can provide comprehensive care for anybody and any care for the many people who would be grateful for even fragmented health services. Within the context of this larger question, I wonder if we can ever reframe women's health without questioning some of the most basic prevailing assumptions about health and about women.

Reframing is the art of transforming meaning, by shifting the content and/or the context of phenomena (Watzlawick, Weakland, & Fisch, 1974). Nearly 30 years ago, the women's movement provided a healing explanatory framework for many personal experiences for which most of us had few words and fewer outlets. The simple phrase *the personal is the political* reframed a private, invisible, and isolating litany of questions into a visible social reality/framework that could be analyzed (deconstructed) and ultimately connected to potential solutions/actions at both the personal and the social levels. The lens through which we see a phenomenon, then, changes the meaning of women's experience by changing the context or frame in which it is understood. Consequently, the theories we use and the assumptions inherent in those theories become much more than an academic exercise.

However, as a constructivist concept, reframing also assumes the simultaneous existence of multiple truths and multiple realities (Dowd & Pace, 1989). The naming of phenomena causes us to focus on a particular reality and, in a very fundamental way, *creates* a reality that remains otherwise invisible.

SOURCE: This chapter originally appeared in modified form in *Journal of Women's Health,* Vol. 2, No. 1, 1993, pp. 81-84; used by permission of Mary Ann Liebert, Inc., 1651 Third Ave., New York, NY 10128.

In so doing, it can create the content as well as changing the context. Indeed, the concept of "consciousness-raising" refers to bringing into awareness a particular reality that could not previously have been seen, recognized, or named. Even the concept of "women's health" has the power to make visible what has been invisible.

Reframing Interstitial Cystitis

Reframing is also a powerful therapeutic technique that acknowledges and takes advantage of the inherent paradoxes in situations (Watzlawick et al., 1974). It is in the context of struggling with the tensions and paradoxes inherent in a women's health perspective that I will focus on a women's health problem that has only recently been brought to the attention of women's health advocates. Interstitial cystitis (IC) is a relatively rare, but probably underdiagnosed, condition, which affects 10 times more women than men. It is estimated that as many as 450,000 people in the United States suffer from this chronic bladder inflammation, which appears to be of noninfectious origin. Characterized by urinary urgency, frequency, and suprapubic pain, the constant or intermittent pain and urination sometimes as often as every 15 minutes can result in sleep deprivation and physical and emotional debilitation, along with disturbed relationships and role performance (Held, Hanno, Wein, Pauly, & Cahn, 1990).

Currently, the diagnosis of interstitial cystitis is made based on clinical presentation and following a cystoscopic bladder biopsy under general anesthesia. The biopsy provides for exclusion of histologic evidence for other sources of bladder inflammation, such as infection, bladder cancer, radiation cystitis, or tuberculosis. For those with IC, the hydrolic hyperdistention of the bladder during the procedure results in bleeding of the bladder walls. The etiology of the condition is unknown and treatments, which are only palliative, vary widely in effectiveness across individuals as does consistency of response within individuals. The characteristic and often unpredictable exacerbation and remission pattern of the disease makes it particularly difficult to attribute improvement to single or multiple precipitants or interventions (Sant, 1991).

The continued elusiveness of an etiology for IC is certainly not for lack of hypotheses, although interest in generating them is of fairly recent origin. The efforts of a consumers group, the Interstitial Cystitis Association (ICA), is primarily responsible for bringing about a serious effort to understand and more effectively treat this problem. Etiologic theories range from fastidious infection, autoimmune, allergic, hormonal, neuropathic, traumatic, and psychosomatic explanations to those involving toxic urine, a defect in the bladder lining, or an interaction effect between the bladder and urine. Although many physicians are reluctant to diagnose IC unless they can visualize a "Hunner's ulcer" in the bladder wall or a severely shrunken and scarred bladder, it is now recognized that the disease may range from mild to severe and age of onset and bladder size may vary considerably (Sant, 1989).

The medical and surgical treatments for IC reflect the variation in theories about the disease as well as the desperation of those who have it or try to treat it. Antispasmodics, bladder antiseptics, antidepressants, antihistamines, narcotic antagonists, steroidal and nonsteroidal anti-inflammatory agents, and anticoagulants are among the less invasive treatment approaches. Other widely used treatments include stretching the bladder under anesthesia, or bladder instillations, singly or in combination with DMSO (an industrial solvent with anti-inflammatory properties), anticoagulant substitutes for mucin in the bladder lining (sodium pentosanpolysulfate), cortisone, or a strong bleach (oxychlorosene sodium), which may be effective either for its germicidal properties or for its destructive effects on bladder nerves and/or the bladder lining. In 1%-2% of cases, women eventually have to have their bladders removed (Sant, 1991).

Despite the increased interest in understanding and treating IC, probably most physicians and nurses know little about it, and many simply do not believe it exists. For the 1,000 IC patients surveyed by the Urban Institute Study, it took an average of 4.2 years and visits to a mean of 4.9 physicians before they obtained an accurate diagnosis (Held et al., 1990). One reason may be that, of those who accept its existence, many believe it to be a psychiatric problem. This perspective is perhaps best described by the following quote from a 1978 urology text: "Interstitial cystitis—a disease that is taunting in its evasion of being understood—may represent the end stage of a bladder that has been made irritable by emotional disturbance . . . a pathway for the discharge of unconscious hatreds" (Bojar & Reich, 1978, p. 1907).

Considering that the major treatments at that time for this painful condition included either instilling caustic silver nitrate into the bladder or shoving increasingly large dilators into the irritated urethral opening, it would seem quite reasonable to assume that these patients, indeed, harbored considerable and justifiable *conscious* hatreds. Before eventually obtaining an accurate diagnosis, many were told it was "just nerves" and that they should "find a lover," "get married," "have a baby," or "get a life" (Chalker & Whitmore, 1990; Ratner, Slade, & Whitmore, 1992). My own research found that, even after obtaining a diagnosis, many are told, "There is nothing more I can do for you. You'll just have to learn to live with the pain" (Webster, n.d.).

The long-awaited development of a national database for IC appears to be on the horizon. While this is a major victory in the recognition of the problem and improves the probability of finding enlightening symptom and treatment response patterns, there were several discomforting additional questions added to the database questionnaire. The questions are discomforting not because they are unimportant but because it is never clear how such information will be interpreted. Although most research in interstitial cystitis defines it as a urologic problem, most women in my study (and others) had additional symptoms, which included dyspareunia, vaginal inflammations, and abdominal pain. Theories about any chronic pain, and especially chronic pelvic pain, bring different theories, and therefore different assumptions, to the mystery. Chronic pain is estimated to affect between 25% and 30% of the population in industrialized countries (Bonica, 1990). Multiple theories explain chronic pain; however, the biomedical or disease model, as the most familiar model, tends to prevail in medical settings. Weiner and Fawzy (1989) describe this model as materialistic and mechanistic in its focus on single causes of disease, which can only be understood in biophysical or biochemical terms. Health in this model is the absence of disease and disease means an identifiable pathology at the cellular level, usually associated with a single organ. Without an identifiable disease, there can be no legitimate illness (Weiner & Fawzy, 1989). Within this model, those who have chronic pain without sufficient physical evidence of disease are seen as malingering and may be dismissed and/or are at risk from multiple procedures to identify and treat the presumed cause.

Chronic Pelvic Pain

Chronic pelvic pain is a subset of chronic pain that is described by Reading (1982) as a major source of headaches—for gynecologists. Particularly seen as a problem are patients having what is called "pelvic pain without obvious pathology." A widely referenced 1960 study reported that such patients had considerable psychopathology, evidence for which included ambivalent attitudes toward homemaking, conflicts toward their femininity, sexual problems, relationship difficulties, depression, anxiety, and rage, with 34 of 40 women having diagnoses of schizophrenia or borderline syndrome. It was noted that many came from large families and had suffered from a lack of maternal warmth (Gidro-Frank, Gordon, & Taylor, 1960).

Many sources also describe chronic pelvic pain as a somatiform disorder—either somatization disorder or somatiform pain disorder. With the diagnosis of somatization disorder, the problem is placed squarely in the bailiwick of psychiatry. The current *DSM-III-R* criteria for somatization disorder lists 35 physical symptoms. If one has 13 of these symptoms, or only 2 of 7 "highly suspicious" symptoms, without evidence of a related organic pathology or pathophysiologic mechanism, the diagnosis is confirmed. However, it can also be given if one *does* have evidence of organic pathology and the degree of complaint about it, or difficulty in meeting role obligations, is deemed "in excess of what would be expected." Amazingly, somatization disorder is reported to occur almost exclusively in women, and more often among blacks, lower socioeconomic groups, and those less formally educated (American Psychiatric Association, 1987; Smith, 1990). In fact, the mnemonic aid for recalling the seven major symptoms is "somatization disorder besets ladies and vexes physicians." The suspicious symptoms include shortness of breath, dysmenorrhea, burning in sex organs, lump in throat, amnesia, vomiting, and painful extremities (Othmer & DeSouza, 1985). Among the other somatization symptoms are pain during intercourse, sexual indifference, excessive menstrual bleeding, menstrual irregularity, and urinary problems of retention, hesitancy, or painful urination. From this description it becomes clear that those professionals who either do not know about interstitial cystitis or "don't believe in it" (and would not therefore be likely to look for or identify organic pathology) would conclude that the reported symptoms represented somatization disorder (Webster, 1993).

Somatization disorder is one of several "disorders" containing a collection of signs and symptoms that until recent years was called "hysteria." The other former hysteria categories include hysterical and borderline personality disorders and the dissociative disorders. What all of these classifications are now known to have in common is a high incidence of history of sexual abuse (Krishnan & France, 1988; Spiegel, 1991; Stone, 1990). But the questions about sexual abuse in the history of IC patients make me uncomfortable.

Sexual Abuse and IC

I profoundly believe a history of abuse is an important risk factor for all kinds of problems and I routinely ask clients about any abuse, in the context of our growing awareness of how widespread it is. And yet here I find myself perched unsteadily on the horns of several dilemmas.

As a feminist, I believe women must be supported to find our voices and to speak our truths. The truth about sexual abuse is ugly and has serious consequences. It has been, for far too long, ignored, distorted, diagnosed, and medicated out of existence. However, I also find theories that continue to define women almost exclusively by our sexuality to reflect a historical and ever-present view that women are to be valued for our ability to provide sexual pleasure for men and to reproduce. If we don't do either, or resent doing either, we *are* a problem. The view is also a reflection of the time-honored position that all women's problems are the result of too much or too little sex.

As a therapist, however, I am also acutely aware of the range of responses that women who describe abuse histories present. For many it is devastating, while for others it seems either one aspect among many difficult factors or to have had a minimal effect on their ability to grow and find meaning in their lives. I also am very concerned about the growing number of women who have been referred to therapy for sexual and other abuse problems, which were either not defined as problems by the women themselves or had never—to their knowledge—occurred. These referrals do not come exclusively from other health care professionals. Many have been "diagnosed" by their friends, based on observations of some aspects of their behavior. They were told they "must have been sexually abused" as a child. I do not believe they were simply "denying" their abuse; nor am I convinced that the friends had special knowledge unavailable to my clients as a result of presumed amnesia. I take very seriously the possible consequences of abuse, and I also believe that to pathologize another's behavior and redefine her life history for her is violence of the highest order. Not only are such women left with a shattered trust in their own memories, but they are often painfully estranged from families as well as friends whom they had previously seen as support persons.

As a nurse, I believe in the bodymindspirit; in health and illness as holistic experiences (Benner, 1989; Newman, 1986; Watson, 1988). The above descriptions of chronic pain do not in any way address the spiritual, and yet many incest survivors indicate that the worst aspect of sexual abuse is the damage to one's soul (Shengold, 1990). As a nurse, I focus on health as well as illness; I try to learn about a person's values, individual needs, strengths, and patterns of response over and above knowledge of whatever pathology may or may not have precipitated contact with the health care system. As a nurse, I view people in a context of developmental, social, and cultural systems.

As a hypnotist, I've learned that body-mind phenomena are the norm (Rossi, 1986). Emotions are called feelings because they tend to be perceived with our senses, and they are often encoded. While we tend to think of memory as associated with mind, memory also can be embodied (Lynch, 1985). Because sexual abuse is usually experienced as being much less about sex than it is about violence and the distortion of love, post-traumatic stress disorder (PTSD) is a more empathic, useful, and accurate description of the many psychological and physical sequelae (Herman, 1992). I am also aware that words can be as traumatizing as physical assault, sexual or otherwise. And, in many instances, as we are learning from psychoneuroimmunology, words and beliefs can be profoundly healing (Dolan, 1991; Rossi & Cheek, 1988).

As a researcher, I question how one could interpret the findings of questions about sexual abuse, because it would be difficult to accurately estimate the incidence and prevalence of sexual abuse in the general population. Courtois (1988) cites a figure of 20% for women, but that percentage could be considerably higher or lower, depending on the definition of abuse and such factors as social stigma and memory. I question the assumption that similar events are perceived, consciously or unconsciously, in the same way by everyone having that particular experience. I also question the use of measurement tools that are developed to root out evidence of psychopathology, because any instrument is capable of finding only what it seeks. Such instruments necessarily provide a skewed picture of all respondents.

As we all now know, Freud originally linked hysteria with sexual abuse/incest but he later reframed his theory, basing it not on actual abuse but on fantasy and intrapsychic conflict between the wish for and fear of an illicit sexual relationship (Masson, 1984). I wish to honor the naming of the tragic interruption of childhood suffered in silence by so many women for so many years. At the same time I do not want to be party to the resurrection, in all its glory, of the specter of hysteria because I don't trust that it will be honored as a source of wonder at the capacity of the human spirit to survive ordeals. I fear it will, again, be used as a reason to dismiss women's physical and emotional pain. Neither do I want to see women who are already suffering with the pain of interstitial cystitis confronted with a theoretical connection that, unless it is a connection they have made for themselves, may be far more damaging than healing.

I have concluded, then, from my own conflict around these issues, that what is needed in women's health is a lot fewer experts and a lot more students. We need considerably less certainty, and considerably more curiosity and compassion. We badly need more interdisciplinary opportunities to share knowledge from many different perspectives, while respecting that, above all, it is the theories of the person who has the problem that are of the greatest importance. We also need theories and research about women and about health that go beyond making intellectually satisfying connections to those that illuminate ways to prevent and heal the damage we have experienced and inflicted on each other at all levels: personal, social, and cultural. Ultimately, women's health is about all of us and the need to find better ways to live together in peace on this fragile planet.

Before my many personalities sit down, I cannot resist sharing with you my favorite personal story about experts. Several years ago I was sent for an expert second opinion prior to a surgical procedure. Following a cursory gynecological examination, I was informed, with piercing sincerity, that, based on the appearance of my cervix, I could not possibly have delivered two children.

References

American Psychiatric Association. (1987). *Diagnostic and statistical manual* (3rd ed., rev., pp. 255-267). Washington, DC: Author.

Benner, P. (1989). *The primacy of caring: Stress and coping in health and illness.* Menlo Park, CA: Addison-Wesley.

Bojar, S., & Reich, P. (1978). Psychosomatic aspects of urology. In J. Harrison, R. Gittes, A. Perlmutter, T. Stamey, & P. Walsh (Eds.), *Campbell's urology* (4th ed., pp. 1906-1909). Philadelphia: W. B. Saunders.

Bonica, J. (1990). General consideration of chronic pain. In J. Bonica (Ed.), *The management of pain* (Vol. 1, 2nd ed., pp. 180-196). Philadelphia: Lea & Febiger.

Chalker, R., & Whitmore, K. (1990). *Overcoming bladder disorders.* New York: Harper & Row.

Courtois, C. (1988). *Healing the incest wound: Adult survivors in therapy.* New York: Norton.

Dolan, Y. (1991). *Resolving sexual abuse: Solution-focused therapy and Ericksonian hypnosis for adult survivors.* New York: Norton.

Dowd, E. T., & Pace, T. (1989). The relativity of reality: Second-order change in psychotherapy. In A. Freeman, D. M. Simon, L. Beutler, & R. Arkowitz (Eds.), *Comprehensive handbook of cognitive therapy* (pp. 213-226). New York: Plenum.

Gidro-Frank, L., Gordon, T., & Taylor, H. C. (1960). Pelvic pain and female identity: A study of emotional factors in 40 patients. *American Journal of Obstetrics and Gynecology, 79,* 1184.

Held, P. J., Hanno, P. A., Wein, A. J., Pauly, M. V., & Cahn, M. A. (1990). Epidemiology of interstitial cystitis. In P. M. Hanno, D. R. Staskin, R. J. Krane, & A. J. Wein (Eds.), *Interstitial cystitis* (pp. 29-48). London: Springer-Verlag.

Herman, J. (1992). *Trauma and recovery.* New York: Basic Books.

Krishnan, K. R., & France, R. D. (1988). Chronic pain syndromes of idiopathic and organic origin. In R. France & K. Krishnan (Eds.), *Chronic pain* (pp. 142-193). Washington, DC: American Psychiatric Association Press.

Lynch, J. (1985). *The language of the heart: The body's response to human dialogue.* New York: Basic Books.

Masson, J. M. (1984). *The assault on truth: Freud's suppression of the seduction theory.* New York: Harper.

Newman, M. (1986). *Health as expanding consciousness.* St. Louis, MO: C. V. Mosby.

Othmer, E., & DeSouza, C. (1985). A screening test for somatization disorder (hysteria). *American Journal of Psychiatry, 142,* 1146-1149.

Ratner, V., Slade, D., & Whitmore, K. (1992). Interstitial cystitis: A bladder disease finds legitimacy. *Journal of Women's Health, 1*(1), 63-68.

Reading, A. (1982). Chronic pain in gynecology: A psychological analysis. In J. Barber & C. Adrian (Eds.), *Psychological approaches to the management of pain* (pp. 137-149). New York: Brunner/Mazel.

Rossi, E. (1986). *The psychobiology of mind-body healing: New concepts of therapeutic hypnosis.* New York: Norton.

Rossi, E., & Cheek, D. (1988). *Mind-body therapy: Methods of ideodynamic healing in hypnosis.* New York: Norton.

Sant, G. (1989). Interstitial cystitis: Pathogenesis, clinical evaluation and treatment. *Urology Annual, 3,* 171-196.

Sant, G. (1991). Interstitial cystitis. In T. Stamey (Ed.), *Monographs in Urology, 12*(3), 37-63.

Shengold, L. (1990). *Soul murder.* New York: Fawcett-Columbine.

Smith, G. R. (1990). *Somatization disorder in the medical setting* (DHHS Pub [ADM] 90-1631). Rockville, MD: Public Health Service.

Spiegel, D. (1991). Dissociative disorders. In A. Tasman & S. Goldfinger (Eds.), *Review of psychiatry* (Vol. 10). Washington, DC: American Psychiatric Association Press.

Stone, M. (1990). *The fate of borderline patients*. New York: Guilford.

Watson, J. (1988). *Nursing: Human science and human care*. New York: National League for Nursing.

Watzlawick, P., Weakland, J., & Fisch, R. (1974). *Change*. New York: Norton.

Webster, D. (1993). Interstitial cystitis. In L. Andrist (Ed.), *AWHONN's Clinical Issues in Perinatal and Women's Health Nursing, 4*(2), 236-243.

Webster, D. (n.d.). [Unpublished findings of ongoing research].

Weiner, H., & Fawzy, F. (1989). An integrative model of health, disease and illness. In S. Cheren (Ed.), *Psychosomatic medicine: Theory, physiology, and practice* (Vol. 1, pp. 9-44). Madison, WI: International Universities Press.

Epilogue: An Invitation

Alice J. Dan
Jessica A. Jonikas
Zylphia L. Ford

A Broader Perspective

The chapters included in this book have provided a comprehensive, often provocative, view of the directions needed to reframe women's health. The authors have described a variety of attempts in research and practice to resolve inequities in health knowledge about and health care for women. What do we know about this new framework? Certainly that it is complex, with many voices finding expression in it. It contains a critique of 20th century medicine and visions of alternative models. A key value in the framework is the words of women themselves, their perspectives on their own lives. Therefore, a key criterion for work in women's health is that it listens to—connects with—women in particular contexts as they tell their experience (see Heilbrun, 1988). Listening to the voices of women, one hears their strength and resilience, their strategies for meeting the demands of their lives. Not only must we attend to the problems of women, but we have so much to learn about the nature of these difficulties, how health is compromised and what caring systems are needed. This entails respect for women's agency, no matter how victimized they are. In many situations (examples abound in this volume) listening to women points our attention to their context: their relationships, their access to resources, and a host of other factors, including age, race, ethnicity, religion, sexual preference, (dis)abilities. . . .

Just as adult development in the human species means taking responsibility for creating one's own life, perhaps the maturity of a movement is signaled by its acceptance of responsibility for helping to create a context to nurture its vision. Whether our primary identity is in research, education, professional health care, informal care, or advocacy, the need to influence context brings us into the policy arena. In this epilogue, each of these themes—the critique, the assertion of women's voices, and implications for policy in research, education, and health care—will be briefly reviewed, for the purpose of seeing what tasks lie before us.

The Critique

As noted by several authors in this volume, the critique of the medical model has two components: criticism of the hierarchical organization of health institutions, and second of biomedical science as it is applied to women's health. These are related but distinct aspects of 20th century medicine. The critique of biomedical research is part of a more general attack on positivist models of science for their reductionism, and their over-emphasis on universal truth, an objective stance that mystifies the values and interests behind the scientist mask (Harding & O'Barr, 1987; Longino, 1990). Post-modernist theory, particularly as expressed by feminist writers (e.g., Haraway, 1989, 1991; Harding, 1991), is especially helpful in understanding the multiplicity of what we call reality, how it is knit together from fragmentary experience, and that *who* does the knitting determines the design. We want to create a many colored quilt (like the Hot Flash Fan described by Ann Stewart Anderson, 1993), a collage, a tapestry or a dinner party to which we all contribute (Chicago, 1979).

Systematic observation, documentation and analysis remain at the heart of scientific consensus (Longino, 1990). Because of the historical context in which Western science developed, it speaks most directly to white European male experience. Men of color and European women share more of that experience; women of color perhaps less. This means that scientifically speaking, we may have the most to learn from women of color. Finally, we honor such womanist writers as Toni Morrison, Alice Walker, bell hooks (1992).

Another important lesson from post-modernist theory is the relationship of power to definitions of reality. Hierarchical systems, like doctor-patient or doctor-nurse relationships, define reality from the standpoint of the dominant group. This means that "health" for the subordinate is defined as what looks good to the dominant. (Read, "women's health has been defined by men.") In feminist legal thought, this has been referred to as "positionality" (Bartlett, 1991).

Social psychology (attribution theory) teaches us that causal attributions are made differently by an observer of someone than they are by the self. I am more likely to credit environmental events, contextual factors outside myself, with influencing my own behavior; while I am more likely to see your behavior as reflecting something about you, some personal quality (e. g., personality, gender). Both of these views are partial, both can be shown to have validity in some situations. Because in the dominant reality women have been "objects" of description (Beauvoir, 1972), rather than describing their own experience, we don't know as much about the context of women's lives. Medical theories about health/illness in women have tended to "blame the victim" by attributing to her the causes for her own problems. The diagnosis of "self-defeating personality" proposed by the American Psychiatric Association (but which fortunately defeated itself) is a particularly apt example of this tendency. (It was to be used most frequently to label women who were repeatedly abused. It was in fact used by NIMH as a label for a young psychiatrist who complained of sexual harassment there.)

In order to include women's perspectives more fully in our understanding of health, power relationships have to change. Otherwise, the insights we are gaining now by listening to women will be lost, as has happened many times before in history (e. g., Spender, 1982). Unless social institutions can change from hierarchical to egalitarian organization, we will all lose the wisdom of women again. Self-in-relation theory, and other feminist writings are critically important to our understanding of how to accomplish this shift toward mutuality and reciprocity in relationships, including health care relationships between providers and patients. We are still a long way from making this happen. Even within the medical profession, the women are marginalized, their medical power devalued because of their gender.

One effect of patriarchal practices such as sexual harassment is to make it more difficult for women to collaborate across professions, or other groups. For example, a recent report of sexual harassment of female doctors by patients (Phillips & Schneider, 1993, p. 1939), noted that, "At a time when physicians are criticized for magnifying the inevitable differences in power that separate them from their patients, it is ironic that female doctors see the reinforcement of a physician's power as a means of protection." In fact, the article concludes, "The vulnerability inherent in their sex . . . override[s] their power as doctors, leaving female physicians open to sexual harassment." Making sexual harassment a visible aspect of women's lives can be part of a collaborative effort that unites women of many groups around a common goal. Similarly, a commitment to valuing the views of women from many different situations can provide the basis for mutual support across the new framework of women's health.

The Assertion

It would be a mistake to assume that just because we recognize the need to value women's voices, things will change. The job of articulation is immense, and must be contributed to by so many of us. In the meantime, it is all too easy to slip back into the rut of "how things are always done." Two concepts that can guide us in supporting the process of articulation are *totality* and *centrality*, as suggested by Helen Rodriguez-Trias (1992). Totality refers to a holistic concept of health, in which mental and physical aspects are equally important, in which the health problems of women are seen as "deeply implanted in the statuses that derive from their multiple social relations." Whether we are serving an individual woman, or thinking about a women's health policy issue, the question is, are we looking at the larger picture? Women occupy not only reproductive roles, but also are productive workers; not only consume health care as patients, but also provide health care in families, in communities, and as health professionals. As many authors in this book have demonstrated, experiences of violence, poverty, discrimination, and the socialization of girls in ways that lead to low self-esteem, have critical impact on women's health.

Centrality requires that women's experiences, the ways in which they view their own health and illness, must be the basis for developing new knowledge in women's health. One consequence of centrality is to focus our attention on understanding women's experiences, which have been omitted in many analyses of health issues. In other words, health practitioners and researchers must take seriously the experience of women as women themselves describe it, not as the practitioners and researchers imagine it to be (see, e.g., West, 1993; Fonow & Cook, 1991). Such important issues as weight control and eating disorders can be illuminated by understanding women's experiences with their bodies and what bodily experiences mean to women (e.g., Young, 1990). Understanding the impact of chronic conditions and morbidity on women's lives, as opposed to the usual health research focus on mortality, is another example of a "woman-centered" perspective. Centrality also refers to the recentering of health relationships, away from the hierarchical model of the "expert" professional who has all the knowledge to care for an ignorant patient, toward the recognition that the patient brings important information to the interaction and that decision making needs to be shared. Many of the authors in this book have provided examples of how health practice and research have not started from where women are, often to the detriment of women. These authors also provide directions that practitioners and researchers might take to integrate the concept of centrality into the health care system by including women in all aspects of their own health care.

What Next? Strategies
to Achieve Excellence in Women's Health

In planning a summer institute to further the work of "reframing women's health," we have outlined seven objectives to focus our efforts.

1. *Reconnecting the women's health movement. Gathering resources and exploring alternatives for women's health practice, education and research.* We need to recognize that the visibility of women's health in 1994 is largely the result of the work of many grassroots groups around the country, since the late 1960s. On the one hand, it is important to credit those who have worked long and hard in the past, and on the other hand, to extend ourselves, to be more inclusive in the future.

2. *Outlining the guiding concepts underlying the principles of women's health.* This book offers a beginning for this objective, but beyond identifying what we hold in common, we also need to apply these concepts to each of our own disciplines and situations.

3. *Stimulating and fostering multidisciplinary collaboration in women's health.* Awareness of the principle of *totality* leads to the acceptance that no one approach or profession can solve all health problems. Trust and communication among disciplines need to be nurtured.

4. *Enabling the development of curricula or programs according to the needs of specific situations and populations.* By coming together with a wide range of resources and perspectives, we can support each other's work toward change.

5. *Including women of all communities and their self-identified health concerns in the development of programs.* Whether we are planning new health services, education, or research, women as potential participants in our programs should be included in the planning. It may not always be easy to hear the ideas of community women, especially when they say that they do not want what we are offering, but it is necessary that their views be part of the dialogue. We have much to learn about how to make this happen.

6. *Setting directions for policy development in women's health.* This is the action piece. How do we assess the larger picture to use women's knowledge and insight to improve health for all? The *Copenhagen Conference Statement* (presented in the Introduction) is one formulation from an international women's health perspective. Another example of the development of policy by representatives of many professions and community organizations is the recent *Urban Women's Health Agenda* by the Mayor's Task Force on Women's Health, a project of the Department of Health of the City of Chicago. Under the leadership of Sheila Lyne, R.S.M., Commissioner of the Department of Health, and Hedy Ratner, Co-Director of the Women's Business Development Center, this agenda describes "systemic obstacles to better health for women and girls." These include social attitudes and discrimination affecting all women, barriers having

a disparate negative impact on poor women, unique challenges to healthy lives for young women, as well as institutional problems in the health care delivery system itself.

7. *Exploring options and mechanisms for promotion of excellence in women's health.* What are the choices confronting us, and how will different alternatives influence women's health? You are invited to join in this discussion, at the Summer Institute of 1994, and beyond. How can we get connected, maintain our diverse backgrounds, interests, abilities, and communicate across them to improve health in all our communities? What forms of communication and organization will best facilitate our efforts to put into practice our new knowledge in women's health? How can we expand our knowledge in the areas of greatest need for women's health?

This is a time of historic change in health care in the United States, and we can be sure that what happens here will affect other areas of the world. It is particularly appropriate to insist on the full representation of women's voices as health care reform is developed. The processes by which we continue this work, the relationships we form, are as critical to its success as the choices we make. We extend this invitation to become part of the conversation.

References

Anderson, A. S. (1993). Afterword: Creating a visual image of menopause. In J. Callahan (Ed.), *Menopause: A midlife passage.* Bloomington: Indiana University Press.

Bartlett, K. T. (1991) Feminist legal methods. In K. T. Bartlett & R. Kennedy (Eds.), *Feminist legal theory: Readings in law and gender* (pp. 392-393). Boulder, CO: Westview Press.

Beauvoir, S. de (1972). *The second sex.* Harmondsworth, UK: Penguin. (originally published in 1949)

Chicago, J. (1979). *The dinner party: A symbol of our heritage.* Garden City, NY: Anchor Books.

Fonow, M. M., & Cook, J. A. (1991). *Beyond methodology: Feminist scholarship as lived research.* Bloomington: Indiana University Press.

Haraway, D. (1989). *Primate visions: Gender, race, and nature in the world of modern science.* New York: Routledge, Chapman, & Hall.

Haraway, D. J. (1991) *Simians, cyborgs, and women: The reinvention of nature.* New York: Routledge, Chapman & Hall.

Harding, S. (1991). *Whose science? Whose knowledge? Thinking from women's lives.* Ithaca, NY: Cornell University Press.

Harding, S., & O'Barr, J. F. (Eds.). (1987). *Sex and scientific inquiry.* Chicago, IL: University of Chicago Press.

Heilbrun, C. G. (1988). *Writing a women's life.* New York: Ballantine Books.

hooks, bell (1992). *Black looks: Race and representation.* Boston, MA: South End Press.

Longino, H. E. (1990). *Science as social knowledge: Values and objectivity in scientific inquiry.* Princeton, NJ: Princeton University Press.

Phillips, S. P., & Schneider, M. S. (1993). Sexual harassment of female doctors by patients. *The New England Journal of Medicine, 329*(26), 1936-1939.

Rodriguez-Trias, H. (1992). Women's health, women's lives, women's rights. *American Journal of Public Health, 82*, 663-664.

Spender, D. (1982). *Women of ideas (and what men have done to them).* London: Routledge & Kegan Paul.

Urban Women's Health Agenda. (1993, June). Mayor's task force on women's health: A project of the Department of Health of the city of Chicago.

West, R. (1993). *Narrative, authority and law.* Ann Arbor: University of Michigan Press.

Young, I. M. (1990). The breasted experience. In *Throwing like a girl, and other essays in feminist philosophy and social theory.* Bloomington: Indiana University Press.

Index

About the Contributors

Carmen Barroso is the Director of the Population Program of the John D. and Catherine T. MacArthur Foundation. She has a Ph.D. from Columbia University and has published numerous books and articles, mostly in Brazil, where she taught in the Sociology Department of the University of São Paulo and did research at the Carlos Chagas Foundation. She has been active in the women's movement in Brazil and was one of the founding members of DAWN (Development Alternatives with Women for a New Era).

Ruth Behar, an anthropologist at the University of Michigan, is the author of *The Presence of the Past in a Spanish Village* and *Translated Woman: Crossing the Border with Esperanza's Story*. She is at work on a coedited anthology, *Women Writing Culture/Culture Writing Women*, an exploration of feminist approaches to anthropology.

Lucy M. Candib is a family physician teacher at an urban neighborhood health center in Worcester, Massachusetts. She has practiced and taught a feminist perspective toward women's health in this multicultural setting for 20 years.

Joan C. Chrisler is Associate Professor of Psychology at Connecticut College. She specializes in health psychology and the psychology of women and has written extensively on women's health issues. She is known for her work on weight and eating and on psychosocial aspects of the menstrual cycle.

Mardge Cohen (M.D.) is the director of the Women and Children's HIV Program at Cook County Hospital. She has been an internist since 1976 and is on the Board of Directors for the Chicago Woman's AIDS Project.

Susan M. Cohen (D.S.N., R.N.) is Associate Professor at the University of Texas—Houston. She is a nurse practitioner in women's health.

Alice J. Dan, a psychologist, is Professor and Director of the Center for Research on Women and Gender, University of Illinois at Chicago. A founder of the Society for Menstrual Cycle Research, she also edited *Menstrual Health in Women's Lives* (1991).

Mary Driscoll (R.N., M.P.H.) is the Primary Care Administrator at the HIV Center of Cook County Hospital. She is also the President of the Illinois Maternal and Child Health Coalition plus a researcher, advocate, and policy expert for women and children's health issues.

Sue Fisher, Associate Professor at Wesleyan University, is a sociologist with a long-standing interest in the delivery of health care to women. In her earlier work, *In the Patient's Best Interest* (1986), she pays close attention to the ways language is used during medical consultations to encourage some women patients to have treatments (hysterectomies) that are not medically necessary while, for others, important preventive procedures (Pap smears) are not recommended. In her new work, *Re-producing Identities*, she focuses on how gendered and professional identities are reproduced and undermined during medical and nursing encounters.

Zylphia L. Ford (MPH) is a Project Coordinator at the Center for Research on Women and Gender at the University of Illinois at Chicago. She is also an active member of the Chicago Women's Health Center collective.

Carol J. Gill (Ph.D.) is a clinical and research psychologist specializing in disability issues. She is President of the Chicago Institute of Disability Research, Willowbrook, Illinois.

Ann Pollinger Haas (Ph.D.) is a sociologist and Professor of Health Services at Lehman College of the City University of New York. She is affiliated with the Center for Lesbian and Gay Studies at the CUNY Graduate Center and also with New York Medical College. Her current research interests center on women who experience sexual orientation and sexual identity changes later in life.

Jean A. Hamilton (M.D.) is Professor in Psychology, Social and Health Sciences, and Women's Studies at Duke University. Her interests include the psychology of women, women's health, and public policy related to women's health.

Michelle Harrison (M.D.) a family physician and psychiatrist, has been an articulate and prolific spokesperson for changes in the health care of women.

She is the author of *A Woman in Residence* (1982; 1993) and *Self-Help for Premenstrual Syndrome* (1985). She currently practices in Highland Park, New Jersey. She is the Clinical Associate Professor of Family Medicine at the Robert Wood Johnson Medical School—UMDNJ and the Director of the Women's Health Fellowship Program.

Lori L. Heise directs the Violence, Health and Development Project, a research and advocacy initiative of the Pacific Institute for Women's Health, Washington, DC. The project's mission is to assist organizations working against gender violence in the developing world by mobilizing the resources, technical know-how, and research capacity of the international health and development community.

Eileen Hoffman (M.D.) is an internist in private practice in New York City, Clinical Assistant Professor of Medicine at New York University School of Medicine, and cofounder of the Women's Health Project. She is the author of an upcoming book: *In Her Own Image: Women Centered Health Care.*

Jean Hunt, a longtime health activist, was formerly the Executive Director of the Elizabeth Blackwell Center in Philadelphia. She currently consults for a number of nonprofit health groups.

Carole Joffe is Professor of Sociology and Women's Studies at the University of California, Davis. She is the author of *The Regulation of Sexuality: Experiences of Family Planning Workers* (1986) and is completing a book on physician involvement in abortion before and after *Roe v. Wade.*

Karen Johnson (M.D.) is a feminist psychiatrist, Clinical Scholar in Women's Health at Stanford University, Assistant Clinical Professor of Psychiatry at the University of California, San Francisco, Assistant Editor of *Women's Health Forum*, cofounder of the Women's Health Project, and author of *Trusting Ourselves: The Complete Guide to Emotional Well-Being for Women* (1991).

Jessica A. Jonikas is a graduate student in the School of Social Service Administration and the Graduate Program in Health Administration and Policy at the University of Chicago. Currently, she is an intern with the Center for Research on Women and Gender at the University of Illinois at Chicago. She also works in research and training in the field of psychiatric rehabilitation, with a special interest in feminist clinical practice and the life experiences of women who have psychiatric disabilities and/or are homeless.

Patricia Kelly (R.N., F.N.P., M.P.H.) is currently teaching in the community nurse practitioner program at Rush University. She has done extensive work directing and implementing research studies for women with HIV.

Kristi L. Kirschner (M.D.) is Assistant Professor in the Department of Rehabilitation Medicine, Northwestern University Medical School, Assistant Director of the Stroke Program, and Co-Director of the Health Resource Center for Women with Disabilities at the Rehabilitation Institute of Chicago.

Mary P. Koss (Ph.D.) is Professor of Family and Community Medicine with joint appointments in the Departments of Psychology and Psychiatry at the University of Arizona in Tucson. She is coauthor of the book *The Rape Victim: Clinical and Community Interventions* (1991). She is cochair of the American Psychological Association Task Force on Violence Against Women and the recipient of a research career development award from the National Institute of Mental Health. She is Associate Editor of *Psychology of Women Quarterly* and *Violence and Victims* and also on the editorial boards of eight other journals.

Diane Lauver (Ph.D., R.N., C.S.), Assistant Professor, University of Wisconsin—Madison School of Nursing and Women's Studies, has been a nurse practitioner in women's health for several years. She is coeditor of *Sexual Health Promotion*. As a researcher, she has focused recently on women's behaviors for the early detection of breast cancer.

Sara Segal Loevy is a consultant in health care, specializing in program evaluation, survey research, and needs assessment. She holds a Dr.P.H. from the University of Illinois and has taught epidemiology and evaluation research while on the faculty at Rush-Presbyterian-St. Luke's Medical Center. In addition, she served as a Research Associate at the Center for Health Administration Studies at the University of Chicago and, as a Senior Survey Director at NORC, managed large-scale health surveys for the federal government.

Angela Barron McBride is Dean and Distinguished Professor at Indiana University School of Nursing; in keeping with her interdisciplinary interests, she also holds adjunct faculty status in psychology, psychiatry, and women's studies within her university. She is best known for having written the first critically acclaimed book to look at motherhood in light of the women's movement, *The Growth and Development of Mothers* (1973).

William Leon McBride is Professor of Philosophy at Purdue University. He has had a long-standing interest in social philosophy, including the theoretical underpinnings of women's studies, which he has written about in *Women & Health, Hypatia,* and *the Journal of Women's Health.*

Ellen O. Mitchell (Ph.D., R.N.C.) is an Associate Professor in the women's health graduate track at the University of Washington. She is a nurse practitioner.

GiGi Nicks is the Administrative Assistant and an HIV/AIDS peer health educator for the Cook County Women and Children's HIV Program. As an HIV positive person, she has spent most of her time educating others on HIV/AIDS.

Judy Norsigian is a coauthor of *Our Bodies, Ourselves* and *The New Our Bodies, Ourselves* and a codirector of the Boston Women's Health Book Collective. She also served on the Board of the National Women's Health Network for 12 years.

Michelle Oberman is Assistant Professor of Law, DePaul University College of Law, and Assistant Professor of Medical Humanities, University of Illinois at Chicago College of Medicine. She is a graduate of Cornell University (B.A.) and the University of Michigan Schools of Law and Public Health (J.D., M.P.H.). Her background ranges from the in-house hospital setting to state government consulting, where she has assisted in drafting AIDS-related legislation. She specializes in health law, women's health and the law, bioethics, and public health policy.

Mary Utne O'Brien is Associate Professor of Epidemiology at the University of Illinois at Chicago, where she is also Research Director of the AIDS Community Outreach Intervention Projects. She holds a Ph.D. in sociology from the University of Wisconsin, Madison, and taught graduate and undergraduate social research methods courses while on the faculty of the University of Chicago (1978-1987).

Virginia Olesen (Ph.D.) is Professor at the University of California, San Francisco. She teaches in the Women, Health and Healing Program in the Department of Social and Behavioral Sciences and was an early force in the formation of women's health as a specialty discipline.

Ellen Olshansky (D.N.S., R.N.C.) is Associate Professor and Director of the Women's Health Primary Care graduate track at the University of Washington. She is a women's health care nurse practitioner.

Judith Panko Reis (M.A.) is the Administrative Director of the Health Resource Center for Women with Disabilities at the Rehabilitation Institute of Chicago. She is the recipient of a Robert Wood Johnson Community Health Leadership award regarding her work with disabled women.

Beth E. Richie (M.S.W., Ph.D.) is a member of the faculty in the Program in Community Health Education at Hunter College of the City University of New York. She has been an activist on the issues of violence against women, an advocate for incarcerated women in prison, and a consultant and trainer on issues related to the health of women of color for the past 15 years.

Sue V. Rosser (Ph.D., zoology) is Director of Women's Studies at the University of South Carolina at Columbia and Professor of Family and Preventive Medicine in the medical school there. She has edited collections and written numerous journal articles on the theoretical and applied problems of women and science. Author of the books *Teaching About Science and Health from a Feminist Perspective: A Practical Guide* (1986), *Feminism Within the Science and Health Care Professions: Overcoming Resistance* (1988), *Female-Friendly Science* (1990), *Feminism and Biology: A Dynamic Interaction* (1992), *People Friendly Medicine* (in press), and *Teaching the Majority* (in press), she also served as the Latin and North American Coeditor of *Women's Studies International Forum* (from 1989 to 1993).

Renee Royak-Schaler (Ph.D.) is Associate Professor, Department of Health Sciences, Towson State University, and author of the book *Challenging the Breast Cancer Legacy: A Program of Emotional Support and Medical Care for Women at Risk.* She is currently a National Cancer Institute Cancer Prevention and Control Research Fellow at the University of North Carolina Lineberger Comprehensive Cancer Center.

Nanette Silva is the Director of the Women's Health Initiative Program at the Chicago Foundation for Women. She administers the grant-making, education, and community relations work related to the women's health partnership with the John D. and Catherine T. MacArthur Foundation. She is an appointed member of the Mayor of Chicago's Task Force on Women's Health and a founding member of the Illinois Council for the Prevention of Violence and of the battered women's shelter Rainbow House/Arco Iris in Chicago. She is an M.P.H. candidate at the San Diego State University School of Public Health. She has extensive experience in prevention and health promotion in the areas of woman battering, HIV/AIDS, teen pregnancy, child health, mental health, reproductive health, and smoking.

Nada L. Stotland (M.D.) received her college, medical, and psychiatric education at the University of Chicago, where she is currently on the faculty in the departments of psychiatry and obstetrics/gynecology. She is the author or editor of four books on psychosocial aspects of women's reproductive health care.

Deane Taylor is Director of Prevention and Education for the Cook County Hospital Women and Children's HIV Program. She is the founding and continuing facilitator of the support group, "The Evolution of Dignity."

Diana L. Taylor (Ph.D., R.N.) is Assistant Professor and Director of the Women's Health Primary Care graduate track at the University of California, San Francisco. She is a women's health care nurse practitioner.

Leonore Tiefer earned a Ph.D. in 1969 in comparative and physiological psychology from the University of California, Berkeley, and then respecialized at New York University as a clinical psychologist in the 1980s. All along, though, she has been a research and theory-oriented feminist-activist-sexologist.

Lila A. Wallis (M.D., F.A.C.P.) is Clinical Professor of Medicine, Cornell University Medical College, Past President of the American Medical Women's Association, Chair of the Task Force on Women's Health Curriculum, and Founding President of the National Council on Women's Health.

Carole Warshaw (M.D.) is Director of Behavioral Science for the Primary Care Internal Medicine Residency at Cook County Hospital, is Co-Director of the Hospital Crisis Intervention Project, which provides training for health care providers on domestic violence and on-site intervention and advocacy for battered women, and has a part-time private practice in psychiatry.

Gail Webber (M.D.) is a family medicine resident at Queen's University at Kingston, Ontario, Canada. She has an M.A. in women's studies from the University of York, England.

Denise C. Webster has been involved in women's health for nearly 30 years as a nurse clinician, nurse educator, and nurse researcher. Her interests include women as consumers and providers of health care. She is currently teaching in the graduate program in psychiatric nursing at the University of Colorado as well as completing research on women's self-care for interstitial cystitis. She also maintains a small private practice in psychotherapy for women.

Mildred Williamson (B.A., M.S.) is the Project Administrator for the Women and Children's HIV Program. She is a Ph.D. candidate at the University of Chicago.

Judith Wuest is Associate Professor at the Faculty of Nursing, University of New Brunswick, in Fredericton, New Brunswick, Canada. She received her basic nursing education at the University of Toronto and her M.A. at Dalhousie University, and is presently a doctoral student in the College of Nursing at Wayne State University. She has served as the Chair of the International Committee of the Canadian Nurses Association and is currently the President-Elect of the Canadian Nursing Research Group. She is primarily interested in qualitative research methods, particularly grounded theory conducted from a feminist perspective.